Third Edition

FUNDAMENTALS OF ATHLETIC TRAINING

Lorin A. Cartwright, MS, ATC
Ann Arbor Pioneer High School

William A. Pitney, EdD, ATC, FNATA
Northern Illinois University

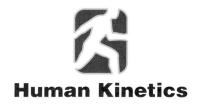
Human Kinetics

Library of Congress Cataloging-in-Publication Data

Cartwright, Lorin, 1956-
    Fundamentals of athletic training / Lorin A. Cartwright, William A. Pitney. -- 3rd
ed.
        p. cm.
    Includes bibliographical references and index.
    ISBN-13: 978-0-7360-8373-7 (hard cover)
    ISBN-10: 0-7360-8373-1 (hard cover)
    1. Athletic trainers. I. Pitney, William. II. Title.
RC1210.C36 2011
613.7'11--dc22

ISBN-10: 0-7360-8373-1 (print)
ISBN-13: 978-0-7360-8373-7 (print)

The Web addresses cited in this text were current as of October 2010, unless otherwise noted.

Acquisitions Editor: Loarn D. Robertson, PhD; **Developmental Editor:** Judy Park; **Assistant Editors:** Elizabeth Evans and Brendan Shea; **Copyeditor:** Alisha Jeddeloh; **Indexer:** Bobbi Swanson; **Permission Manager:** Dalene Reeder; **Graphic Designer:** Joe Buck; **Graphic Artist:** Yvonne Griffith; **Cover Designer:** Keith Blomberg; **Photographer (cover):** Human Kinetics; **Photo Asset Manager:** Laura Fitch; **Visual Production Assistant:** Joyce Brumfield; **Photo Production Manager:** Jason Allen; **Art Manager:** Kelly Hendren; **Associate Art Manager:** Alan L. Wilborn; **Illustrations:** © Human Kinetics; **Printer:** Courier Companies, Inc.

Printed in the United States of America   10 9 8 7 6 5 4 3 2 1

The paper in this book is certified under a sustainable forestry program.

Human Kinetics
Web site: www.HumanKinetics.com

United States: Human Kinetics
P.O. Box 5076
Champaign, IL 61825-5076
800-747-4457
e-mail: humank@hkusa.com

Canada: Human Kinetics
475 Devonshire Road Unit 100
Windsor, ON N8Y 2L5
800-465-7301 (in Canada only)
e-mail: info@hkcanada.com

Europe: Human Kinetics
107 Bradford Road
Stanningley
Leeds LS28 6AT, United Kingdom
+44 (0) 113 255 5665
e-mail: hk@hkeurope.com

Australia: Human Kinetics
57A Price Avenue
Lower Mitcham, South Australia 5062
08 8372 0999
e-mail: info@hkaustralia.com

New Zealand: Human Kinetics
P.O. Box 80
Torrens Park, South Australia 5062
0800 222 062
e-mail: info@hknewzealand.com

E4851

To educators everywhere who take a vested interest in introducing the profession of athletic training to students. *You are expanding the knowledge and horizons of future certified athletic trainers.*

Contents

List of Anatomical Drawings

Shoulder

Elbow

Wrist and Hand

Lower Extremity

Hip, Pelvis, and Thigh

Knee

Foot, Ankle, and Lower Leg

Preface

The world of athletic training is ever evolving and expanding. Writing the third edition of *Fundamentals of Athletic Training* has been an opportunity to include recent changes to keep the reader updated on the latest information in the field of athletic training.

This one-of-a-kind book is designed to introduce the world of athletic training to students getting their first exposure to the profession. We present basic information for those exploring the field of athletic training, and we provide detailed information for student assistants who want to learn more about what occurs in the athletic training room or who aspire to a career as a certified athletic trainer (AT). This textbook will help students become familiar with the practices of the AT and also understand their own role.

A student assistant's most important role is to learn as much as possible. Although they cannot perform many of the AT's tasks, this text can help students understand what they will observe during their experience in the athletic training room. It will also enable them to ask the AT intelligent questions.

In this book we address the concepts, injuries, and illnesses that we have dealt with at the high school level as certified ATs. Our hope is that the material will encourage students to consider athletic training or another medical field as a profession.

HOW THIS BOOK IS ORGANIZED

The text is organized so that each unit can stand alone and be comprehended without reading previous units. We suggest, however, that units II through VI be covered to provide a solid understanding of anatomy and physiology before reading about specific injuries. Learning about injuries that occur to the body as well as the associated anatomy is necessary before learning about rehabilitation and treatment.

The book is divided into nine units:

- Unit I gives an overview of the athletic training profession and the administrative tasks important to success in the field.
- Unit II is a discussion of the body's anatomy and the physiology of injury and tissue healing.
- Units III, IV, and V explain specific anatomy, injuries, and treatment for injured athletes.
- Unit VI discusses the fundamentals of rehabilitation and returning athletes to competition, including the psychological aspects of their return.
- Unit VII discusses how to plan and deal with emergency situations.
- Unit VIII explains injury prevention through the use of taping, wrapping, and protective equipment.
- Unit IX covers various conditions, illnesses, disabilities, communicable diseases, common drugs, and nutritional aspects that affect athletes.

SPECIAL CHAPTER ELEMENTS

A number of special features are contained within the text. At the front of the book you will find a list of all anatomical drawings and their locations within the book for quick reference. Each chapter begins with a list of objectives that the reader will be able to answer after completing the chapter. The objectives will help students focus their attention when reading the material. The Real World features share actual experiences of ATs. What Would You Do If . . . segments act as discussion openers and allow students to prioritize their thinking about the situation; these dilemmas show that being an AT involves not only medical challenges but also challenges of responsibility. FYI boxes provide more information about a particular topic that may be challenging. We have added content related to current NATA position statements, and we have also added a segment called *Understanding Diversity* to facilitate students' thinking about various cultures and races that ATs may work with.

At the end of each chapter is a wrap-up section, which includes a summary, key terms, questions for review, activities for reinforcement, and activities for going above and beyond. The key terms are bolded within the text where they are defined and are also listed at the conclusion of each chapter. The questions for review reflect major topics and objectives. Defining the key terms and answering the questions for review allow readers to check how well they are learning and serve as a review for chapter tests. The activities for reinforcement are just that: recommended hands-on experiences that enable students to apply the theory in the chapter in practical ways. These activities clarify and reinforce the facts and techniques presented in the text. We challenge the student who wants to dig deeper with suggested projects in the Above and Beyond segments.

NEW TO THIS EDITION

In this edition, new topics include working with athletes with specific conditions or disabilities, design features of athletic training facilities, modality safety, balance activities, working with athletes of diverse cultures, and the role of the AT in school emergencies. We have added content to the chapters on the profession and professional preparation, reconditioning, primary care, environmental situations, protective equipment, drug use, and nutrition. The appendixes have been updated as well.

NOTES FOR INSTRUCTORS

The text is designed for people receiving their first exposure to content found in the athletic training profession. The information presented, therefore, is fundamental. At the end of each chapter, however, we include exercises to help students explore topics at a greater depth when necessary.

The test pacckage contains a large question bank primarily composed of multiple-choice questions. Questions are organized by chapter and answers are provided. The instructor guide includes a lecture outline to guide the presentation of material as well as worksheets for students to complete to ensure they are engaged and self-directed in their learning.

To fine-tune your presentations, the image bank includes the art and photos of the text. This will allow you to use graphics in PowerPoint presentations and help link information in your presentations to the text that the students have read.

eBook
available at
HumanKinetics.com

This book and its features will make readers the best student assistants possible in support of the AT. This is the beginning of the possibility that the students may become intrigued by this field and set a goal to make a living caring for athletes.

Acknowledgments

To my friends and family for your love, support, and encouragement. To my writing partner, Bill, for great ideas and common sense. To Barb Hansen for her patience, suggestions, wisdom, balance, and support. You are the best.

Lorin A. Cartwright

To Liam and Quinlan for helping me understand my priorities in life. My students at NIU . . . you have taught me more than you will ever know! To Lorin, who is the most dedicated professional I know—it is always a pleasure working with you. To my best friend, my soul mate, my everything, Lisa, for her love and devotion. I am surely the luckiest man alive . . . did I ever tell you you're awesome?

William A. Pitney III

UNIT I

Professional and Administrative Aspects of Athletic Training

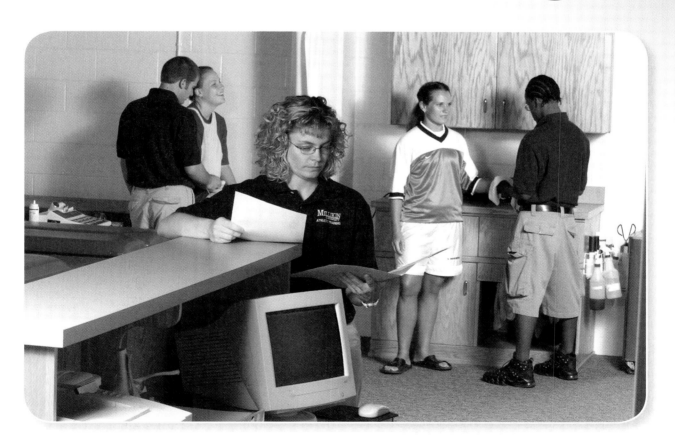

chapter 1

Athletic Training as a Profession

Objectives

Upon completing this chapter, the student will be able to do the following:

- Define *athletic training.*
- Describe the roles of the certified athletic trainer.
- Describe the roles of other health care providers and the sports medicine team.
- List the requirements for becoming a competent certified AT.
- Describe the job opportunities available to certified ATs.

Athletic training is a profession dedicated to maintaining and improving the health and well-being of the physically active population and preventing athletics-related injuries and illnesses. The credential for the **certified athletic trainer (AT)** is the **ATC**. The credential *ATC* after one's name is evidence that the person has the appropriate education and training to work as a certified AT. Although individuals have provided health care to injured athletes for centuries, it was not until 1991 that the American Medical Association formally recognized athletic training as an allied health care profession. The **National Athletic Trainers' Association (NATA)**, which is responsible for setting professional standards, was formed in 1950. The NATA **Board of Certification (BOC)** is responsible for conducting the national certification process.

ROLES OF THE ATHLETIC TRAINER

The BOC has studied and established the various roles of the AT, which include the following practice domains:

- *Injury prevention.* The prevention of athletic injuries includes preparticipation physical exams;

proper strength and conditioning programs; proper equipment and equipment fitting; taping, bandaging, and bracing; and good nutrition.

● *Clinical evaluation and diagnosis.* The AT must be able to recognize the type of injury and its severity so that she will know how to treat it or when to refer the athlete to a physician.

● *Immediate care of athletic injuries.* When an athlete is injured, the AT must be ready to respond. He must maintain first aid and cardiopulmonary resuscitation (CPR) certification through such organizations as the **American Red Cross** and the **National Safety Council**.

● *Treatment, rehabilitation, and reconditioning of athletic injuries.* After initial treatment, the AT directs the athlete through exercises and treatments to help her return to normal function. This is called **rehabilitation**. **Reconditioning** is getting the athlete back into physical shape for athletic participation.

● *Organization and administration.* ATs are often responsible for managing state-of-the-art facilities, so they must have the administrative skills necessary for preparing work and purchase orders and scheduling staff. Additionally, injuries, treatments, and rehabilitation progress must be documented accurately.

● *Professional development and responsibility.* Technology changes rapidly, and ATs must continue their education to remain current with the latest developments in health care. To do so, they attend seminars, read journals, write articles and books, and conduct research. ATs must conduct themselves professionally and with integrity. No one likes receiving medical treatment from someone who is unprofessional. A professional understands that she cannot accomplish everything by herself, so she works as part of a sports medicine team.

THE SPORTS MEDICINE TEAM

In this book, **sports medicine** refers to the care of physically active people who have suffered athletic injury or illness. The sports medicine profession includes ATs, medical doctors, physical therapists, dentists, chiropractors, coaches, sport psychologists, strength and conditioning specialists, school

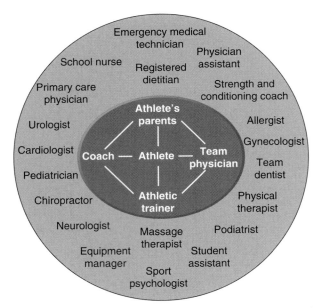

Figure 1.1 The sports medicine team consists of central and peripheral members, each of whom has specific responsibilities and areas of expertise.

nurses, sport nutritionists, and student assistants (see figure 1.1). A sports medicine team may include any or all of these people.

As with any team, the sports medicine team must work cooperatively. If a football running back runs wherever he wants with the ball regardless of where the blockers are, his team will never win. The team must coordinate its plays if it is ever to be successful. This is how an effective sports medicine team works.

Central Team

Ideally, the central team is composed of the injured athlete, the athlete's parents, the AT, the team physician, and the coach. The central team works together to make initial decisions about injuries, illness, and even sport performance.

● *The athlete.* The athlete is the center of the team. She provides other members with vital information about the injury.

● *The athlete's parent or guardian.* Because the sports medicine team is concerned about making decisions in the athlete's best interest, both the athlete and her parent or guardian must be involved in the central team.

● *Team physician.* The team physician is the medical authority who oversees the sports medicine team effort. The physician examines the athlete for injuries and illnesses and performs tests such as **X rays** (electromagnetic waves used to make a picture of a body part) or blood tests to help determine an athlete's problem. The AT acts under the direction of the team physician, who is typically an orthopedic specialist. **Orthopedists** deal primarily with injuries to the musculoskeletal system.

• *Certified AT.* The AT communicates with the injured athlete, the athlete's parent or guardian, the team physician, and the coach. The AT is onsite at a game or practice, and he often makes the initial injury assessment, provides emergency injury care, and provides follow-up treatment or referrals to other sports medicine team members as needed. Because of these multiple roles, the AT is a critical link in the chain of professionals that composes the sports medicine team.

The Real World

We had a freshman football receiver who was unable to catch the ball. He was fast, but he dropped everything. His position coach recommended an eye exam and was sure that the results would be subpar and that we would recommend glasses or contacts to improve his performance. The exam revealed the player's vision to be 20/10, which is exceedingly better than average. I recommended that the coach work with the young man on the skills necessary to perform well at the position. The player became one of the school's all-time statistical leaders and has had a long and successful career in the NFL as a receiver.

Paul W. Schmidt, MS, PT, ATC

• *The coach.* Because the coach has daily contact with the athletes, he may know them better than the rest of the sports medicine team does. The coach often has close contact with the parents or guardians of the athletes as well. This allows him to play a vital role in communicating with the injured athlete and her parents. When an athlete returns to

Principles of Medical Ethics

Physicians provide supervision and direction of ATs and are critical central members of the sports medicine team. A physician's care is guided by the principles of medical ethics (American Medical Association 2001):

1. A physician shall be dedicated to providing competent medical care, with compassion and respect for human dignity and rights.

2. A physician shall uphold the standards of professionalism, be honest in all professional interactions, and strive to report physicians deficient in character or competence, or engaging in fraud or deception, to appropriate entities.

3. A physician shall respect the law and also recognize a responsibility to seek changes in those requirements that are contrary to the best interests of the patient.

4. A physician shall respect the rights of patients, colleagues, and other health professionals and shall safeguard patient confidences and privacy within the constraints of the law.

5. A physician shall continue to study, apply, and advance scientific knowledge; maintain a commitment to medical education; make relevant information available to patients, colleagues, and the public; obtain consultation; and use the talents of other health professionals when indicated.

6. A physician shall, in the provision of appropriate patient care, except in emergencies, be free to choose whom to serve, with whom to associate, and the environment in which to provide medical care.

7. A physician shall recognize a responsibility to participate in activities contributing to the improvement of the community and the betterment of public health.

8. A physician shall, while caring for a patient, regard responsibility to the patient as paramount.

9. A physician shall support access to medical care for all people.

competition following rehabilitation, the coach, in consultation with the AT, can modify the training, exercises, and drills the athlete performs so that she can safely progress to peak performance.

Peripheral Team

Although members of the central sports medicine team work together to manage an athletic injury, they often rely on peripheral team members to provide specialized care or assistance.

- Many injured athletes have a **primary care physician**. Because this doctor has worked with the athlete before, the sports medicine team must include the primary care physician in their decisions. The primary care physician may refer the athlete to a specialist such as a podiatrist, allergist, urologist, gynecologist, cardiologist, neurologist, pediatrician, and so on.

- A **podiatrist** examines and diagnoses problems below the knee and performs foot surgeries. She can prescribe corrective devices such as orthotics (shoe inserts).

- An **allergist** determines whether someone has an allergy, and if so, how to treat it. An **allergy** is an immune response, which may include red, swollen tissue or a runny nose, to a substance that normally should be tolerated.

- A **urologist** treats problems of the urinary tract.

- A **gynecologist** deals with conditions and care of the female reproductive system.

- A **cardiologist** treats heart disease and heart abnormalities.

- A **pediatrician** specializes in the medical treatment of children.

- A **dentist** may be involved if the athletic injury is to the facial area. The team dentist may also provide properly fitting mouth guards to prevent dental injuries.

- A **physical therapist** provides rehabilitation for bone and joint injuries, head injuries, and muscle injuries and imbalances so that patients may return to normal physical function and active daily living.

- A **physician assistant** works under the supervision of a physician and conducts examinations, orders diagnostic tests, writes prescriptions, and diagnoses and treats injuries and illnesses. Assistants typically specialize in a particular form of medicine. They free up physicians to deal with more critical patients.

- A **neurologist** is a physician who specializes in conditions of the nervous system and may examine an athlete who has suffered a head injury.

- A **student assistant** assists the AT with many daily tasks. For example, a student assistant may enter treatment data into a computer program, tape athletes before practices and games, stock medical cabinets and bags, organize the sidelines before games, hydrate the athletes during practices in hot weather, and prepare for rehabilitation procedures (e.g., organizing weights, whirlpools, and equipment). Also, because they are often the same age as the athletes, student assistants can identify with the athletes and may develop strong bonds with them. This can be especially helpful because the athletes often feel comfortable enough to ask questions and clarify information they have received. It is important to keep in mind that *student assistants can only function under the direct supervision of an AT.* In some states the student assistant is referred to as an *athletic trainer aide.* Also, it is important that student assistants not violate state practice acts and attempt to act in the capacity of an AT.

- A **chiropractor** is a health professional who takes a holistic approach to patient care by focusing on spinal misalignments. Although chiropractors are not physicians, they may treat musculoskeletal disorders and restore normal function by manipulating bones, specifically at the spinal column.

- The **school nurse** is a health care professional trained to identify and care for illnesses and disorders. The school nurse is a valuable educational resource for the AT and can help the athletic training team deliver safe, effective health care.

- A **registered dietitian** is a nutritional specialist who can help an athlete, and sometimes the entire athletic team, construct a proper diet based on the level of activity and dietary needs. He can also tailor meals for athletes who have specific problems, such as diabetes.

- An **emergency medical technician (EMT)** is an emergency medical service (EMS) specialist who is certified to provide acute care for those who have a critical injury or illness. EMTs are often called upon to provide acute care and transportation of a victim to a nearby hospital. The National Registry for Emergency Medical Technicians recognizes varying levels of certification. These include EMT-Basic, EMT-Intermediate, and EMT-Paramedic.

- A **massage therapist** is a health care professional who specializes in working with muscles and tendons. This role is important because tissue that is in spasm, needs to be warmed, or needs improved circulation can be aided by massage techniques.

- A **sport psychologist** works with athletes who may need help with goal setting, anxiety, frustration, self-esteem, family issues, and more. This work is essential to help athletes be mentally prepared to participate at their best.

- A **strength and conditioning coach** works with athletes to ensure that each is in shape to meet the demands of athletic competition. Programs are designed to be sport specific and to improve the athlete's areas of weakness.

- The **equipment manager** purchases and maintains appropriate protective and supportive athletic equipment. This is a significant role because many athletic injuries can be prevented with proper equipment. Equipment managers stay current on the latest and best types of padding, headgear, and clothing.

BECOMING A CERTIFIED ATHLETIC TRAINER

To become an AT, you must earn either a bachelor's or entry-level master's degree from a college or university that has an athletic training education program accredited by the Commission on Accreditation of Athletic Training Education (CAATE). The athletic training program must offer a major in athletic training. Students enrolled in an undergraduate athletic training program are expected to receive clinical experiences that provide supervised, hands-on experience as well as specified courses related to athletic training. After graduation, a student must pass the BOC certification exam and earn the ATC credential before practicing as a certified AT. Many states have laws that require state licensure in addition to national certification. Practicing without a license or certification could result in legal action,

What Would You Do If...

An athlete was hit in the head during practice. He was evaluated by the AT and the team physician, both of whom wanted another opinion. The athlete complains to you, saying, "I don't understand why I have to see a neurologist. I've already been seen by our team physician."

including arrest. The regulations for athletic training vary greatly from state to state. Three common forms of credentials are licensure, certification, and registration.

States that have **licensure** requirements generally specify who is allowed to practice athletic training and what duties they are allowed to perform. **Certification** ensures that an individual has achieved basic knowledge and skill to practice athletic training, and **registration** requires an individual to register with the state before practicing athletic training.

When a student enters an athletic training education program, she must receive formal instruction in specific subjects. The required subject matter is identified by NATA in the *Athletic Training Educational Competencies*. The fourth edition contains the latest required content that includes the following 12 areas:

1. Risk management and injury prevention
2. Pathology of injury and illnesses
3. Orthopedic clinical examination and diagnosis
4. Medical conditions and disabilities
5. Acute care of injuries and illnesses
6. Therapeutic modalities
7. Conditioning and rehabilitation exercise
8. Pharmacology
9. Psychosocial intervention and referral
10. Nutritional aspects of injuries and illness
11. Health care administration
12. Professional development and responsibility

Each of these subjects is further clarified next.

- *Risk management and injury prevention* refers to the principles and strategies for minimizing the risk of injury as well as the risk of legal liability.

• *Pathology of injury and illnesses* refers to the cause of an injury or illness and the functional changes that occur in the body as a result.

• *Orthopedic clinical examination and diagnosis* refers to understanding and identifying an athlete's musculoskeletal injury and determining his readiness to participate in physical activity. This content area also involves identifying athletic injuries and assessing an athlete's progress during the rehabilitation of an athletic injury.

• *Medical conditions and disabilities* include disease processes and the disabilities that result from athletic injuries. They also include disabilities that may exist as preexisting conditions in active people. These issues must be understood before they can be managed.

• *Acute care of injuries and illnesses* involves systematically managing acute injury and illness in an emergency situation.

• *Therapeutic modalities* refer to methods of facilitating the healing process. ATs must understand the **physics** behind energy absorption, dissipation, and transmission as energy is applied to the body in the various modalities.

• *Conditioning and rehabilitation exercise* refers to preparing an athlete for the demands of a sport or activity by helping her to attain an appropriate level of fitness and function. An AT must understand the principles and techniques of the exercises used.

• *Pharmacology* refers to the science of drugs and drug interactions in the body. Although ATs cannot administer medications to athletes, they must understand prescription and nonprescription medications. For example, if an athlete should not be exposed to the sun when taking certain medications, the AT can recommend moving practice to a shaded area or see to it that the athlete wears appropriate clothing.

• *Psychosocial intervention and referral* involves understanding both the psychological and sociological aspects of an injury or illness and knowing how to intervene and refer an athlete for appropriate care. From a psychological perspective, students study the variables that affect human behavior. For athletes who have dedicated a tremendous amount of time to their sport, injuries are not only devastating physically but also emotionally. The AT can use what she learns of psychology to understand an athlete's behavior after an injury and to differentiate symptoms of an injury or illness from an emotional problem. Moreover, ATs need to understand how to help athletes through the difficult task of rehabilitation after a serious injury. In addition, the AT must know when and where to make referrals and how to develop alcohol- and drug-abuse prevention programs.

• *Nutritional aspects of injuries and illness* include the way that food fulfills the metabolic needs of the body. Athletes have slightly different nutritional demands than those of people who do not exercise. ATs must have a basic understanding of **nutrition** in order to provide accurate advice and to refer athletes to specialists if advanced nutritional help is needed.

• *Health care administration* refers to the management aspects of athletic training and athletics. Many ATs develop policies and procedures for operating various facilities. They also need to understand the legal issues that ATs often face in athletics.

• *Professional development and responsibility* refers to an AT's obligation to continually learn and to conduct himself in a professional manner.

Besides the content areas that must be addressed in an athletic training curriculum, students must learn several foundational behaviors of professional practice. The foundational behaviors documented in the 2006 NATA Educational Competencies are fundamental behaviors and values that affect all aspects of patient care (see table 1.1).

The Real World

Although I originally went to college to become a physical educator, I have always been interested in health care. Thus, I selected athletic training as a health profession because it deals with sport and because it is one of the few health professions where you are trained to prevent injuries, give immediate care to an injury, and rehabilitate an injury. We have the privilege of working with people from the moment they are injured until the moment they return to their sport. This is a claim that few health professions can make.

Bill Pitney, EdD, ATC

Table 1.1　Fundamental Concepts in Professional Practice

Fundamental	Explanation
Primacy of the patient	Putting the care of the patient first and providing the best possible care to the patient
Teamed approach to practice	Understanding that the central and peripheral sports medicine teams both play a role in rendering quality care to a patient; understanding the scope of practice in athletic training and having an ability to work with others
Legal practice	Following the laws that guide the practice and understanding what constitutes illegal practice
Ethical practice	Following the NATA code of ethics at all times and working to follow appropriate practice guidelines as a health care professional
Advancing knowledge	Examining evidence from research to guide one's practice as an AT and engaging in continuing education to improve the quality of patient care
Cultural competence	Understanding and valuing patients' differences and working responsibly with diverse patient populations
Professionalism	Acting in a compassionate manner and behaving with honesty and integrity; promoting the AT profession

After becoming an AT, an individual must recertify every three years by obtaining emergency cardiac care certification and participating in at least 75 hours of continuing education activity. Continuing education can take many forms, but a common method is to attend workshops and conferences that offer educational content.

ATHLETIC TRAINING CAREERS

ATs have opportunities for employment in a variety of settings. The following describes various job settings, including organized athletics and clinical and industrial venues. Information from NATA about average salaries is also presented.

Organized Athletics

Organized athletics includes high schools, colleges or universities, professional or semiprofessional athletic teams, and youth sport leagues.

● *High school environments.* Considering the fact that many high schools may offer anywhere from 10 to 28 sports, these settings can be challenging. Some high schools have full-time ATs, but many high school ATs teach academic courses and receive a stipend for providing athletic training after school. Most high school ATs work 10 months of the year. Some ATs do similar work in middle school or

junior high schools. According to the September 2009 NATA membership statistics, about 16.5% of ATs work in the secondary school setting. In terms of salaries for this setting, the 2008 NATA salary survey showed that the average range for ATs was $44,811 (private high schools) to $47,822 (public high schools).

● *Universities and colleges.* Nearly every college athletic program hires ATs to provide health care to its athletes. College athletic training contracts can range from 9 to 12 months, and some college ATs also act as instructors for the athletic training education programs. Positions vary greatly in the college setting because programs come in many sizes, from large universities with many teams to small colleges with only a few athletic teams. The NATA membership statistics in September 2009 showed 22.7% of ATs working in the college setting. The 2008 NATA salary survey revealed that the average salary for a college or university staff AT was $39,285.

● *Professional and semiprofessional teams.* Although many students want to become an AT with a professional sport team, this goal is difficult to achieve. Compared with the number of positions in colleges, high schools, and clinical settings, there are few positions in the professional ranks. As of September 2009, the NATA membership data revealed that only 3% of ATs work in the professional sport setting. Also, ATs with professional teams often

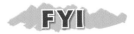

Medical Ethics and Legal Issues

The moral aspects of health care as well as the legal statutes that dictate what ATs are allowed to do as professionals.

Human Anatomy

How the body is organized; the study of bones, joints, muscles, and organs and their structure and location. The AT cannot recognize injuries unless he understands human anatomy.

Human Physiology

Human bodily functions. The treatments rendered to athletes by ATs must be based on sound physiological principles. For example, after an athlete is injured, the tissue heals in several stages. The AT must understand what happens during each stage in order to prescribe exercises that won't reinjure the tissue.

Exercise Physiology

The processes that occur in the body during activity. When a person exercises, she places demands on her body, and her body adapts to them. An exercising person's heart and breathing rates will be higher than when she is at rest. Understanding the changes that exercise causes in the body is essential for recognizing signs and symptoms of illness or injury.

First Aid and Emergency Care

Systematically managing acute injury and illness in an emergency situation.

Strength Training and Reconditioning

Preparing athletes for the demands of a sport or activity by helping them attain an appropriate level of strength, endurance, flexibility, and cardiorespiratory fitness. An AT must understand the principles and techniques of these programs.

Biomechanics

The science of movement mechanics, **biomechanics** also called **kinesiology**. ATs are responsible for teaching athletes how to properly perform exercises that will help them recover from injuries. In addition, ATs often apply tape and braces to prevent athletes from performing certain movements that might cause injury. These treatments cannot be effectively applied unless one first understands biomechanics.

Statistics and Research Design

Ways of collecting and analyzing data. An AT must understand these fields in order to obtain accurate evidence related to injury treatment strategies, injury prevention programs, and so forth.

have a grueling travel schedule. The reward is the opportunity to work closely with elite athletes and coaches in an extremely competitive environment. The 2008 NATA salary survey is limited in the number of professional sports represented, but overall the average salary range for this setting was $36,858 to $73,423. Pro football ATs averaged $64,266 annually.

• *Youth sport leagues.* Some organized youth sport leagues have taken the initiative to hire full-time ATs to care for their athletes. The primary role of ATs in youth sport is the prevention and care of athletic injuries, and the reward is working with young athletes as they develop their athletic ability. The 2008 NATA salary survey revealed that ATs working in the youth sport, amateur, and recreational settings earned an average of $42,887 per year.

Clinical and Hospital Settings

Clinical settings include sites such as outpatient rehabilitation or sports medicine centers, clinical-outreach positions whereby an AT works in a sports medicine center part time and at a secondary school part time, and physician-owned clinics. Hospital settings involve ATs working in the emergency room, in orthopedics, or even in administration.

• *Sports medicine centers.* Although most ATs fill diverse roles ranging from emergency care to health care administration, the clinical AT tends to focus on rehabilitation. Many clinical ATs enjoy the one-on-one relationships they build with patients during their rehabilitation programs.

• *Clinic outreach.* Many programs have combined the traditional and clinical settings and created new positions and job opportunities for ATs. For example, it is not uncommon for a sports medicine center to have ATs who work part of a day (usually the morning) in a clinic and then go to a local high school in the afternoon to cover practices and events.

• *Physician-owned clinics.* Many physicians have found value in hiring an AT to examine patients, assist with medical procedures, and treat athletic injuries. Many ATs are also hired by physicians to provide durable good care, meaning the AT fits

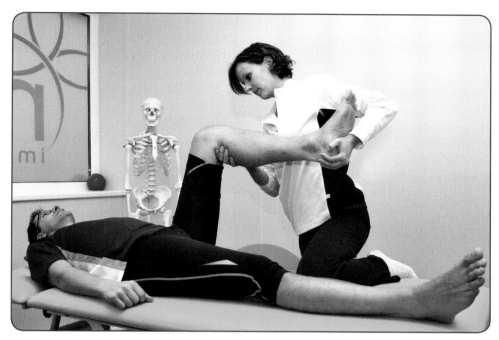

ATs also work in clinical settings such as sports medicine clinics.

patients with walking boots, splints, braces, and so on.

According to the 2008 NATA salary survey, average salaries for ATs working in clinical and hospital settings ranged from $37,052 for clinic-outreach ATs to $73,366 for ATs working in hospital administrative roles.

Industrial and Occupational Settings

Industrial and occupational settings for ATs include health and fitness centers. They also include industrial and manufacturing sites.

• *Health and fitness centers.* Many companies and health centers have come to realize that ATs are a business asset. Not everyone who enters a health center or corporate fitness program is completely healthy. Some may even be under a physician's care for a particular injury and therefore may need an AT to get started on a safe fitness routine that will not aggravate the injury. The NATA 2008 salary survey identified the average salaries for ATs working in the health and fitness setting as $50,503.

• *Industrial and manufacturing sites.* Businesses spend billions of dollars annually for health care. In an attempt to reduce health care

costs, many companies are beginning to see the advantages of having a full-time AT on staff to help prevent and treat work-site injuries. ATs are often able to treat these injuries at the workplace under the supervision of a physician, decreasing the amount of work time lost to the industrial athlete.

In the industrial setting, the supervisor takes the place of a coach, and the employee replaces an athlete. The peripheral team may add an **ergonomics specialist** to the other allied medical professionals. An ergonomics specialist measures and adapts a work environment to prevent and treat musculoskeletal disorders. For example, rather than forcing workers to stand on a hard concrete floor and work at a bench that is so low they have to bend over for eight hours a day, executives may hire an ergonomics specialist to recommend changes in the physical environment that will reduce the wear and tear on workers' bodies. Such modifications may be as simple as providing higher workbenches, special chairs, and cushioned floor mats.

Military and Law Enforcement Settings

A new and emerging practice setting for ATs is with the military and law enforcement. Administrators in these settings have recognized that many injuries

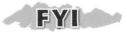

suffered in combat are similar to those suffered by athletes. Moreover, soldiers and law officers must make a quick recovery and return to their jobs in excellent physical condition; otherwise their lives are at serious risk. According to the NATA salary survey, ATs working in military settings earned an average salary of $54,494 in 2008.

Job Outlook

The United States Department of Labor (USDL) documents that the job growth for athletic training looks good, expecting a 24% growth for athletic training from 2006 to 2016. The USDL expects job growth to be concentrated in hospital settings and the offices of health care practitioners.

NATIONAL ATHLETIC TRAINERS' ASSOCIATION

The athletic training profession is directed by its professional association, NATA. This organization is composed of voluntary members, including ATs, athletic training students, and associate members. NATA guides the advancement of the profession and sponsors the publishing of important information that affects how athletes are treated. Among these important publications are the *Journal of Athletic Training*, the *Athletic Training Education Journal*, and various professional statements that provide timely and important information related to injuries, illnesses, and diseases. NATA and the BOC also provide ethical guidelines that guide the practice of ATs. These are covered in chapter 2.

The NATA statements are important aspects of the profession because they provide ATs with standards of care and guidelines for treating those in need. NATA position statements include the following:

- Acute management of athletes with cervical spine injuries
- Environmental cold injuries
- Emergency planning in athletics
- Exertional heat illnesses
- Fluid replacement for athletes
- Head-down contact and spearing in tackle football
- Lightning safety for athletics and recreation
- Management of asthma in athletes
- Management of sport-related concussion
- Management of athlete with type 1 diabetes mellitus
- Prevention, detection, and management of disordered eating in athletes

March is National Athletic Training Month. The purpose of this month is to make the public aware of the athletic training profession. NATA encourages all ATs to participate in the grassroots effort by sponsoring contests and doing presentations to parents, school boards, and legislative groups. Many students create signs and advertisements promoting the profession, and others create Web sites to further describe what the profession is all about.

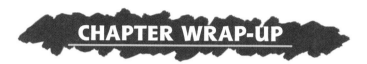

Summary

The AT plays a vital role in providing health care to the physically active population. A successful AT recognizes that the best health care is given through a team approach that draws on the strengths of a variety of professionals. ATs provide health care in many places, including high schools, colleges, professional sport teams, sports medicine clinics, and industrial settings. To become an AT, one must complete a bachelor's or entry-level master's degree and have studied specific subjects, including human anatomy and physiology, athletic-injury assessment, pharmacology, rehabilitation and reconditioning, and biomechanics.

Key Terms

Define the following terms found in this chapter:

allergist
allergy
American Red Cross
ATC
athletic training
biomechanics
Board of Certification (BOC)
cardiologist
certification
certified athletic trainer (AT)
chiropractor
dentist
dietitian (registered)
emergency medical technician (EMT)
equipment manager
ergonomics specialist
gynecologist
kinesiology
licensure
massage therapist
National Athletic Trainers' Association (NATA)

National Safety Council
neurologist
nutrition
orthopedist
pediatrician
pharmacology
physical therapist
physician assistant
physics
podiatrist
primary care physician
reconditioning
registration
rehabilitation
school nurse
sports medicine
sport psychologist
strength and conditioning coach
student assistant
urologist
X rays

Questions for Review

1. What is athletic training?
2. Name the members of the central sports medicine team, and describe their roles and responsibilities. When would members of the peripheral team become involved? Give an example.
3. Describe the ways to become a certified athletic trainer (AT). Explain the advantages and disadvantages of each.
4. Explain the domains of practice that an AT is responsible for.
5. Consider the job opportunities available to ATs. What personal attributes do you think would be necessary for success with each type of job? Justify your answer.

Activities for Reinforcement

1. Invite an AT to come to class and discuss the setting in which she works.
2. Invite several ATs who each work in a different setting to come to class and give a panel discussion.
3. Discuss which job opportunities in athletic training most interest you and why.
4. Go to www.nata.org/sites/default/files/code_of_ethics.pdf and read the NATA code of ethics. How does it guide the practice of an AT? In what ways does the code limit practice?

Above and Beyond

1. Visit the NATA Web site at www.nata.org to find the latest information about athletic training. Write a report about the structure of the professional organization.
2. Examine the NATA position statements, official statements, consensus statements, and support statements located at www.nata.org/statements/. What do you believe are the primary differences between the types of statements?
3. Visit the BOC Web site at www.bocatc.org for the latest information about the ATC credential and continuing education.
4. Go to www.caate.net and select Accredited Programs to view a list of programs accredited by the Commission on Accreditation of Allied Health Education Programs (CAAHEP).
5. Visit the American Academy of Physician Assistants (AAPA) at www.aapa.org to learn more about the role of physician assistants.
6. Visit the National Registry of Emergency Medical Technicians at www.nremt.org to learn more about the educational requirements of the EMS industry.
7. Visit the USDL Web site and learn more about the jobs of ATs:

   www.bls.gov/oco/ocos294.htm#outlook.
8. Find a modern version of the Hippocratic oath for physicians. How does this oath guide the practice of a physician? Does the oath limit what a physician can or cannot do?
9. Investigate the salaries of ATs in various career settings. You may use the most recent survey information at www.nata.org/NR110705. Outside of salary, what are the benefits of working in each setting? To do an effective investigation, you may have to interview ATs in each setting.

2

Administration and Professional Development

Objectives

Upon completing this chapter, the student will be able to do the following:

- Describe the concept of negligence, and explain ways to prevent being negligent.
- Understand the types of medical paperwork and record keeping necessary for organizational and administrative purposes.
- Describe why insurance is necessary.
- Explain why preventing injuries is the best defense against legal liability.
- Describe the typical organization of a preparticipation physical exam.
- Understand the concept of professional practice in athletic training.
- Describe the standards of professional practice in athletic training.
- Explain the importance of continuing education and the NATA requirements.
- Explain the elements of leadership.
- Describe characteristics that are helpful to being a future professional.
- Describe the primary aspects of an athletic training facility.

In addition to caring for and preventing athletic injuries, ATs must perform a variety of administrative duties. Moreover, they must be aware of certain legal issues that will greatly affect how they choose to administrate their athletic training program.

LEGAL ISSUES

When athletes choose to participate in sport, they risk becoming injured or even permanently disabled. Because ATs may be subject to legal liability as a result of athletes' injuries or illnesses, they must understand certain legal terminology.

Duty of Care

Duty of care means that an AT has an official job responsibility to render treatment and procedures related to the health and well-being of an athlete. An AT's duty of care is often outlined in an official job description. If an AT has a duty of care but fails to perform that duty, negligence may result.

Negligence

Negligence is a legal wrong characterized by the failure to act as a reasonably prudent person would act in a similar situation. For example, if an AT provides care below the standard of the law, he may be found negligent in certain circumstances. Picture an AT who has noticed an extremely large hole on the field a couple of hours before a field hockey game. A reasonably prudent person would think that this hole could cause an injury, and he would take reasonable action. For example, the AT could contact appropriate personnel such as the grounds crew, athletic director, or maintenance department to attempt to fill in the hole before game time, or he could place an orange cone in the hole to alert players of the danger.

Gross Negligence

Gross negligence has been described as a step beyond negligence; that is, an AT fails to provide even a slight amount of care when needed. To distinguish negligence from gross negligence, let's look at an example. If we were to use basic first aid to care for a victim whose finger is bleeding severely, we would provide reasonable care for controlling bleeding by applying direct pressure, elevating the arm, using a pressure bandage if necessary, and applying pressure at a pressure point. If the AT who helped the victim only told her to elevate her arm and eventually decided that perhaps he should put a dressing around the finger because it was still bleeding, he may be negligent. A grossly negligent AT, on the other hand, might fail even to provide instructions to the bleeding athlete. Although an AT may not want to come into contact with someone's blood for fear of disease transmission, he can at least give instructions to the person so she can start giving care to herself, and he can also seek additional help.

Assumption of Risk

Not warning athletes of the hazards involved in sport can leave the AT open to charges of negligence. This is part of a concept called **assumption of risk**. An athlete must fully understand that by participating in sport, she may be injured; that is, she assumes the risk of being injured after being fully warned of the dangers. Thus, an organization such as a high school must warn athletes and parents of the dangers that are common in the sports that the athletes will play. To make sure that athletes and parents understand the dangers, many programs require athletes to read and sign an assumption-of-risk form (see appendix A). Many coaches and ATs go even further and have the teams watch injury movies that explain the rules of the game and potential consequences of playing, such as injury or death. In addition, they use well-organized practice plans that document the day, time, and names of athletes who were given specific instructions about rules and technique.

Informed Consent

Before an AT can perform any medical procedure, he must obtain the consent of the athlete (or parent if the athlete is a minor). Failure to do so may make him liable for negligence. Therefore, the athlete or parent must be given enough information to make an intelligent decision about granting permission for care. Many schools have rules addressing this particular issue. See appendix B for an example of a form giving permission to treat (i.e., **informed consent**). This example also includes a medical information card. Many ATs put the permission to treat and the medical information on opposite sides of an index card. If the information is organized in this manner, it is easy to transport in a file folder or medical bag. The hospital staff is often thankful to have this information as well.

Proximate Cause

Proximate cause is described as a close connection between the way an AT acted and the resulting injury to an athlete. Noticing that an action will lead to a certain result and potentially harm someone is a component of proximate cause. For example, suppose an AT evaluates an athlete's injured neck and determines that there is considerable weakness and a lack of movement when the athlete attempts to look up or down. Also, the athlete is in some pain. If the AT were to allow the athlete to continue playing and this resulted in further injury and permanent neck damage, proximate cause could be shown. That is, the AT's action (letting the athlete continue playing) may be directly linked to the further injury (permanent neck damage).

Because ATs use many products for the prevention and care of athletic injuries, they must be aware of the established guidelines for use of certain products. For example, the sports medicine team should only purchase football helmets approved by the National Operating Committee on Standards for Athletic Equipment (NOCSAE). Failure to do so may lead to injury or even death. We recommend that an AT or an athletic program buy top-of-the-line products and look at available research to be sure that the product is of high quality.

AVOIDING LEGAL PROBLEMS

Several authors in the literature on athletic training have offered numerous suggestions for avoiding legal liability. These suggestions can be summarized as follows:

- *Have a written contract.* ATs, coaches, and other pertinent personnel should have a detailed contract with their employer that includes a job description. Either in this contract or in a separate document, the relationship between the head AT and students or assistants should be explained. At the high school and college levels, student assistants are under the direct supervision of an AT, which means that anything a student does in the athletic

training room should be monitored. Students are able to observe and learn, which is a valuable experience. They can also assist the AT with procedures if it is deemed appropriate by the AT.

- *Use equipment that meets established safety standards.* Use equipment only for its intended purposes, and be sure it is properly fitted.

- *Require preparticipation physical examinations.* Preparticipation exams help identify existing conditions that may lead to injuries. If these conditions can be identified, injuries can potentially be prevented, which limits the chance of liability.

- *Have all athletes and their parents or guardians sign an assumption-of-risk form.* Participants must understand the risks involved with sport and know that a potential for injury or illness exists.

- *Maintain CPR and first aid certifications.* The AT should practice these skills regularly.

- *Have a crisis plan.* The AT must have an effective crisis plan in writing for all home and away contests. The crisis plan should explain the procedures to be carried out, and all who are involved should have a copy and know their role.

- *Document all injuries and procedures.* An AT should not only detail all injuries that occur but also all rehabilitation procedures, treatments, and follow-up care on the appropriate administrative forms. See appendix D for a sample treatment log to document daily procedures.

- *Maintain confidentiality.* ATs are required by law to keep medical information confidential. The Health Insurance Portability and Accountability Act (HIPAA) of 1996 requires that personal health-related information be secured and kept private. In other words, ATs can only share information if permission is granted. If an athlete is younger than 18, her parent or guardian must give permission to the AT to share information to necessary individuals such as coaches. The concept of confidentiality involves not only oral information but also written documents such as injury reports and other forms used in the athletic training room. It is important not to divulge medical information to anyone who is not authorized. For example, as a student assistant, you may be approached by a reporter looking for information about an injured athlete to print in a newspaper. Be sure to avoid disclosing any information.

•*Build trust.* An effective line of communication and good rapport within the athletic training team allows the AT to build trust and respect with everyone involved with an athletic injury.

•*Check for hazards.* Regularly examine athletic fields, courts, and equipment to identify potential hazards. If an AT finds a hazard, he should remove it or have it removed and document his actions.

•*Stay educated.* ATs have a responsibility to continue their education and stay current on the latest information in the allied medical field. An AT must also understand her qualifications and know her limitations. Moreover, because state laws differ, it is important for ATs to understand their state regulations.

ATHLETIC TRAINING FACILITIES

When it comes to evaluating athletes, conducting prevention procedures, treating injuries, and providing first aid, ATs fulfill their professional obligations in athletic training rooms. As health care providers, ATs have an obligation to make sure the athletic training room meets the patients' needs and allows for proper care.

The Real World

During an intercollegiate game, a goalie from a visiting soccer team received a blow to the head from one of his teammates while trying to scoop up a soccer ball. He was hit so hard that his skull was fractured. The host AT attended the athlete and called for an ambulance immediately. The athlete's condition was worsening even as he was being taken to the emergency room, and a helicopter was called because the athlete needed to be transferred to a trauma center in another city. Unfortunately, the visiting team had no medical information about the athlete or any emergency contact information. Treatment was initiated because the athlete was unconscious; permission to treat was implied. Because the athlete had recently walked on to the team, even his full name was a mystery—thankfully, a rare occurrence. It took many phone calls to the school before the athlete's name was determined and then more detective work to figure out how to reach his parents. The moral of the story is to always have appropriate medical information—complete with emergency contact numbers—with the team at all times.

Phil Voorhis, MSEd, ATC

Athletic training room facilities should be well organized, clean, and well illuminated. Also, each athletic training room should contain the following areas:

•*Private examination room.* Team physicians will need a secured, quiet area to conduct examinations of athlete's injuries. In instances where a private examination room does not exist, at least a curtained-off section of a treatment area should be available.

•*Treatment area.* ATs will need plinths, or tables, available to treat athletes with ice or heat applications and other modalities.

•*Game and practice preparation area.* Game and practice preparation often involves taping and bracing limbs and helping to apply protective padding. Because many athletes need to use only this area because they do not receive other treatments, it should be close to an entrance.

•*Wound care and first aid area.* When athletes are wounded and in need of emergency care, an area with quick access to bandages, emergency equipment, and proper disposal containers for blood-stained items is necessary. Preferably athletes shouldn't have to walk through a treatment or taping area to access the wound care station. The wound care area should have a sink so ATs can wash their hands immediately after treatment.

• *Hydrotherapy area.* Any whirlpools and ice machines should be sectioned off and located over an appropriate drainage area. This area is necessary to prevent water from flowing into other regions of the room.

• *Rehabilitation and reconditioning area.* Space is needed for athletes to perform therapeutic exercises so they can regain strength, flexibility, balance, and range of motion. The rehabilitation space is often large because various types of equipment are needed to facilitate exercise.

• *AT office or record-keeping area.* An AT must keep adequate injury reports and records of treatments. A quiet and secure location is necessary to complete the various forms and maintain the records in locked cabinets.

Not every facility will have every area available for use, and some level of adaptability will likely be necessary to adequately treat athletes. Regardless of the size and quality of the facility, it should be kept organized and sanitized. Tables should be cleaned after an athlete has been treated, and floors, whirlpools, and equipment must be disinfected daily with appropriate solutions.

A training room should be designed to create the best facility to serve the student population. Most often ATs find themselves in a converted closet that was not designed for the type of work they do. If you are able to design a new facility, research many articles and AT training rooms to ensure you get what is necessary. For those who find themselves making do with what they have, adding items as funding becomes available may be all that can be done.

Location

The training room should be centrally located near locker rooms and the gyms. It is best for the training room to have an exterior wall with an exit to the outdoors. If the training room has a golf cart, it should be located within a storage room near the training room for easy access. The training room should be on the first floor unless there is an elevator (although the first floor is still ideal). All doors must be wide enough to allow for EMS to bring in stretchers. The exterior door should allow EMS access and parking in proximity.

Electrical

The training room must have ground fault interrupters for each outlet. This will prevent overload and electrocution. The outlets should not be lower than 3 feet (91 cm) from the floor (Ray 2000). Between each treatment table there should be an electrical outlet for modalities. Ray (2000) also states that outlets should be placed every 4 feet (123 cm) along the wall.

Plumbing

Plumbing is essential in the whirlpool room. There should be a mixing valve and a drain for each whirlpool. To ensure that whirlpools will work with the plumbing design, it's best to get the specifications for each whirlpool ahead of time. The ice machine requires only an old water outlet and a drain. In some instances the water will need to be filtered

to prevent breakdown of the machine. The hand-cleaning sink should have a sensor to start the water flow so that hands do not have to touch hot or cold handles.

Ventilation

A ventilation system must heat and cool effectively. The whirlpool area must have ventilation to reduce the humidity that may build up. Finally, the training room must have its own thermostat (Ray 2000).

Lighting

Ray (2000) suggests that 30 to 50 foot-candles (323-538 lux) are appropriate for the athletic training room. If natural lighting is available, the lighting should come from overhead. The lighting in the whirlpool room must be sealed to prevent humidity from entering the fixtures.

Office

The office should be big enough for all AT staff to have a desk space. It needs to be isolated so that private calls can be taken and not overheard. Athletic files, records from physicals, and injury reports have to be in locked cabinets. The office could have windows so that there is privacy yet a view of the training room as a whole. There should be Internet access within the office.

Whirlpool Room

The whirlpool room has to be large enough to allow for all of the whirlpools and flow of traffic through the room. The room must be visible from as many areas of the training room as possible. In some cases convex mirrors can be placed to reflect the whirlpool area to make it easier to see. The whirlpool room should be closed off from the rest of the training room to keep the noise level down and to keep the water within the room. The floor must have an antislip surface and drains in the floor in the event of an overflow.

Rehabilitation

In a high school setting, there may not be enough space for a rehabilitation area within the athletic training room. For some, the rehabilitation room may be the weight room. If the rehabilitation area is within the training room, it's best to have either a rubberized or carpeted floor. The area will have to be large enough for all machines, rehabilitation tables, mirrors, weights, balls, and open floor space for stretching and exercises.

Taping

The taping area is determined by the number of staff members who will be working and the number of students the AT will be dealing with at peak times. Because the taping area is the busiest, it should be located close to the door to provide quick entry and exit for athletes. Between each taping table there should be a countertop for extra supplies.

Treatment

The treatment area is designed for athletes who may require ultrasound, muscle stimulation, intermittent compression, or evaluation. Therapy equipment is found on moveable carts between each treatment table. Some treatment tables are adjustable for the purpose of moving the athlete up or down to ergonomically accommodate the AT's needs during treatment.

Storage

The storage room should be located close to the taping area. The size of the room will depend upon whether a year's worth of supplies will be stored or whether supplies will be delivered more than once a year. The availability of cabinets that can store supplies will also influence the size of the storage room. If tape will be stored in the closet, it needs to be in a cool, dry room. Supplies that are expensive should be held in a locked cabinet. If old injury files are to be kept in storage, they must be kept in locked file cabinets. If possible, the size of the storage room should be slightly larger than what was calculated as necessary.

PREVENTING ATHLETIC INJURIES

Reducing the risk of legal liability includes practicing comprehensive injury prevention. A comprehensive injury prevention program includes education, rule enforcement, proper matching of participants during practice, and elements of physical fitness. We will highlight some of the components involved in each of these elements of injury prevention.

What Would You Do If...

While in the athletic training room, you notice that several athletes from the basketball team have failed to write their names on the treatment log.

- *Educating the athlete.* Education includes both teaching athletes about the dangers involved with sport and the proper technique of their particular sport. For example, the AT and the coaching staff should educate a football player that his helmet is for protection and is not to be used as a weapon. When these educational sessions are completed, the coach should document which athletes were in attendance as a way to ensure that all athletes have been educated. Additionally, football players should be educated in proper technique several times a year. Failure to provide proper instruction leaves the AT potentially liable for negligence.

- *Rule enforcement.* Many rules are designed to prevent injuries. In football, for example, spearing was banned in 1976. Enforcement of this rule is necessary to prevent an athlete from using his head as a weapon. Coaches must enforce these rules in practice settings as well, because most athletic injuries occur during practice.

- *Proper matching.* Participants should be matched according to several factors, especially in contact sports such as wrestling, boxing, football, field hockey, and hockey, to help reduce the risk of injury. These factors include weight, age, physical maturity, and skill level. For example, if a 132-pound (60 kg) wrestler were matched with a 232-pound (105 kg) wrestler during practice, the smaller wrestler would be at a definite disadvantage in terms of size. The larger opponent could easily use his weight to inflict injury.

- *Physical fitness.* Participants who are physically fit can reduce their risk of injury. Being physically fit means that the elements of muscular strength, flexibility, cardiorespiratory and muscular endurance, and body composition have been addressed through a comprehensive program.

ADMINISTRATIVE ISSUES AND DOCUMENTATION

It is essential that the members of the sports medicine team document all the procedures they perform in order to prevent lawsuits and to provide the best care possible. For example, ATs need to be able to compare current physical findings of an injured athlete with previous findings from a physical examination or injury report. Moreover, it may be essential to review past injury treatments to determine the best type of care for an athlete.

Preparticipation Examinations

Preparticipation physical examinations are performed by a medical doctor to determine if an athlete is able to participate in a sport without extra risk of injury or illness. Additionally, preparticipation physical examinations give baseline information from which to make comparisons if an injury or illness does arise (see the highlight box on the following page). For example, if the AT is examining an athlete who is complaining of dizziness and her blood pressure seems a bit low, the AT can compare the value with the measurement recorded from a previous physical examination. The preparticipation physical examination should document an athlete's height and weight, blood pressure, and pulse. Also, the ears, nose, throat, heart, lungs, abdomen, flexibility, joint stability, and posture should be examined.

In many high schools, the AT and the team physician organize a large-scale physical examination for their athletes. These physical examinations often include a set of stations, and the athletes move from one station to the next until they have visited each station. The athletes could progress through the stations as follows:

1. Registration
2. Height, weight, and skinfold measurements
3. Blood pressure
4. Flexibility and joint stability
5. Posture
6. Ear, nose, and throat
7. Heart, lungs, and abdomen
8. Checkout with team physician in charge
9. Postregistration

When the athlete first enters the exam area, he registers for the physical and receives his paperwork. He fills out his name, address, and past medical history. He then progresses through the height, weight, skinfold, and blood pressure stations. When the athlete arrives at the flexibility, joint stability, and posture screening station, one of several ATs works with him individually to assess past athletic injuries and to see if he has joint problems, postural defects, or a lack of flexibility that may cause an injury. If a problem is found, the AT makes a note of it for the team physician to check at the end.

The athlete then moves to one of several physicians who will check his ears, nose, and throat. Next, the athlete is examined by one of several physicians who will listen to his heart and lungs for any abnormalities. His abdomen is checked at this time as well. The team physician is the last doctor that the athlete sees. At this point, the team physician checks any noted conditions from the previous stations to determine whether the athlete can play. The athlete then progresses to the postregistration booth. Here he can pick up information regarding the findings. For example, suppose an AT found that an athlete had much less strength in one leg than in the other. Knowing that this lack of strength could create problems and increase the athlete's risk of injury, the athlete would be given an instruction sheet for a lower-body strengthening program to improve his condition.

Medical Information Forms

The preparticipation physical examination is a good time for parents to fill out a medical information card along with the medical history. It is a good idea for an AT to keep with her at all times an informed consent form (permission to treat), an athlete's insurance information, and medical information. It is impossible to remember every condition that each athlete has. Therefore, keeping each athlete's medical information card in the medical kit allows the AT or coach to obtain crucial information at a moment's notice. For example, if a coach takes her

Goals and Outcomes of Preparticipation Examinations

The goals of the preparticipation exams are as follows:

1. To build a relationship between the student-athlete and the athletic training staff and the team physician
2. To build a relationship between the student-athlete's parents and the athletic training staff and the team physician
3. To make the AT aware of any conditions, illnesses, or injuries that may require attention when participating
4. To provide an opportunity to strengthen physical deficiencies
5. To allow students with conditions that require further medical care the opportunity to get such care before the season begins
6. To comply with association rules on participation

The outcomes of preparticipation exams are as follows:

1. Passed—this athlete can participate without any restrictions.
2. Passed with conditions—this athlete can participate in some sports but requires additional follow-up. If a physician clears the athlete of the condition, then full participation without restriction can occur.
3. Passed with reservations—the athlete will not be able to participate in contact or collision sports.
4. Failed with reservations—the athlete cannot participate in the sport requested. The physician may allow participation in less intensive sports.
5. Failed with conditions—the athlete has to return to peak health before participating. The athlete must be reevaluated to ensure health.
6. Failed—the athlete cannot participate in any sport at any time.

Adapted from American Academy of Orthopeadic Surgeons (1991) *Athletic training and sports medicine,* 2nd ed. Park Ridge, IL: Author.

tennis team to an away meet where one of her athletes is stung by a bee and suddenly begins to act ill, the coach can look at the medical data form to see if the athlete is allergic to bee stings. If an athlete needs advanced care at a hospital and the parent is not around, the medical data form can provide necessary information for giving proper treatment. As previously mentioned, many high schools keep the permission to treat and medical information on the same card (refer to the permission-to-treat form in appendix B).

Insurance

In most organizations, athletes are required to have some type of medical insurance before they can participate in organized sport. Many athletic programs require that insurance forms be kept with the informed consent (permission-to-treat) forms discussed earlier. Why is this necessary? Say

that an athlete who is traveling with the team on the road gets injured. If his parents are not at the game, the injured athlete can still be treated at a local hospital because permission to treat has been granted and appropriate insurance information has been provided. Unfortunately, insurance coverage is becoming increasingly complicated—ask any AT about the paperwork involved with insurance and watch her reaction. However, insurance is necessary because medical costs can be substantial.

Medical insurance has been described as a written agreement between an insurance company and the person who buys it. This agreement clarifies the terms of reimbursement for medical costs after an athlete has been treated. Many athletic programs purchase supplemental insurance that covers the leftover costs not covered by the primary insurance. The insurance is usually for injuries that occur as a result of athletic participation. Programs carry supplemental insurance so that an athlete's care is completely covered. Many athletic programs also carry catastrophic insurance that is used for injuries that cause permanent disability, such as paralysis.

Several types of insurance exist. These include managed care plans, indemnity plans, and health savings accounts (Anderson and Swann 2009).

Managed care plans include health maintenance organizations (HMOs) and preferred provider organizations (PPOs). Managed care plans are run in such a way that an agreement exists between the insurance company and a group or network of health care professionals. Essentially, restrictions are imposed on a patient and he must see a primary physician within the agreed-upon network to receive health care. A copay is usually required at the time of service. Often the copay is $20, but follow-up costs are limited.

Indemnity plans are sometimes referred to as *reimbursement plans*. They are organized to have an insurance company reimburse a patient for the full or partial amount of the cost of health care (Anderson and Swann 2009).

A health savings account (HSA) is often created by having an employer or individual submit money to a fund that is only used to pay medical claims as they occur. Health care providers are often selected from a larger network. For that reason, HSAs are often similar to HMO or PPO plans.

Reports and Charts

We have already discussed why ATs need to document their procedures. However, exactly which procedures must be documented is often debated. ATs should document any accident of which they are aware (even if it is not due to athletic participation), any treatment that an athlete receives, and the rehabilitation progress that an athlete makes. Many computer documentation or record-keeping systems are available to ATs. These computer systems make it easy to document injury reports, rehabilitation progress, and referral forms.

Accident and Injury Reports

Accident and injury reports contain vital information including the athlete's name, the date of injury, the date of the report, the athlete's sport, the age of the athlete, and the body part that is injured. Additionally, the report must contain information about how the injury or accident occurred, note whether it is a new or previous injury, and include the AT's inspection and assessment information and signature. The report should also contain the AT's thoughts about the injury and record treatment such as ice application, splinting, or medical referral. A sample injury report is shown in appendix C.

Treatment Logs

Any treatment an athlete receives must be documented (see daily treatment log, appendix D). Ice application, heat application, elastic wraps, stretching, strengthening, and so on must all be logged on a specific form.

Rehabilitation Charts

Once an athlete has been injured, her injury assessed, and a proper rehabilitation program designed and implemented, it is essential that the AT document the athlete's progress (see the treatment progress chart in appendix E). The AT must record the exact treatment received by the athlete, the date it was received, any problems or complaints, any changes in treatment, the athlete's response to treatment, and reevaluation data.

Managing and Using Reports

Data from injury reports should not only be recorded to reduce liability but also to track injury trends and make decisions about how best to treat these injuries. Thankfully, there are many programs on the market that allow ATs to enter injury data and generate reports at the end of the year. Examples of data management software include Athletic Injury Management (AIM), SportsWare 2009, and NExTT Solutions Injury Management software, just to name a few.

Using programs such as these allows ATs to identify the most common injuries that occurred and identify appropriate prevention strategies to curtail them. Additionally, ATs can compare their injury data against published reports.

PROFESSIONAL DEVELOPMENT

Professional development refers to the ongoing responsibility of improving one's skills and knowledge in order to deliver appropriate health care to

What Would You Do If...

You are helping the team get ready for practice. You get to the football field and notice that there is a large hole in the ground in the practice area.

injured athletes. The successful AT will behave ethically, stay abreast of the latest medical issues and trends, display good communication skills, and be an effective leader.

Standards of Professional Practice

The AT must treat people fairly to the best of her ability and do what is right. To help its members, NATA has updated its **standards of professional practice**, which are summarized in the NATA **code of ethics** (NATA 2005, 1998).

The principles of this code include the following:

Principle 1: Members shall respect the rights, welfare, and dignity of all.

Principle 2: Members shall comply with the laws and regulations governing the practice of athletic training.

Principle 3: Members shall maintain and promote high standards in their provision of services.

Principle 4: Members shall not engage in conduct that could be construed as a conflict of interest or that reflects negatively on the profession.

Staying Educated

If medical professionals never learned how to use anything new or failed to use the most up-to-date technology, an injured athlete would not get the best care. Therefore, once a person has earned the credential *ATC* after his name, he is required to continue his education. The BOC requires that an AT complete 75 continuing education hours, known as continuing education units (CEUs), every three years. The CEUs are obtained in a variety of ways, such as attending educational workshops, writing and publishing, taking college classes, and completing home study courses. In addition to these professional learning activities, an AT must maintain professional rescuer CPR certification (every three years an AT must show proof of current CPR certification).

Communication

Whether an AT works at a high school, college, or sports medicine clinic, she must have good communication skills. ATs communicate daily with athletes, parents, physicians, coaches, and administrators at every level. Failure to send the right message can result in many anxious hours and negative consequences. Jeff Konin, in a text titled *Clinical Athletic Training* (1997), offers many practical suggestions for ATs to enhance their communication skills. He suggests that as a listener, you should be attentive and open-minded. Establish good eye contact, because direct eye contact sends the message that a matter is important. Also, when you use direct eye contact, people often believe that you spent more time with

BOC Standards of Professional Practice

In addition to the NATA code of ethics, a certified AT must follow the BOC standards of professional practice (BOC 2006). There are seven standards set forth by the BOC:

1. Direction: A physician directs the service provided by an AT.

2. Prevention: An AT must use sound preventive measures to protect each patient.

3. Immediate care: Standards of immediate care procedures are used in all athletic training settings.

4. Clinical evaluation and diagnosis: The AT is to use appropriate assessment procedures and clinical reasoning and decision making to diagnose a patient's injury.

5. Treatment, rehabilitation, and reconditioning: The AT must use proper goal setting, intervention strategies, and assessment measures for the effective treatment of patients.

6. Program discontinuation: The AT will collaborate with a physician to determine when a patient's treatment program can be discontinued.

7. Organization and administration: Any service rendered to a patient is appropriately documented and becomes part of the patient's permanent medical record. Members shall maintain and promote high standards in the provision of services.

them than you actually did. Pay attention to your gestures; they send messages that can be interpreted in unintended ways. For example, if a person crosses his arms, he may be thought of as closed off, as though he isn't really listening.

Leadership

The profession of athletic training has progressed and flourished, undoubtedly because of the leadership of its members. Several principles and qualities of leadership are important for ATs.

• *Integrity* refers to the AT conducting herself in an ethical manner, such as following the standards of professional practice noted earlier.

• *Vision* refers to being able to anticipate the needs of the athletes. Asking questions such as "How can we keep athletes from getting this type of injury?" helps ATs begin looking forward with a vision.

• *Inspiration* refers to being able to persuade people that your vision is appropriate. For example, when an AT rehabilitates an injured athlete, he inspires the athlete to pursue the vision of normal function and return to participation.

• *Competence* refers to having the knowledge and skills necessary to perform effectively.

THE PREMIER MODEL

The **PREMIER model** provides an easy way of thinking about being a future professional. This model is based on the authors' experience as professionals in athletic training. The acronym for this model can be found in figure 2.1.

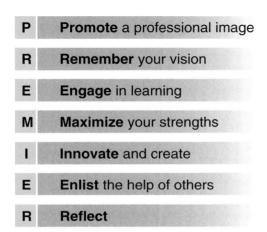

P	**Promote** a professional image
R	**Remember** your vision
E	**Engage** in learning
M	**Maximize** your strengths
I	**Innovate** and create
E	**Enlist** the help of others
R	**Reflect**

Figure 2.1 The PREMIER model gives helpful suggestions for developing yourself as a future professional.

• *Promote a professional image.* As a student assistant, you can project a professional image by the way you dress. An old saying states that you don't get a second chance at a first impression. Although wearing shorts, tennis shoes, and T-shirts may be fine during practice or game coverage for warm-weather activities, it is imperative that you be distinguishable and professional looking in case someone needs to find you for help.

• *Remember your vision.* You must have a good understanding of your career goals and objectives and what type of person you are striving to become. Some people write down their vision statement so they can continually be reminded of their purpose and set appropriate personal goals.

• *Engage in learning.* As a student and future professional, it is important to take initiative to learn new things daily.

• *Maximize your strengths.* We all have limitations. If you dwell too much on them, you may not learn and do the things that can make you successful. Cultivate your strengths and ask yourself how they can support your personal vision.

• *Innovate and create.* Over the past 10 to 20 years, technology has continually advanced. Today's problems cannot be solved with yesterday's solutions. As a future professional, it is important for you to develop new ideas. This will keep you excited about your work.

• *Enlist the help of others.* In the previous chapter you learned about the role of the AT and the sports medicine team. The old saying that there is no *I* in *team* is absolutely accurate. Be a team player.

• *Reflect.* When you become a professional, it will be essential to think back on what you have done and consider the results, whether you are rehabilitating an athlete or performing a tape job on an ankle. Get into the habit now of reflecting on your actions in the athletic training room to help you learn what you might do better in a similar situation in the future.

Tom Abdenour, ATC, states that you should *C* your way to success as a certified AT. The four Cs are conscientiousness, competency, courtesy, and courage. To be successful, be conscientious about the little things, such as following through with treatments, maintaining a clean and safe facility, and being available to the athletes. Being conscientious involves representing yourself, your organization, and your profession in a quality manner and being loyal to your staff and organization. Competency involves being good at what you do and continually learning to expand your horizons. Courtesy involves being a team player, interacting with everyone you work with in a positive manner, and treating people as you would want to be treated. Finally, to be successful, you must have the courage and fortitude to take on challenges.

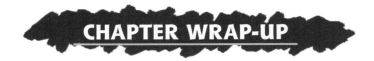

CHAPTER WRAP-UP

Summary

ATs must follow standards of professional practice as set forth by NATA. These standards guide the AT in a quest to deliver professional health care. To maintain an acceptable level of knowledge, the AT is required to participate in 75 hours of continuing education every three years. ATs often find themselves in leadership roles and thus should conduct themselves with integrity, vision, inspiration, and competence. There are numerous administrative considerations for the AT. Not only should proper documentation of injuries and treatments be a concern but also legal liability. An AT should create an environment designed to prevent injury and should take several steps to prevent liability. One such step is to document the occurrence of all athletic and nonathletic injuries and illnesses as well as the treatment or rehabilitation the athlete receives. Clear, concise medical documentation is imperative. Also, a requirement for delivering appropriate services to athletes is having a facility with all the necessary components needed to treat and rehabilitate injuries. These components include a rehabilitation area, whirlpool room, treatment area, taping location, storage room, and secure office.

Key Terms

Define the following terms found in this chapter:

assumption of risk	gross negligence	PREMIER model
code of ethics	informed consent	proximate cause
duty of care	negligence	standards of professional practice

Questions for Review

1. Describe the various medical documentation forms that must be used in an athletic training room.
2. What are the aspects of injury prevention covered in this chapter, and how might they be useful for preventing injuries?
3. List each sport at your school and ways to prevent injuries involved with each.
4. Why does NATA have standards of professional practice? What could potentially happen if they are not followed?
5. List what you believe to be the common qualities involved with leadership. Do you possess all of these? If not, explain how you might begin to improve yourself as a leader.
6. What can a person do to improve his professional image?
7. Describe how insurance works and explain why it is necessary.

Activities for Reinforcement

1. What are your strengths, and how could you maximize them?
2. Reflect on something you observed in the athletic training room this week. What do you think could have been done differently to improve the results?
3. Create various injury report forms, treatment logs, and medical information forms.
4. Volunteer to help with preparticipation examinations.
5. Create a poster that identifies the most important personal characteristics a student assistant should possess.
6. Visit an athletic training facility and identify its service areas. Identify what improvements you might make.
7. Construct a drawing or blueprint of an ideal athletic training room.

Above and Beyond

1. Write a report on legal issues in sport.
2. Go online and find a formula for determining the size of a new training room based on the number of athletes seen per hour.
3. Write a paper on what it means to be a leader.
4. Visit www.acsm.org, search *pre-participation physical exam brochure,* and examine the current comment of the American College of Sports Medicine (ACSM).
5. Visit www.nata.org and find the NATA code of ethics.
6. Visit www.bocatc.org and examine the BOC standards of professional practice.
7. Explore one or more of the following suggested readings:

    Colston, M.A. 2004. Professionalism and ethics. Informed consent: review and implementation. *Athletic Therapy Today* 9(1): 29-31.

    Dick, T. 2004. Professional etiquette: how you show your respect for people. *Emergency Medical Services* 33(4): 91-96.

    Glover, D.W., B.J. Maron, and G.O. Matheson. 1999. The preparticipation physical examination: steps toward consensus and uniformity. *Physician and Sportsmedicine* 27(8).

    Osborne, B. 2001. Principles of liability for athletic trainers: managing sport-related concussion. *Journal of Athletic Training* 36(3): 316-321.

8. Examine the epidemiological study titled "Epidemiological Features of High School Baseball Injuries in the United States, 2005-2007" published in *Pediatrics in Review,* an online journal dedicated to pediatric medicine, by going to http://pediatrics.aappublications. org and searching for the article title. After examining the injury rates, what conclusions can you draw about possible ways to reduce injuries?
9. Visit www.healthinsuranceindepth.com/basics-how-it-works.html and read more about how medical insurance works.

UNIT II
Basics of Human Anatomy and Physiology

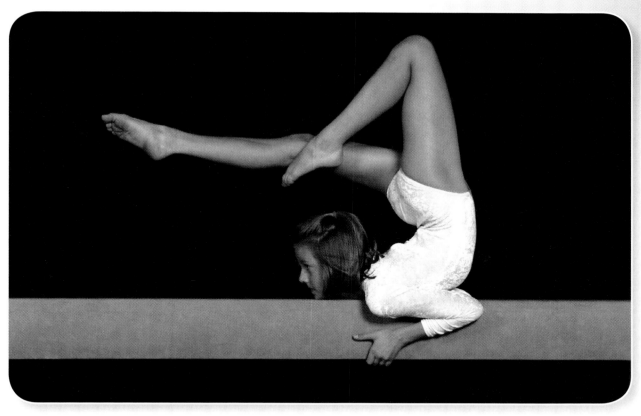

Photodisc/Getty Images

chapter 3

Introduction to Anatomy

Objectives

Upon completing this chapter, the student will be able to do the following:

- Define the anatomical planes and describe the anatomical position.
- Label general muscular and bony anatomy.
- Describe the functions of skin, bone, muscle, ligament, tendon, and cartilage.
- Describe the types of bones and give examples.
- Describe the classification of joints and explain the types of motion produced.

An understanding of human anatomy is the foundation of many health care professions, including that of the certified AT. An AT must have an excellent understanding of anatomy in order to determine what structures have been injured, and she must understand what constitutes normal movements in order to design appropriate rehabilitation and strength and conditioning programs.

ANATOMICAL POSITION

To improve communication between health care professionals and to facilitate a better understanding of human movement, medical professionals have accepted a particular alignment of the body as standard—the **anatomical position**. This position refers to an erect stance with arms at the sides and palms facing forward. The body moves in relation to three planes: **frontal**, **sagittal**, and **transverse**. These can be seen in figure 3.1.

You will need to know several common medical terms that help health care providers explain to one another where an injury is located on the body. There are many terms, and it is beyond the scope of this text to explain them all. Instead, we will present the most common terms that an AT would use in the training room. For instance, you will hear the terms *anterior, posterior, medial, lateral, proximal, distal, superior, inferior, dorsal,* and *ventral*. These terms are all used in reference to the anatomical position. Other common terms include *superficial* and *deep*.

• *Anterior* refers to the front of the body. When you face an athlete, you are looking at the athlete's anterior aspect. If you were to read an injury report stating that an athlete was hit at the anterior aspect of the lower leg, you would know that the front of the leg was injured.

• *Posterior* refers to the back of the body. When you watch an athlete walk away from you, you are looking at the athlete's posterior aspect. If an athlete indicates that the back of the knee hurts, the AT would report that the posterior aspect of the knee is injured.

• The terms **medial** and **lateral** are defined in relation to the sagittal plane, shown in figure 3.1. This imaginary line divides the body into left and right halves and is also called the *midline* of the body. If a body part faces the midline, it is said to be medial, and if it is closer to the midline than another body part, it is said to be more medial. Thus, when you look at the side of an athlete's calf that faces the other leg, you are looking at the medial aspect. On the other hand, if a body part is located away from the midline, it is said to be lateral, and if it is farther from the midline than another part, it is more lateral. Thus, when you look at the side of the calf that faces out, you are looking at the lateral aspect. As another example, your left ear is lateral to your left eye.

• *Proximal* means toward an attachment, such as where a limb attaches to the trunk of the body. Thus, the shoulder is proximal to the elbow, and the hip is proximal to the knee.

• *Distal* means away from an attachment. The knee is distal to the hip. A fingertip joint is distal; one at the base is proximal.

• *Superior* refers to one point, or structure, being higher than another. For example, the knee is superior to the ankle. The term **cephalic** means toward the head and is synonymous with *superior*.

• *Inferior* refers to one point, or structure, being lower than another. For example, the pelvis is inferior to the ribs. The term **caudal** is synonymous with *infererior*.

• The terms **dorsal** and **ventral** are synonymous with the terms *posterior* and *anterior*, respectively,

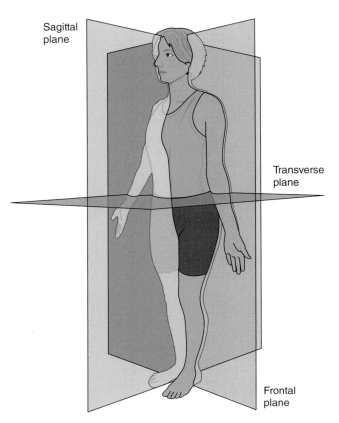

Figure 3.1 Anatomical planes. The anatomical position refers to a standing alignment with the arms at the sides and the palms of the hands facing forward. Note the planes that slice through the body.

Reprinted, by permission, from NSCA, 2008, Biomechanics of resistance exercise, by E. Harman. In *Essentials of strength training and conditioning*, 3rd ed., edited by Thomas Baechle and Roger Earle (Champaign, IL: Human Kinetics), 73.

but are often used in reference to the hand and foot. *Ventral* refers to the anterior aspect of a structure. *Dorsal* refers to the posterior aspect of a structure.

• *Superficial* means close to the body's surface; **deep** means away from the body's surface.

BODY TISSUES

Athletics-related injuries typically involve injuries to the skin, bones, cartilage, muscles, tendons, and ligaments. Before we can understand the specific injuries that occur to these tissues, we must first understand the basic function of these structures.

Skin

Skin is the outermost surface of the body. It provides the first line of defense against external forces such as insects, air, dirt, bacteria, and blows. The skin keeps bodily fluids in, it picks up sensations, and it secretes an oily substance. The skin is made of several layers (see figure 3.2). The most superficial layer is called the **epidermis**. The epidermis is thin and connects to the thicker **dermis** layer that is just below it. Below the dermis is the hypodermis. The hypodermis is not technically considered part of the skin, but it helps to hold the skin to underlying bone and muscle tissue. The hypodermis is sometimes called the *subcutaneous layer* and is responsible for storing about 50% of the body's fat (Seeley, Stephens, and Tate 1992). A break in the skin is a wound.

> **Understanding Diversity**

Vitiligo, a skin condition where pigmentation is absent, is more common in African Americans (Purnell and Paulanka 2005).

Skin has the ability to expand; for example, it expands to accommodate an increase in muscle **girth** (the distance around a body part) from weightlifting. Stretch marks are lines on the skin where the dermis was stretched excessively until elastic fibers ruptured. If the athlete loses girth, the skin will recover to a small extent.

> **Understanding Diversity**

Skin cancer resulting from overexposure to the sun is more often found in fair-skinned people (Purnell and Paulanka 2005).

Bones

Bones have three primary functions.

1. They protect vital organs and structures from trauma. Consider the brain. It is packaged in a hard shell (the skull) filled with fluid (cerebrospinal fluid), which helps to absorb shock and protect the brain. Similarly, the lungs and heart are surrounded by the rib cage, which supports and protects them.

2. Bones are the stiff structures that are acted on by muscles to create movement.

3. Bones are metabolically active; that is, they produce blood cells and store minerals such as calcium and phosphorus.

Bones also protect the nerves and blood vessels that travel alongside them.

The human body has approximately 206 bones and an astounding number of muscles. The skeleton is categorized into the **axial skeleton**, which includes the bones of the spine, thorax, and skull, and the **appendicular skeleton**, which includes the bones of the extremities. Although we will discuss specific bones in more detail in later chapters, here we present a general discussion of bony anatomy, bone types, and joint classification. See figure 3.3, *a* and *b*, for a look at the bones of the body.

> **Understanding Diversity**

African Americans have greater bone density and are less likely to have osteoporosis (Purnell and Paulanka 2005).

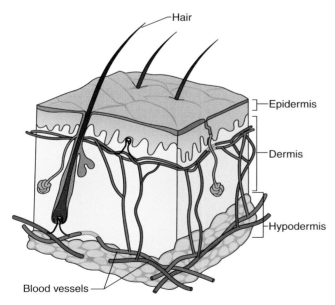

Figure 3.2 Cross section of skin tissue.

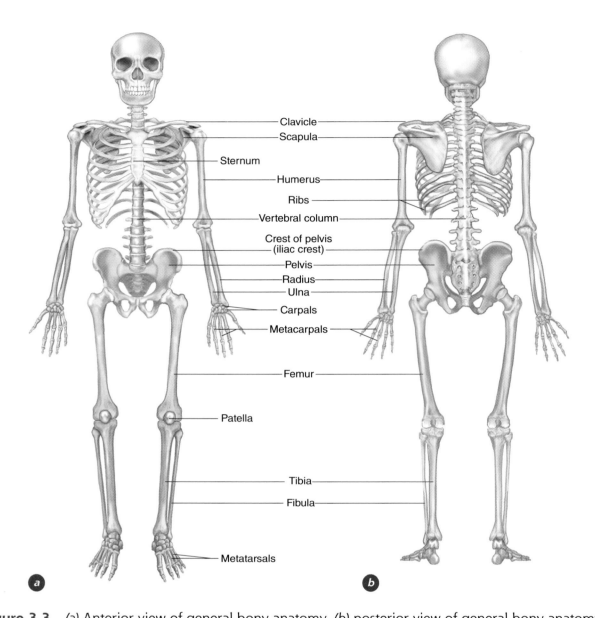

Figure 3.3 *(a)* Anterior view of general bony anatomy, *(b)* posterior view of general bony anatomy.

Reprinted, by permission, from J. Watkins. 2010. *Structure and function of the musculoskeletal system,* 2nd ed. (Champaign, IL: Human Kinetics), 33.

Bones come in several shapes and sizes, including long (e.g., femur), short (e.g., metacarpal), flat (e.g., scapula) and irregular (e.g., vertebra). Long bones possess an interesting feature. At the end of each long bone is an area where growth primarily takes place; this area is called an **epiphysis**, or *growth plate*. The area is somewhat spongy during adolescence and can be problematic for the adolescent athlete. The AT working in a high school setting should know that these growth plates are vulnerable to injury—a bone will often fracture at the growth plate.

Cartilage

Cartilage covers the ends of long bones and can be found between bones. Although cartilage comes in various forms, it typically functions to join structures (for example, the ribs and sternum), absorb shock, and permit smooth bone movement.

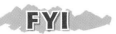

Muscles, Tendons, and Ligaments

Muscle contractions allow the body to accelerate, decelerate, stop movement, and maintain normal postural alignment. Moreover, they produce heat. Ligaments and tendons are both composed of connective tissue. **Tendons** attach muscle to bone and transmit the force that a muscle exerts. **Ligaments** connect bones and help to form joints.

Skeletal muscles are made of fibers. Each fiber has the ability to contract when a nerve impulse tells it to move. These fibers have to have the correct chemical balance to move properly. Skeletal muscles are attached to bones to create movement. A tendon is a strong fibrous cord that attaches the muscle to the bone. As a person ages, the skeletal muscles degenerates and is replaced by fibrous connective tissue, which limits range of motion.

Sphincter muscles reduce the size of an opening in the body. There are sphincter muscles in the eyes, stomach, bladder, and rectum.

Cardiac muscle is found in the walls of the heart. It is muscle that contracts on its own. Smooth muscle is found in hollow organs such as the stomach, intestines, and blood vessels.

CLASSIFICATION OF JOINTS

There are three classifications of joints:

- Diarthrodial
- Amphiarthrodial
- Synarthrodial

Diarthrodial joints are also known as *synovial joints*. They have fantastic mobility and consist of a **joint capsule** (a sleevelike ligament that surrounds the entire joint), a **synovial membrane** (a slick lining on the inside of the capsule), **hyaline cartilage** (a thin layer of cushioning at the ends of the bones), and ligaments. Diarthrodial joints are divided into several types, including hinge and multiaxial joints. Examples of **hinge joints** are the elbow and knee, which move back and forth like a

hinge on a door. Examples of **multiaxial joints** are the hip and shoulder. These joints can be moved in multiple directions (along many axes). The shoulder and hip joints are also commonly referred to as **ball-and-socket joints**; that is, the end of the long bone is rounded like a ball and is set into a cuplike socket of the other bone. Generally, these joints have a great deal of mobility compared with other joints.

Amphiarthrodial joints have cartilage attaching two bones together. They are also known as *cartilaginous joints*. An example of an amphiarthrodial joint is found where the ribs join the sternum. **Synarthrodial joints** are also called **fibrous joints**. These joints are held together by tough connective tissue, and the joints are basically immovable. This type of joint joins the bones of the skull and the tibia and fibula in the lower leg.

MOVEMENT

Without muscles, the body would not be able to move. An understanding of general muscular anatomy is essential for assessment of an athletic injury and rehabilitation following an injury. Therefore, an AT must learn where muscles are located and what actions they perform. Figure 3.4 illustrates the muscles located just underneath the skin. We talk more about specific muscles in later chapters.

Muscle tissue is divided into two categories, voluntary and involuntary. The movement of voluntary muscles is controlled by the person, whereas the movement of involuntary muscles is automatic. Involuntary muscles include the heart, intestines, and blood vessels.

Skeletal muscles generally attach at two points, the origin and insertion. The origin is the attachment to

What Would You Do If...

You are in the athletic training room and the AT has stepped out to speak with a coach. You notice an athlete reading his medical report, and he asks you to explain what the report means when it states, "Limited forearm pronation and supination as well as swelling at the distal end of the radius."

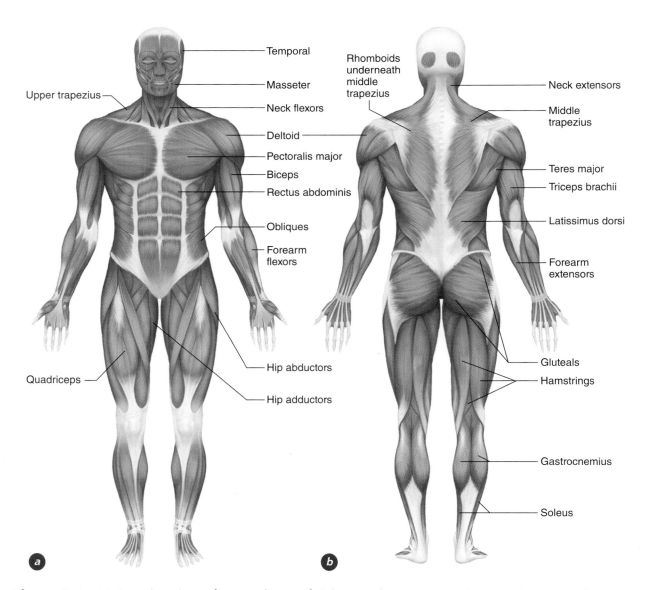

Figure 3.4 *(a)* Anterior view of general superficial muscular anatomy, *(b)* posterior view of general superficial muscular anatomy.

Reprinted, by permission, from NSCA, 2008, Biomechanics of resistance exercise, by E. Harman. In *Essentials of strength training and conditioning*, 3rd ed., edited by T. Baechle and R. Earle (Champaign, IL: Human Kinetics), 68.

a joint that is usually at the proximal end of a bone, and the insertion is at the distal end of a joint. The bulk of a muscle lies proximal to the joint it moves.

The muscle that is most responsible for a movement is called a *prime mover*. The muscle that relaxes to allow the prime mover to cause movement is called the *agonist*. If both muscles become part of the primary movement, they are commonly called *synergists*.

As muscles contract and produce movement, bony segments are moved in specific directions. Movement results from the angle at which the muscle pulls on the segment and the type of joint that joins the bones. Directional terms most commonly used by ATs and other medical professionals are *flexion* and *extension*, *abduction* and *adduction*, *pronation* and *supination*, *inversion* and *eversion*, *protraction* and *retraction*, *rotation*, *elevation*, *opposi-*

tions, and *circumduction* (figure 3.5, *a-j*, illustrates these movements). They are discussed in the following text.

- *Flexion* of a hinge joint is the bending·of the joint. The anatomical position (elbows and knees straight) shows those joints in **extension**. However, hinge joints such as the knee, elbow, fingers, and toes are not the only ones capable of flexing and extending. The shoulder, neck, trunk, hip, and wrist also flex and extend.

- Movement of a body segment away from the midline (the line of the sagittal plane) is termed **abduction**. For example, moving one leg outward from the anatomical position is abduction of the hip. Subsequently returning it toward the midline is termed **adduction**.

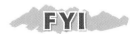

Axis

An axis is an imaginary line around which a segment such as an arm or leg rotates. For example, if you flex your hip (bring your knee toward your chest), you can say that the axis of motion is where the thigh (femur) joins the hip (pelvis).

- *Pronation* and **supination** occur at the wrist and ankle. At the wrist, for example, if you turned your palm toward the sky as though you were going to hold a bowl of soup, you would be supinating your wrist. Conversely, if you turned your wrist so the palm faced the ground as if you were pouring out the soup, you would be pronating

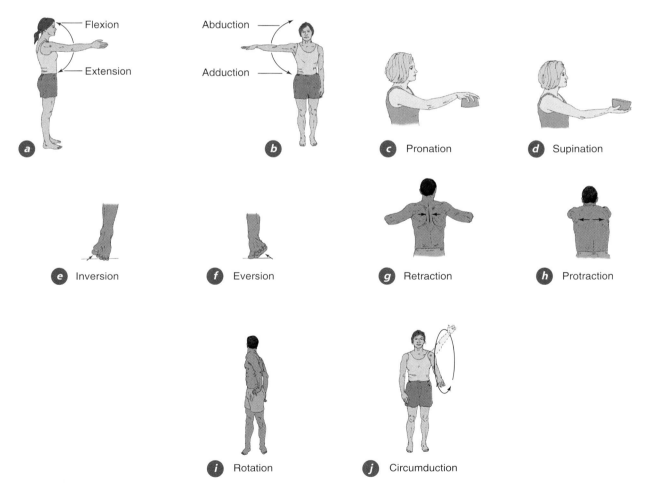

Figure 3.5 Illustrations of directional terms most commonly used by ATs.

a, b, e, f, i, and *j*: Adapted, by permission, from J. Griffin, 2006, *Client-centered exercise prescription* 2nd ed. (Champaign, IL: Human Kinetics), 119.

your wrist. In the anatomical position the wrist is supinated.

• *Inversion* and **eversion** of the ankle can be seen in figure 3.5. Inversion occurs when the sole of the foot is turned inward, and eversion is when the sole of the foot is turned outward.

• *Protraction* occurs when a segment glides forward, as when the lower jaw pushes outward until the chin sticks out. **Retraction** is gliding a segment backward, as when the scapulae squeeze together.

• *Rotation* occurs when a bony segment (or series of segments) spins or turns on an axis. An example of rotation is turning your head to look over your shoulder. Rotation can also occur either internally (toward the midline of the body) or externally (away from the midline of the body). For example, if you rotate your humerus with the elbow bent so that your hands move away from your body, you are performing external rotation.

• *Circumduction* occurs when a ball-and-socket joint, such as the shoulder or hip, encompasses several directions with one movement. In so doing, the joint is moved in a circular fashion around its axis.

• *Elevation* occurs when a bony segment is moved in a superior direction. When you shrug your shoulders, you are elevating them. **Depression** occurs when a bony segment is moved in an inferior direction. When you lower your shoulders after shrugging, you are depressing them.

• *Opposition* occurs when you move your thumb across your hand to meet your smallest finger, or fifth digit.

• *Reposition* means simply returning your thumb and fifth digit to their starting position.

The Real World

As an AT, I have had the opportunity to work with a great number of physicians who come regularly to our school to evaluate injured athletes. I typically examine the athlete before the physician arrives in order to give the doctor information about how the athlete was injured and to brief the doctor on the problem. One afternoon I told our team physician that an athlete was having pain at the fourth lumbar vertebra in his low back. After his examination, the team physician felt we should get an X ray of the spine to make sure there wasn't a fracture. The physician thought, however, that the pain was at the third lumbar vertebra. I found it odd that we disagreed about which vertebra was injured. After receiving the X rays, we found two interesting facts—the athlete did not have a fracture, but he did have a rare extra vertebra in his spine. Given the circumstances, we agreed that we were both right about which vertebra was involved!

Anonymous

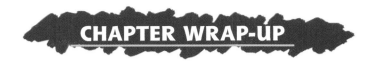

CHAPTER WRAP-UP

Summary

Understanding basic human anatomy is essential for understanding athletic injuries. The AT will use precise medical terminology when talking about a body area, and the student assistant should be familiar with this terminology in order to understand exactly what the AT is discussing. The body is made of several tissue types: skin, cartilage, bone, ligaments, tendons, and muscle. Bones come in a variety of shapes and sizes. A joint is a point of contact between bones, and joint structure determines the type of movement possible. Muscles move the bones through the planes of the body. The ligaments, cartilage, and tendons help hold the joints together and produce smooth movement.

Key Terms

Define the following terms found in this chapter:

abduction	epidermis	opposition
adduction	epiphysis	posterior
amphiarthrodial joint	eversion	pronation
anatomical position	extension	protraction
anterior	fibrous joints	proximal
appendicular skeleton	flexion	reposition
axial skeleton	frontal plane	retraction
ball-and-socket joint	girth	rotation
caudal	hinge joint	sagittal plane
cephalic	hyaline cartilage	superficial
circumduction	inferior	superior
deep	inversion	supination
dermis	joint capsule	synarthrodial joints
depression	lateral	synovial membrane
diarthrodial joints	ligaments	tendons
distal	medial	transverse plane
dorsal	multiaxial joint	ventral
elevation		

Questions for Review

1. What are the three anatomical planes of the body?
2. How does the function of a ligament differ from that of a tendon?
3. Give two examples each of a long bone, an irregular bone, and a flat bone.
4. Describe a synovial joint and give two examples.
5. What term describes the growth plate of a bone?
6. What are the three layers of skin called?

Activities for Reinforcement

1. Working with a partner, move each joint through its various positions, and give the proper term for each movement.

2. Point to a body part and have your partner name it. Include muscle groups and bones.

3. Working with a partner, point to a body part and have the other person describe its location using medical terminology. For example, when you point to the forearm, your partner might state that the location is proximal to the wrist and distal to the elbow.

4. Using an anatomical chart, identify the major bones of the body.

Above and Beyond

1. If you are interested in learning more about the various anatomical systems of the body, visit the following Web sites, click on a system, and have fun learning:

   www.nlm.nih.gov/research/visible/visible_human.html

   www.innerbody.com/htm/body.html

2. Go to http://anatomy.med.umich.edu/atlas/atlas_index.html, which contains an atlas of various parts of the human body. The site allows you to view to see the anatomical structures in great detail.

3. Visit the following Web site to find charts you could use as learning tools:

   www.enchantedlearning.com/subjects/anatomy/titlepage.shtml.

4. Students who are interested in learning more detailed anatomy can investigate the following Web sites:

   www.getbodysmart.com/

   www.innerbody.com/htm/body.html

   www.gwc.maricopa.edu/home_pages/crimando/Tutorial_Big.htm

5. Visit www.human-anatomy.net and examine the detailed images of human anatomy.

Basics
of Tissue Injuries

Objectives

Upon completing this chapter, the student will be able to do the following:

- Explain the types of soft-tissue injuries.
- Explain tissue repair and healing.
- Explain the various bone injuries.
- Explain bone repair and healing.

The body is made up of various tissues, each of which has unique characteristics and functions. In this chapter we discuss the body tissues in both healthy and injured states.

SOFT-TISSUE INJURIES

Soft-tissue injuries are often called *wounds*, *sprains*, and *strains*. These types of injuries are commonplace in athletics. When a soft tissue is injured, it may bleed, become inflamed, or produce extra fluid. These injuries are often classified as acute because they occur suddenly as a result of a high amount of force applied to the tissue over a short time.

Wounds are injuries to the skin. The soft-tissue injuries form (figure 4.1 on pages 42-43) describes the types of wounds that occur.

Sprains and **strains** are injuries that bleed internally, which may cause fluid buildup. Sprains are injuries to ligaments—the strong pieces of tissue that hold adjoining bones together. A strain is an injury to a muscle or tendon. A tendon attaches a muscle to a bone and transmits the force that a muscle exerts.

Sprains and strains are categorized in order of severity as first-, second-, or third-degree injuries. If the tissue is overstretched and there is no loss of motion in the injured body part, the sprain or strain is first degree, or mild. If the tissue is partially torn and there is some loss of motion and swelling, the injury is second degree, or moderate. If the tissue is completely or nearly ruptured (pulled apart), the injury is considered third degree, or severe. With a third-degree injury, the athlete typically cannot

Incision

An incision is an open wound made by a cutting object such as a scalpel. It is rarely seen in athletics.

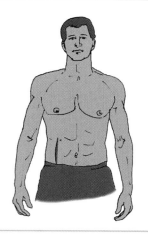

Abrasion

An abrasion results from scraping off a layer of skin. It may or may not bleed, depending upon its depth. A base runner in softball or baseball may acquire an abrasion when sliding into base.

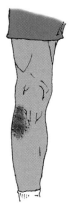

Contusion

A contusion is a closed wound, commonly called a *bruise*. It bleeds under the skin, which can cause swelling and discoloration. An athlete receives a contusion from running into something, such as another person's elbow.

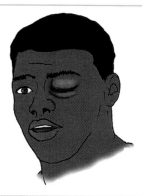

Laceration

A laceration is a jagged, irregular open wound created by a noncutting object such as a steel pole or a wall. For example, a lacrosse player who runs into the goalpost may receive a laceration.

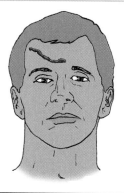

Figure 4.1   Soft-tissue injuries.

Contrecoup: Adapted, by permission, from W. Whiting and R. Zernicke. 2008. *Biomechanics of musculoskeletal injury,* 2nd ed. (Champaign, IL: Human Kinetics), 250.

Avulsion

An avulsion is a partial tearing away of a body part. An avulsion of a finger may occur if one catches a ring on the basketball hoop when dunking a basketball.

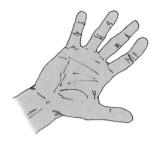

Amputation

An amputation is an open wound in which a body part is completely cut away from the body. Cutting off a finger with an ice skate is an example of an amputation.

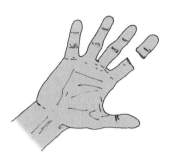

Puncture

A puncture wound occurs when a pointed object enters the body, such as stepping on a nail. Puncture wounds do not bleed much, so they are more likely to become infected than freely bleeding wounds.

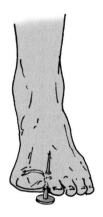

Contrecoup

A contrecoup injury occurs on the opposite side of the initial injury. This usually occurs in the brain when the head hits an unyielding object or surface. The impact to the back of the head, for example, forces the brain against the anterior part of the skull, resulting in a contrecoup injury.

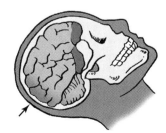

function well. For strains, this means an inability to move the body part because the muscle cannot pull on the bony levers. For sprains, this means an inability to bear weight and move a joint because of pain and looseness of the joint.

Another soft tissue that can be injured is a nerve. Nerve tissue connects the brain and spinal cord with all parts of the body. Nerves transmit the sensations of touch, pain, heat, and cold, and they relay messages from the brain to signal a muscle to contract or relax. Therefore, when a nerve is injured the athlete may experience a lack of sensation and even of movement. A stretched nerve can send a message of extreme pain. A nerve injury takes a long time to heal, and if the damage is severe, it will not heal.

One specific nerve injury is a neuroma. A neuroma is an enlarged nerve tissue that develops most often in the foot. The enlargement is caused by constant compression and irritation of the nerve.

Chronic Soft-Tissue Injuries

Soft-tissue injuries can also be chronic. Chronic injuries are the result of lesser forces being applied to the body over a long time. For example, a distance runner who trains extensively every day for several months without getting enough rest may load the soft tissues enough to cause damage.

There are several types of chronic soft-tissue injuries, including synovitis, bursitis, myositis, and fasciitis. **Synovitis** is a chronic injury to the synovial lining of a joint. The cause can be an acute injury that is never treated properly or rested, but more often the injury is chronic and the result of repeated joint injury.

Bursitis is the chronic inflammation of a bursa sac. Bursa sacs are located near joints where soft-tissue structures may rub near a bone. When a bursa becomes irritated, it tends to swell and can create a pocket of swelling at the joint.

Myositis is chronic inflammation of the muscle tissue. The condition is characterized by soreness, tenderness, and mild swelling in the muscle. The injury is particularly sore when trying to contract the muscle.

The fascia is a thick, tough connective tissue that surrounds the muscles and helps to loosely bind the skin to the underlying fat and muscle tissue. When fascia becomes strained due to overuse, it can become thickened, swollen, and painful. Chronic inflammation is called **fasciitis**.

Stages of Soft-Tissue Healing

When soft tissue is injured, it progresses through three stages of healing: acute inflammatory, repair, and remodeling. We describe each stage in the following text.

● *Stage I: Acute inflammatory.* When a body part is injured, cells within the area die both from being ripped apart and from being cut off from their food and oxygen supply. In the acute inflammatory stage, an increased flow of blood to the injured area brings cells and chemicals to begin the healing process. **Phagocytes** are specialized cells that engulf and eat the dead cells. **Leukocytes** are infection-fighting white blood cells. **Platelets** carry blood-clotting materials. The acute stage lasts for about two days after the initial injury.

● *Stage II: Repair.* The injured area has now been filled with blood, cells, and chemicals to rebuild the area. The **fibroblasts** (fiber-building cells) begin building fibers across the area of injury. Fibroblasts form a scar, which takes from six weeks to as long as three months depending on the extent of the injury.

● *Stage III: Remodeling.* Remodeling takes up to a year or more to accomplish. It is the body's way of building tissue strength in the tendons, ligaments, and muscles to withstand the stress applied to the body during activity.

> ### Understanding Diversity
>
> African Americans have a higher incidence of keloid scar formation (Purnell and Paulanka 2003) and are more likely to have excessive scar formation.

In general, the greater the injury to the tissue, the longer the healing time, although it depends on the degree of the injury, the location of the injury, the blood supply to the injury, and the age of the athlete. If blood supply to an area is poor, such as in the eyeball, the healing process will take longer.

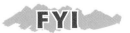

FYI

The Suffix *itis*

The suffix *itis* denotes an inflammatory reaction. In chronic conditions, the inflammatory response does not resolve, preventing the body from moving on to the next stages of healing.

Corticosteroids

Corticosteroids are chemicals made in the body that help reduce inflammation. When an injury occurs, a synthetic corticosteroid may be used as a medication to help reduce inflammation, but it can also increase the healing time.

Skin Closures

A skin closure is a thin, tough piece of material that can bring together the edges of a wound and close a deep wound effectively. A skin closure may also be called a *butterfly*.

Other factors that significantly slow the healing process are poor nutrition, illnesses such as diabetes, medications such as corticosteroids, and infections. Some athletes believe that eating certain foods will hasten healing, but no research supports this.

One complication of healing is excessive scar tissue (keloid) that results when more tissue is laid down than is necessary to repair the wound. Excessive scar tissue can delay healing and interfere with function, especially if it forms deep within joints. In some instances, scar tissue must be surgically removed so that proper movement can occur.

Large wounds whose edges are far apart take longer to heal. Keeping the wounds closed with stitches or skin closures will help the healing.

If activity is resumed too soon after an injury, healing time will be longer because the early activity can cause more cellular injury. Although athletes are always anxious to get back to competition, the AT must use good judgment early in the healing process to ensure proper healing.

BONE INJURIES

ATs must be familiar with the types of bone injuries and their stages of healing. Dislocations and fractures are common athletic injuries. Why do bones break? How much force must be applied before a bone will break? The answers to these questions vary depending on the athlete, the location where the force is applied, the bone type, the body position, and so forth.

Dislocation

When bones come together at a joint, they are said to **articulate**. A **dislocation** occurs when a significant force displaces bone so that the two bone ends in the same joint no longer line up. A dislocation can also cause avulsion fractures (see page 46), strains, sprains, disruption of blood flow, and disruption of nerve conduction. Dislocations present with deformity and pain and are not easily moved. Dislocations are cared for by the team physician and are not put back in place by the AT.

Understanding Diversity

The long bones in Alaska Natives are less dense, making them more prone to fractures (Schrefer 1994).

Fracture

The amount of energy required to cause a **fracture**—a broken bone—is called the **failure point**. Failure points vary with the athlete, age, and bone structure. For example, an athlete with a bone-deteriorating condition such as osteoporosis will have a lower failure point than an athlete with healthy bones.

Fractures are named according to the type of impact and how failure of the bone occurs; for example, we say a bone has been *broken, cracked,* or *chipped,* or we may say it has a *hairline fracture.* All of these terms mean that the bone has been compromised and weakened. With any fracture injury the athlete will be in a splint or cast for six to eight weeks, which is the amount of time required for healing. However, some fractures can be splinted, and the athlete can resume participation immediately. A student assistant should be familiar with the various types of fractures (see figure 4.2).

Avulsion

An avulsion occurs when a ligament or tendon pulls so hard at its bony attachment that a portion of the bone is torn away. Avulsion fractures are common with sprains, strains, and dislocations.

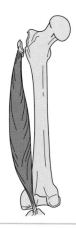

Stress

A stress fracture, also known as a fatigue fracture, occurs in a bone that has been subjected to a repetitive stress. That athlete will complain of a persistent sore spot over the bone. Stress fractures are microscopic and cannot be viewed on an X ray.

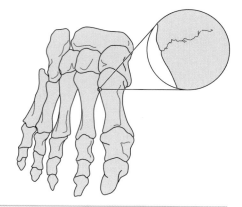

Spiral

A torsional force along the length of a bone causes a spiral fracture. Imagine that you are in-line skating and you are not very good. If your foot moves to the right while the rest of your body goes to the left, the stress may cause a spiral fracture. On an X ray, the spiral fracture looks like the stripe on a candy cane.

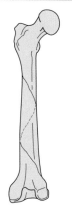

Longitudinal

A longitudinal fracture runs the length of a bone and is usually caused by an impact. A pole-vaulter who misses the mat and lands on her feet is likely to suffer a longitudinal fracture.

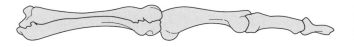

Figure 4.2 Types of fractures.

Spiral, oblique, and transverse: Adapted, by permission, from W. Whiting and R. Zernicke, 2008, *Biomechanics of musculoskeletal injury,* 2nd ed. (Champaign, IL: Human Kinetics), 163.

Compression

A compression fracture occurs when opposing forces are applied to a bone from both ends at the same time. Compression fractures often occur in the spine. For example, a compression fracture may result when an athlete lands on his feet or buttocks from a height. The impact from the ground is one force, and the weight of the falling body is the other. The opposing forces cause a compression fracture in the vertebrae.

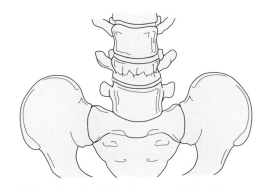

Oblique

Imagine a diagonal line across a bone from one side to another. You have just visualized an oblique fracture. An oblique fracture in a weight-bearing bone, such as a leg bone, takes longer to heal because the diagonal angle of the bone ends makes it easy for the bones to move out of alignment, even in a cast.

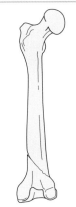

Comminuted

When a bone is crushed into smaller pieces, it is comminuted—think of a baseball catcher whose bare hand is hit by a bat.

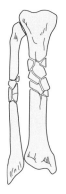

Greenstick

Adolescents' and children's bones are soft; that is, their bones still have some of the properties of cartilage. These bones tend to bend and fracture only partway through, and this is known as a greenstick fracture.

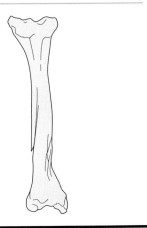

(continued)

Figure 4.2 *(continued)*

Transverse

A fracture that travels across and perpendicular to a bone is transverse. Transverse fractures occur from impacts perpendicular to the bone. A lacrosse player who brings his stick down across another player's forearms can cause a transverse fracture.

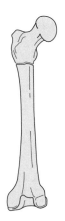

Depressed

A depressed fracture usually occurs from a direct impact to the skull, which indents. This indentation is called a *depression*.

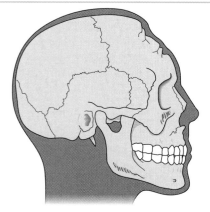

Blowout

A blowout fracture occurs when an eye is pushed hard backward and down into the eye socket. The small bones under the eye are crushed and embedded into the muscles of the eye. A blowout can occur when a hard object such as a baseball strikes the eye.

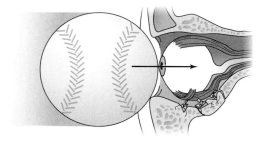

Pathological

A disease process such as a bone tumor can weaken the bones so that a little stress will cause a fracture. Improper nutrition and eating disorders are the most common causes of pathologic fractures among teenage athletes. The bones weaken because minerals are taken from them to support vital functions.

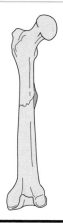

Figure 4.2 *(continued)*

Epiphyseal

The area of a bone where bone growth occurs, the epiphysis, is susceptible to fracture because the bony tissue is stronger than the epiphysis. In adolescents and children, many epiphyseal fractures occur, especially in the long bones. Adults do not get epiphyseal fractures because their growth areas are closed; that is, they do not have active growth centers. An X ray will not reveal a fracture of the epiphysis because epiphyses are clear on film.

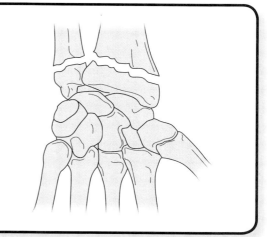

Figure 4.2 *(continued)*

Stages of Bone Fracture Healing

Similar to soft-tissue injuries, bone fractures go through the acute, repair, and remodeling stages of healing.

• *Stage I: Acute.* An injury to the bone causes the bone to break, and bleeding occurs in the area. Osteoclasts begin to eat the debris or resorb it into the body. Osteoblasts begin to add new layers to the outside of the bone tissue. This continues for about four days.

• *Stage II: Repair.* During the repair stage, osteoclasts and osteoblasts continue to regenerate the bone. A bony splint, or fibrous **callus**, forms (figure 4.3). The fibrous callus, which extends both

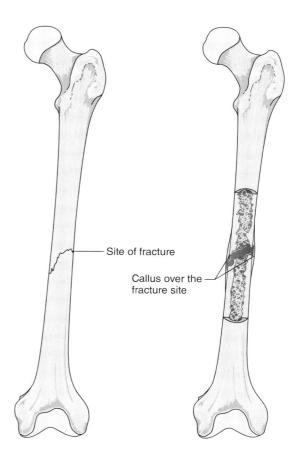

Site of fracture

Callus over the fracture site

Figure 4.3 When the bone heals, a callus forms.

What Would You Do If...

An athlete who has had a contusion under his toenail notices that the nail is pulling away from the nail bed. He says the nail is getting stuck on his sock. He has heard that pulling the nail off will make the new nail grow faster. He hands you a pair of pliers and asks you to pull it off.

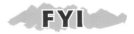

Deformity

Deformity refers to a misalignment of a body part.

Team Physician

The team physician is the medical authority of the sports medicine team. The doctor's role is to work with the AT to oversee the entire sports medicine team.

Osteoporosis

Osteoporosis is a condition in which bones are porous and fragile. In a young person it is caused by lack of calcium in the diet or by the inability to absorb minerals, especially calcium.

Osteogenesis

The process of laying down new bone, which provides a thickening of the bony structure, is called *osteogenesis*. Bone cells are called *osteocytes*, and a bone-forming cell is an *osteoblast*, whereas a cell involved in bone resorption is an *osteoclast*. As an athlete grows, osteoblasts replace cartilage and form bone tissue by laying down a new layer on the outside of bones. Osteoclasts eat at the interior layer of the bone. This normal process allows bone growth, removes older bone cells, and helps control the weight of a bony structure.

Cartilage

Cartilage is a tissue found at the ends of long bones and between bones. It absorbs shock and permits smooth bone movement at joints.

internally and externally to hold the bone ends together, is transformed into a sleeve of hard callus (i.e., bone). The process of transforming callus to bone begins at about week 3 and continues for 3 months. In most cases, after 6 weeks in a cast the fracture is strong enough to allow participation with protection, and the athlete is able to return to competition. However, the athlete must remember that the healing process is far from complete.

• *Stage III: Remodeling.* Stage III takes several years to complete. During this phase the callus is reabsorbed and replaced with a fibrous cord of bone that is formed around the fracture site. Growth of this fibrous cord of bone can be stimulated through surgically implanted electrodes when the bones are not healing. Bones contain minerals that have an electrical charge, and adding electrical stimulation increases the layering of the bone. If a bone never heals, the fracture is referred to as a **nonunion** fracture. A nonunion fracture in a weight-bearing bone, such as a leg, means that the athlete will not walk. A common nonunion fracture of the wrist occurs in the scaphoid bone. Such fractures are painful and may lead to arthritis and the inability to move the wrist.

The Real World

While working in a physician's clinic I had an opportunity to work with diabetic patients. A common symptom exhibited by diabetics is that it takes longer for wounds to heal than it does for people without diabetes. One physician with whom I worked found that applying low amounts of electrical current to diabetics' wounds helped them heal faster. For example, one of his patients had an open wound (an ulcer) on her foot. He ran a controlled amount of current into the patient's foot and took a picture after each session to document the healing process. He found that the healing time was much faster when he used the electrical current than when he used more traditional forms of treatment.

John Robinson, ATC

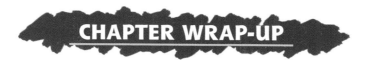

CHAPTER WRAP-UP

Summary

The body can get injured and, being a miraculous thing, repair itself. Indications of an injury to soft or bony tissue most commonly include pain, swelling, and bleeding. A soft-tissue injury may keep an athlete sidelined for longer than it takes a broken bone to heal. A fractured bone requires making new bone and fibers and reabsorbing the injured bone tissue. Healing time depends on the athlete's health at the time of injury and the care given during the healing process.

Key Terms

Define the following terms found in this chapter:

articulate	fibroblasts	platelets
bursitis	fracture	sprain
callus	leukocytes	strain
dislocation	myotosis	synovitis
failure point	nonunion	
fasciitis	phagocytes	

Questions for Review

1. Make a list of the types of fractures and determine who is most likely to suffer from each (e.g., adolescent, adult, male, female) and why.
2. What is the difference between a sprain and a strain?
3. How is a first-, second-, or third-degree sprain or strain defined?
4. Name the stages of soft-tissue healing and describe what happens in each one.
5. Name the stages of bone healing and describe what occurs during each one. Compare and contrast the healing of soft tissue and bony tissue.
6. What is the typical healing time for a fracture?

Activities for Reinforcement

1. Gather pictures of various wounds.
2. Have a physician demonstrate closing wounds with stitches and butterflies.
3. Make a picture showing how tissue repair and healing occur.
4. Make a picture showing how bone repair and healing occur.

Above and Beyond

1. Using the following materials, write a report about the healing process and some of the procedures that may enhance it.

    Bahr, R., and S. Maehlum, eds. 2004. *Clinical guide to sports injuries.* Champaign, IL: Human Kinetics.

Kloth, L.C., and J.M. McCulloch, eds. 2002. *Wound healing: alternatives in management.* 3rd ed. Philadelphia: Davis.

Whiting, W., and R. Zernicke. 1998. *Biomechanics of musculoskeletal injury.* Champaign, IL: Human Kinetics.

2. Interview a physician. Determine when and why the physician uses certain casting materials and bandages to treat fractures and wounds.

3. Visit the following Web site, review information related to sprains and strains, and view the types of fractures that occur in sport: www.sportsinjuryclinic.net.

UNIT III

Understanding Athletics-Related Injuries to the Axial Region

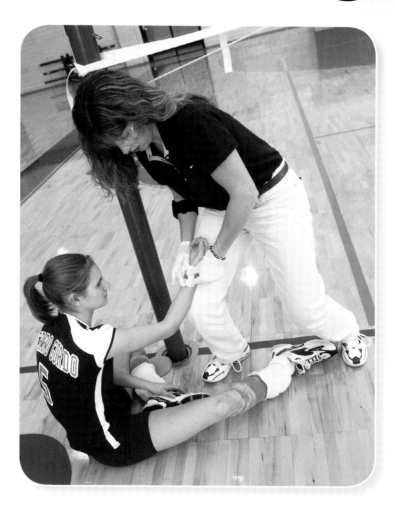

chapter 5

Head Injuries

Objectives

Upon completing this chapter, the student will be able to do the following:

- Describe the anatomy of the head.
- Understand that head injuries can be prevented.
- Understand the urgency involved with caring for brain injuries.
- Describe the types of head injuries.

When an athlete has a head injury, the AT must act quickly to lessen the chance of death and permanent injury. In this chapter we provide information to assist the student in understanding head injury and its prevention.

ANATOMY OF THE HEAD

The skull is composed of 28 bones that protect the brain (see figure 5.1). A suture line is the area where two bones in the skull come together. The single moveable bone in the skull is the mandible, or lower jaw.

The Brain

The brain is made of billions of cells. It weighs only about 3 pounds (1.4 kg), but it requires 20% of the total body oxygen and 15% of the blood supply. Brain cells grow and develop until age 18. After that, brain cells can be destroyed but not reproduced. Depriving the brain of oxygen will cause unconsciousness and then death—pupils will dilate

within 60 seconds (dilation is an indication of the inability to control the muscle of the iris of the eye). After four to six minutes without oxygen, biological brain death occurs, which means that large numbers of cells are dead.

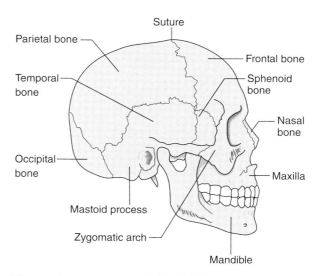

Figure 5.1 Bones of the skull.

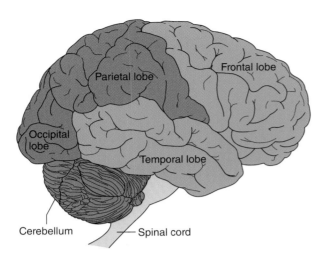

Figure 5.2   Brain areas.

Adapted, by permission, from W.C. Whiting and R.F. Zernicke, 2008, *Biomechanics of musculoskeletal injury,* 2nd ed. (Champaign, IL: Human Kinetics), 243.

The brain is divided into lobes, each named after the bony structure of the skull that covers it: occipital lobe, temporal lobe, parietal lobe, and frontal lobe (see figure 5.2). Each lobe is responsible for specific body functions. The brain attaches to the spinal cord at the brain stem via a crossover, so the right side of the brain controls the left side of the body and vice versa. Preserving brain function is of the utmost importance to injured athletes. Their quality of life—that is, their degree of recovery—depends on how the brain injury is handled.

Cerebrospinal fluid bathes the brain and spinal cord in chemicals for proper functioning, helps maintain regular pressure around the brain and spinal cord, and protects the brain from impacts. The fluid is clear amber in color. In instances of severe head injury, cerebrospinal fluid may drain from an opening in the skull, the nose, or an ear, and it should be allowed to do so. Stopping the drainage will only increase the pressure within the skull and cause more brain damage.

The Scalp

The scalp is the part of the skin that covers the skull, and it contains a large number of blood vessels, muscles, and hair. Skin protects against infections while hair protects the skin from the sun and keeps dirt and sweat away from the eyes. The blood vessels are so numerous in the scalp that even a small laceration will bleed profusely. Cartoonists draw a large lump when a character is hit in the head. This can also happen to athletes; a blow to the head may cause the many blood vessels to break open and bleed under the skin, causing a lump, or **hematoma**.

The scalp has the ability to decrease the force of an impact to the skull due to the additional padding it provides and the increased elasticity created by the tension of the connective tissue between the scalp and the skull. It is believed that without the scalp, the skull could be fractured with as little as 40 pounds (18 kg) of pressure. With the scalp, it may take 425 pounds (193 kg) of pressure before a fracture will occur. An athlete can sustain a serious head injury without a break in the scalp, however, so the AT should not be fooled by a lack of bleeding.

PREVENTING HEAD INJURIES

Head injuries are prevented by helmets, mouth guards, rules, and common sense. A commonly forgotten piece of equipment in the battle to prevent head injuries is the mouth guard, which can prevent not only dental injuries but also concussions. If an athlete is not wearing a mouth guard, an impact to the chin can drive the mandible into the maxilla and cause the brain stem to twist slightly, resulting in loss of consciousness. A mouth guard provides spacing and shock absorption between the mandible

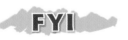

Brain Areas and Functions

The functions of the brain are based on location.

Frontal lobe: voluntary muscle movement, emotion, eye movement

Parietal lobe: sensation

Occipital lobe: vision

Temporal lobe: hearing, speech

Cerebellum: equilibrium, muscle actions, some reflexes.

and maxilla so that the force of the impact will not be transmitted to the brain stem. For a mouth guard to be effective, however, the athlete must be wearing one, and it must be in good condition. A mouth guard that has been chewed up or cut off will not prevent the knockout impact.

Wearing a helmet and face mask is also important in preventing head injuries. In the early years of football, players did not wear helmets. Today, a properly fitted helmet helps protect a player's head from direct impacts. The helmet prevents head injuries but not injuries of the face; thus, the face mask was introduced. With the head and face protected, athletes began to use the helmet as a weapon to punish opposing players. Using the head to make contact with another player is referred to as *spearing*. As spearing continued as a form of tackling, a progressive increase in the number of neck injuries resulting in permanent injury or death occurred—the helmet and face mask protected the head from direct impact but resulted in other forms of injury. Spearing has since been deemed a penalty, an offense severe enough to get a player ejected from the game.

Athletes should be taught the proper skills so that injury can be prevented. Coaches and ATs must teach athletes that they cannot lead with the head when trying to stop an opponent; this is crucial in preventing head injuries. At the beginning of each season, a film outlining sport safety should be shown. The AT should document attendance at this safety film; recording the date and an outline of the discussion should provide some legal protection if an athlete does sustain a serious head injury. The AT should also document days when safety skills are taught at practice, and she should take attendance. She should explain the signs and symptoms of head injuries and proper care of helmets.

HEAD INJURY MECHANISMS

Injury to the brain can be caused by rotation of the head, but the most common mechanism is impact. The region most susceptible in the skull is the temporal region because the bone is thinnest there. **Contrecoup** injuries occur when the head is moving and receives a blow. Upon impact, the

What Would You Do If...

You have been instructed to walk an athlete with a first-degree concussion into the locker room. Another athlete insists you can cure a concussion by cracking his neck. The athlete with the concussion says, "Yes, please make me better."

brain sloshes to the side opposite the blow, where it is stopped by the skull, and that is where the injury occurs. An athlete may complain of a headache opposite the impact, which is evidence of a contrecoup injury. Rotation of the head after an initial impact can cause the brain stem to stop functioning normally. The nerve receptors are overloaded with information to the brain, and brain overload causes unconsciousness. The unconscious state allows for a sorting of the impulses before the athlete returns to consciousness.

TREATING HEAD INJURIES

Potentially life-threatening head injuries include skull fractures, concussions, and intracranial hematomas. This section will discuss the evaluation of each of these types of injuries.

Skull Fracture

Skull fractures occur when there is significant force against the head. Types of skull fractures include depressed, linear, compound, and penetrating. A depressed fracture pushes a portion of the skull inside toward the brain. There will be bleeding under the skin or even a laceration requiring bleeding control. A linear fracture goes across the skull. Although no bones are moved out of place, there are tears in the blood vessels on the inside of the skull. A compound fracture will result in a portion of the skull sticking through the scalp and profuse bleeding. A penetrating fracture involves an object that has gone through the scalp, skull, and likely the brain. A skull fracture will discolor the area behind the ear; this discoloration is called a **battle sign**. Any skull fracture is significant and requires the immediate attention of a physician.

Concussion

A **concussion** is the temporary impairment of brain function caused by impact to the head or by a rotation force. A rotation of the head during the impact will send a massive number of impulses to the brain all at once. The brain, not knowing what to do with all the impulses, is overwhelmed, and the athlete may be confused or dazed or may even lose consciousness. Other symptoms of a concussion include nausea, dizziness, headache, vomiting, difficulty speaking, ringing in the ears (**tinnitus**), loss of balance, unconsciousness, difficulty remembering things before or after the impact (**amnesia**), possible battle sign, and disorientation.

The potential problems related to concussions in sport prompted NATA to create a position statement on the management of sport-related concussions (Guskiewicz et al. 2004). The position statement provides guidelines for ATs, including the idea that ATs must be sensitive to both the causes of concussions and how concussions are presented when an athlete is injured. Also, ATs must not only recognize the common signs of a concussion (balance problems, loss of memory, and difficulty concentrating) but also the symptoms (headache, tinnitus, and nausea).

The NATA position statement also recommends that ATs collect baseline measures of mental function. This preinjury testing often involves using computers to assess an athlete's attention, reaction time, information processing speed, concentration, and memory. The use of computer programs allows an AT to identify even subtle deficiencies in brain function. Such information can help determine when an athlete can safely return to play following a concussion.

A noncomputerized congnitive test that is often used by ATs is the Standardized Assessment of Concussion (SAC) (see McRea 2001). The SAC requires an AT to obtain information from the athlete that relates to orientation (e.g., does she know what day of the week it is?), immediate memory (e.g., remembering five words), concentration (e.g., can she reverse the order of a string of numbers?), and delayed recall (e.g., can she remember the initial five words given during the immediate memory test?). The SAC test also has a neurological screening section whereby the AT examines loss of consciousness, memory loss,

strength, sensation, and coordination. An athlete is given 1 point for a correct response and no points for an incorrect response. The SAC score has 30 possible points. The SAC form creates a record of an athlete's cognitive function and can be used as a pretest so the post-traumatic score can be compared. A score of 25 on the SAC is also used as one criterion for returning an athlete to play.

The severity of concussions is graded the same as sprains and strains—as mild, moderate, or severe. According to the guidelines established by the American Academy of Neurology, the signs and symptoms of a mild, or first-degree, concussion include no loss of consciousness, and the athlete's symptoms (e.g., dizziness) or abnormalities (e.g., loss of balance) are resolved in less than 15 minutes. A moderate, or second-degree, concussion will cause no loss of consciousness, but the athlete's symptoms and abnormalities last longer than 15 minutes. If the athlete is unconscious for any length of time, she has sustained a severe, or third-degree, concussion. The unconscious athlete may experience rapid eye movements that look like fluttering, and her pupils may be unequal in size. The pupil on the side of the head injury will be enlarged if the head injury is serious. The athlete may be in a coma, but she can hear what is being said, and it is important that someone talk to her while the AT is working. The AT will detect increased blood pressure, decreased pulse rate, and signs of shock. A severe concussion can lead to death or paralysis. The AT must be cautious when dealing with a concussion because other injuries may have occurred during the impact. He should also consider the possibility of a neck injury and keep the athlete's head still.

Other grading systems exist for concussions. The Cantu grading system, similar to the American Academy of Neurology, uses a mild, moderate, and severe system. Grade 1 means there is no loss of consciousness, loss of memory lasts less than 30 minutes, and postconcussion signs and symptoms last less than 24 hours. A grade 2 concussion involves loss of consciousness for less than a minute or post-traumatic loss of memory between 30 minutes and 24 hours and postconcussion signs and symptoms lasting one to seven days. A grade 3 concussion will show loss of consciousness of over a minute, memory loss longer than 24 hours, or postconcussion signs and symptoms lasting longer than seven days.

When the athlete is removed from the playing field, it is not uncommon for teammates to hit the player on the head and say, "Hang in there." Although they are trying to be supportive, they're actually contributing to the concussion. Athletes must be instructed ahead of time to keep their hands off so that only the AT touches the injured athlete.

Assessing the level of consciousness should be done using the Glasgow Coma Scale, or GCS (see table 5.1). The scale is used to determine the severity of the brain injury. The scale assesses AVPU, which stands for alert, verbal, pain and unresponsiveness. The scale is broken into three areas: motor response, verbal response, and eye opening. Each category has a grading scale, and the final score is determined by adding all the scales together. The final score is assessed against the chart to determine the athlete's prognosis. The higher the number on the grading scale, the greater the chance of returning to normal.

Head Injury Classification

Severe head injury—GCS score of 8 or less

Moderate head injury—GCS score of 9 to 12

Mild head injury—GCS score of 13 to 15

Adapted from: Advanced Trauma Life Support: Course for Physicians, American College of Surgeons, 1993.

A concussion with or without the loss of consciousness should make the AT wonder about other injuries that may have occurred. It is best to use a backboard for any athlete with a moderate or severe concussion. In the event that an athlete has lost consciousness, he must be referred to a physician the day of the injury.

An athlete who has suffered a concussion will need to be monitored by a physician to determine when

Table 5.1 Glasgow Coma Scale

Response	Grading scale	Score
Eye opening		
Spontaneous eye opening	4	
Eyes open to speech	3	
Eyes open to pain	2	
No eye opening	1	
Verbal		
Oriented	5	
Confused conversation, able to answer questions	4	
Inappropriate words	3	
Incomprehensible speech	2	
No response	1	
Motor		
Obeys commands for movement	6	
Purposeful movement to painful stimulus	5	
Withdraws in response to pain	4	
Flexion in response to pain (decorticate posturing)	3	
Extension response in response to pain (decerebrate posturing)	2	
No response	1	

From the Centers for Disease Control and Prevention.

it is safe to reenter competition. The NATA position statement on concussion management states that an athlete should be monitored every five minutes after the concussion until the condition clears or the athlete is referred for advanced care. In general, an athlete will not be allowed back into competition after the first concussion until there are no remaining signs or symptoms. Specifically, the athlete will have no headache, nausea, dizziness, or amnesia and will have regained full coordination and normal blood pressure. After a second concussion within a year, the athlete must have at least one month free of all signs and symptoms before returning. A third concussion in one year puts the athlete out of competition for one year, starting the day of the third concussion. An athlete who has suffered a concussion should be told about the signs and symptoms of concussions and the implications of repeated impacts. An athlete who has suffered one concussion is four times more likely to suffer another.

What Would You Do If...

The AT has instructed you to take the blood pressure of an athlete with a head injury every five minutes and let her know about any changes. The first blood pressure is 160/92. The athlete is responsive but talks about a headache. The next blood pressure is 126/84. The athlete then vomits.

Decisions about returning to participation should be made by the AT and a team physician. In general, athletes who have suffered a concussion should not return to participation until completing a progression of physical activity and follow-up assessments that begin only after he is free of all concussion symptoms (see table 5.2). Assessments should be compared with previous SAC tests (if

Table 5.2   AT Concussion Assessment and Exertion Progression Log

Original assessment		
Return-to-play decisions		**Criteria for return to play**
Return to play	❑	If athlete had no signs and symptoms of a concussion
Sit out for 15-30 min.	❑	If signs and symptoms lasted fewer than 5 min. and athlete had no more signs or symptoms and had completed exertional testing
Sit out for rest of game	❑	If athlete had all the signs of a concussion and had any episode of blacking out, can wait to refer but must see physician before return to play
Do not return to play	❑	If athlete was unconscious, call 911 for help

Exertional testing			
Activity	**Pass**	**Fail**	**Comments**
Run	❑	❑	
Jog	❑	❑	
Sprint	❑	❑	
3 broad jumps	❑	❑	
3 sets of 10 vertical jumps	❑	❑	
Figure 8	❑	❑	
Box drills	❑	❑	
Balance drills	❑	❑	
Sport-specific activity, treadmill, elliptical	❑	❑	

Based on M. McCrea, 2001, "Standardized mental Status testing on the sideline after sport-related concussion," *Journal of Athletic Training* 36(3): 274-279.

performed). The progression of activity involves engaging in exercises such as stationary biking, push-ups, sit-ups, and low-level running. The AT must reassess the athlete to determine if the concussion symptoms reoccur during activity. If symptoms occur at this time, the athlete is not ready to progress to other activities and more rest is required. If the athlete is symptom free at this time, he can then participate in sport-specific activities that do not pose a risk of further injury, such as noncontact activities. These activities should be done for several days with reassessments performed by the AT. At this point, the athlete can perform **neurocognitive testing** to make sure he is back to normal. Once this is the case, he can return to full sport activity, assuming clearance has been obtained by a physician. In general, a minimum guideline is for an athlete to be symptom free for at least seven days before returning to contact activities.

Understanding Diversity

Some Mexicans believe that touching the head of a nursing infant will cause illness, specifically dehydration and vomiting resulting in a fallen fontanel (Downes, 1997). In reality the dehydration of the child can cause serious illness and death, but the dehydration is more often caused by diarrhea. This illness is called *caida de la mollera* (Downes 1997).

Intracranial Hematoma

An **intracranial hematoma** is severe bleeding within the brain caused by a blow to the head, particularly over the temporal or parietal regions. The hematoma causes a significant increase in pressure on the brain, and rapid death can occur. Sometimes an athlete is thought to have a concussion and is allowed to go home. If she has a hematoma, she may die during the night. If an athlete is found in a coma, the chances of survival are only 40%. Survival depends on early examination by a physician and prompt surgical care. Physicians usually drill a hole in the skull to allow drainage of the blood and attempt to repair the bleeding vessel. If the athlete is not in a coma, the physician must give medication to put

her into a coma. The comatose state keeps the athlete calm and allows the brain to heal without movement.

Symptoms of an intracranial hematoma include headaches, nausea, vomiting, loss of consciousness, paralysis of extremities on the opposite side of the injury, and battle sign. If an intracranial hematoma is suspected, EMS should be contacted for immediate transportation to the hospital. The onset of these symptoms may be gradual, so the athlete must be continually monitored. With the first indication of a condition that is worsening, the athlete must be taken immediately to the hospital. An athlete with a possible head injury should be monitored for at least 24 hours, and he must be awakened every couple of hours to check his status.

The signs of a hematoma are a rise in blood pressure with a drop in pulse rate. The pupil on the same side as the head injury will be enlarged. The athlete may have difficulty speaking, difficulty using the extremities on the side opposite the hematoma, stiffening of posture, rapid eye movements, unconsciousness or coma, and lack of coordination. Depending on the severity of the hematoma, the athlete may fully recover, or she may suffer permanent brain impairment or death.

Postconcussion Syndrome

Postconcussion syndrome is the persistence of symptoms after a concussion. Symptoms may include headache, ringing in the ears, dizziness, and confusion. The athlete should be seen by a physician for a follow-up evaluation. Returning to play too soon following a concussion increases the chance of developing this condition. Postconcussion syndrome usually does not last more than a week or two.

Second-Impact Syndrome

It is thought that damage from concussions and brain injury is cumulative. Therefore, if an athlete is allowed to return to participation before the symptoms of his first concussion have completely subsided and he receives another blow to the head, he can quickly lose brain function and go into a coma. **Second-impact syndrome** can occur when an athlete receives more than one concussion or blow to the head in a relatively short time. Such trauma may disturb the blood supply to the brain and present signs of a minor concussion followed quickly by a semicomatose state. Athletes who have suffered brain injuries must not be allowed to return to participation until they are symptom free and have written permission from a doctor.

Laceration

A laceration to the scalp will bleed profusely because of the number of blood vessels in the scalp. Direct pressure applied to the wound will eventually stop the bleeding, but application of multiple gauze pads is usually necessary. Lacerations of the scalp may require suturing.

The Real World

On September 20, 1993, at 2:35 p.m., our high school dismissed students. My student trainers and I went to work in the training room. It was a fairly busy Monday. My students were preparing athletes for football, soccer, and volleyball, while I was checking a few of the injured athletes. At approximately 2:50 p.m., the athletic director announced over the PA system that I was needed in the parking lot—there had been an accident. By the sound of his voice, I could tell we had a big problem.

I ran out of my training room at full speed. When I hit the doors just outside the athletic office, the athletic director met me, and we ran on together. The accident had occurred at the far end of the parking lot. I surveyed the scene as we approached. Several students were standing around looking at something on the ground. On the right, next to a car, a distraught female student was talking with one of the teachers. I started asking questions as I made my way through the gathering of students. Someone said that a girl had fallen off the hood of the car while it was moving.

The next thing I saw took my breath away. Lying on the ground was a student who had been in my office earlier in the day to arrange for a tutor. She was pale, sweaty, not breathing, and bleeding from her ears, nose, and mouth. I saw a patch of bloody hair on the pavement about 2 feet (.5 m) from us and 8 to 10 feet (2.5-3 m) from the car. All I had to do was look at the athletic director and he got on his radio to his secretary to call an ambulance. Because I suspected both head and neck injuries, I stabilized the student's head and neck. I immediately used the jaw thrust maneuver to open the airway with minimal head movement. When her airway opened, she made a gurgling noise and a bloody froth bubbled from the corners of her mouth. As I continued to stabilize her head and neck, I asked a health teacher, who was at my side, to check the girl's pulse. Her pulse was faint, and her breathing was irregular. She was nonresponsive, and her face was covered with blood. An assistant principal was there with gloves and paper towels, and I had him gently clean her face so I could determine the major source of bleeding. I told the athletic director to keep bystanders back, and I sent the head custodian to the school entrance to direct the ambulance to us. While I was stabilizing the girl's head and neck and maintaining her airway, I was also trying to get a response from her. As we waited for the ambulance I realized that I did not have gloves on, but it was too late to worry about that. We seemed to wait forever. The girl started to choke, and we had to logroll her just as the ambulance made its way into the parking lot.

I continued to maintain the girl's head and neck while the paramedic checked her vitals. While he was doing this, she became combative. The paramedic got a collar on her, and I fought to maintain her head and neck stability while we put her on the backboard and then the stretcher. The paramedic asked me to ride in the ambulance to continue to maintain her head and neck. I held her head between my forearms while a second paramedic tried to get an IV going. In spite of her restraints it took several attempts; she was a lot stronger than I ever could have imagined. We were about a block from the hospital when she started to vomit and she aspirated. Now, clearing her airway became the priority. The paramedic yelled at me to grab the suction line as he turned it on. As he was suctioning the bloody vomit from her mouth, I was trying not to vomit on both of them.

We arrived at the emergency room, and I was still maintaining her head and neck. They did a cross-table X ray, which was negative for cervical spine fracture, and I was allowed to discontinue stabilization. I stayed with the girl in the ER until her parents got there. The doctor told me it was too early to tell how she would be. When I walked out of the ER, I met the athletic director waiting to give me a ride back to school. It was like coming back to the real world. I hadn't even thought about getting back to school or about practice.

The young woman spent two weeks in the ICU being treated for a subdural hematoma. She later returned to school, showing few effects of the injury. I, however, learned that my job extends far beyond the training room—and I always grab a pair of gloves on my way out the door.

Becky Clifton, ATC

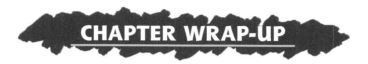

CHAPTER WRAP-UP

Summary

Although the brain is well protected by the skull, it is vulnerable to serious injury—the athlete may suffer intracranial bleeding, concussion, postconcussion syndrome, or second-impact syndrome. If the brain lacks oxygen for any appreciable time, cellular death occurs. Typical signs and symptoms of a head injury include vomiting, unequal pupils, skull depression, increased blood pressure, and unconsciousness, any of which call for immediate EMS attention. An athlete who has suffered a head injury must not have any signs or symptoms of the injury and must have clearance from a physician when he returns to participation.

Key Terms

Define the following terms found in this chapter:

amnesia	hematoma
battle sign	intracranial hematoma
cerebrospinal fluid	neurocognitive testing
concussion	second-impact syndrome
contrecoup	tinnitus

Questions for Review

1. How can head injuries be prevented?
2. What does elevated blood pressure mean when there is a head injury?
3. What are the differences among first-, second-, and third-degree concussions?
4. Compare and contrast the two concussion grading scales presented in this chapter.
5. What is the treatment for a second-degree concussion?
6. If the battle sign is present, what injury has occurred?
7. Why should an athlete be cleared by a physician before returning to participation after a head injury?

Activities for Reinforcement

1. Have an AT demonstrate how to evaluate an athlete with a head injury.
2. Identify the sports offered by your school and list the types of head injuries that are common among athletes in each sport.
3. Have a coach bring a safety film on prevention of head injuries and show it to the class.
4. Make a list of reasons why athletes get head injuries.
5. Visit a head trauma or closed-brain injury center.

Above and Beyond

1. Visit the Web site for the Brain Injury Association of America (www.biausa.org/aboutbitopics. htm) and examine the information related to function of a healthy brain and an injured brain.
2. Visit the Web site for the American Academy of Family Physicians (www.familydoctor.org) and write a report about various brain and nervous system disorders.
3. Examine the information provided at the Brain Injury Resource Center located on the following Web site and give a brief presentation to your peers: www.headinjury.com.
4. Visit www.impacttest.com and examine the ImPACT neurocognitive testing program for concussion management.

5. Visit www.headminder.com and examine the HeadMinder computer neurocognitive testing program for brain injuries.

6. Visit www.sportsconcussion.co.za/Pharos/Computerised_Testing.php and learn about the CogState Sport neurocognitive testing program for sport concussions.

7. Visit each Web site identified in activities 4 through 6 and compare and contrast the features offered by the various programs.

8. Visit the following Web site to learn more about neuroanatomy: http://faculty.washington.edu/chudler/nsdivide.html#pns.

9. Visit the following Web site and read about mouth guards and how they help prevent concussions: www.sportsdentistry.com/concussion.html.

10. The references listed at the end of this section may be used to complete any of the following projects:

    • Draw a side and front view of the brain. Label the parts of the brain, functions, and areas controlled.

    • Locate, compare, and contrast other concussion grading systems found in the literature.

    • Write a report on how long it takes to recover from a concussion.

    • Write a report on the physiological effects of concussions.

Bailes, J.E., and V. Hudson. 2001. Classification of sport-related head trauma: a spectrum of mild to severe injury. *Journal of Athletic Training* 36(3): 236-243.

Broglio, S., and T. Puetz. 2008. The effect of sport concussion on neurocognitive function, self-report symptoms and postural control: a meta-analysis. *Sports Medicine* 38(1): 53-67.

Cantu, R.C. 2001. Posttraumatic retrograde and anterograde amnesia: Pathophysiology and implications in grading and safe return to play. *Journal of Athletic Training* 36(3): 244-248.

Covassin, T., C.B. Swanik, and M. Sachs. 2003. Sex differences and the incidence of concussions among collegiate athletes. *Journal of Athletic Training* 38(3): 238-244.

Guskiewicz, K.M., S.L. Bruce, R.C. Cantu, M.S. Ferrara, J.P. Kelly, M. McCrea, M. Putukian, and T.C. Valovich McLeod. 2004. NATA position statement: Management of sport-related concussion. *Journal of Athletic Training* 39(3): 280-297.

Giza, C.C., and D.A. Hovda. 2001. The neurometabolic cascade of concussion. *Journal of Athletic Training* 36(3): 228-235.

Guskiewicz, K., D. Perrin, and B. Gansneder. 1996. Effects of mild head injury on postural stability in athletes. *Journal of Athletic Training* 31(4): 300-306.

Kaut, K.P., R. DePompei, J. Kerr, and J. Congeni. 2003. Reports of head injury and symptom knowledge among college athletes: Implications for assessment and educational intervention. *Clinical Journal of Sport Medicine* 13(4): 213-221.

Kelly, J.P. 2001. Loss of consciousness: Pathophysiology and implications in grading and safe return to play. *Journal of Athletic Training* 36(3): 249-252.

Mueller, F.O., R.C. Cantu, and S.P. Van Camp. 1996. *Catastrophic injuries in high school and college sports.* Champaign, IL: Human Kinetics.

Putukian, M., and R. Echemendia. 1996. Managing successive minor head injuries. *Physician and Sportsmedicine* 24(11): 25-38.

Susco, T.M. 2003. Injury management update. Establishing concussion-assessment guidelines: on-field, sideline, and off-field. *Athletic Therapy Today* 8(4): 48-50.

Tommasone, B., and T. Valovich McLeod. 2006. Contact sport concussion incidence. *Journal of Athletic Training* 41(4): 470-472.

chapter **6**

Facial Injuries

Objectives

Upon completing this chapter, the student will be able to do the following:

- Describe the basic anatomy of the face.
- Explain the common types of facial injuries, how they occur, and how to prevent them.
- Explain common steps of care for treating facial injuries.

njuries of the face can lead to permanent disfigurement or visual impairment. Immediate action of the AT can lessen the chance of long-term problems, as can protective equipment such as eye guards.

ANATOMY OF THE FACIAL REGION

The face includes bones that are also part of the skull, so the discussion in the previous chapter may clarify the anatomy that follows. There are 18 bones in the face (some are in pairs). Major bones include the maxillae, the mandible, and the zygomatic bones (see figure 6.1). The maxillae are the two bones of the upper jaw, and the mandible is the lower jaw. The nasal bones make up the bridge of the nose. The zygomatic bones are also known as the cheekbones. Within the structure of the sphenoid bone are the sinuses, which become stuffed up when a virus or infection invades the upper respiratory tract. The sinuses are located above and below

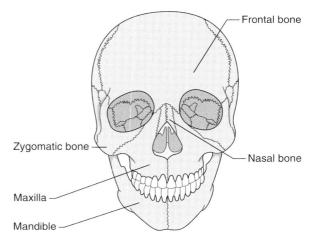

Figure 6.1 Facial bones.

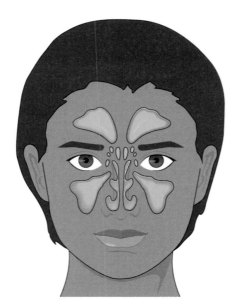

Figure 6.2	Sinuses.

the eyes (see figure 6.2). Some facial fractures may remain hidden because blood runs into the sinuses rather than externally.

The Eye

The eye sits in a socket known as the *orbital foramen*, or *orbit*. Most of the eye is hidden inside the orbital foramen, which protects the eye on three sides and serves as an attachment point for the muscles that move the eye. Lack of eye movement can indicate either a head injury or a serious eye injury (figure 6.3 shows the anatomy of the eye).

The eye itself consists of the anterior and posterior chambers. The two chambers are filled with fluid, which gives the eye its rounded shape. An injury that causes fluid to drain from the eye is likely to cause permanent damage, even blindness.

The covering of the eye has a white area and a clear center. The white outer covering of the eye is the sclera. A change in color of the sclera indicates that the athlete has a problem or an illness, such as liver disease, lack of oxygen, or poisoning. The clear center portion of the eyeball covering is the cornea. The cornea protects other important structures from injury. It covers the iris and pupil and admits light to the interior. The cornea is made up of thousands of tiny cells that can be injured by wearing contact lenses too long or by something that scratches the eye.

The iris is the contractile, colored portion of the eye, and in its center is the pupil, which is the opening in the iris. The iris responds to light, changing the size of the pupil. In bright light, the pupil gets smaller, thus limiting the amount of light entering the eye. In a dark room, the pupil gets larger, allowing all available light into the eye. Also located in the anterior portion of the eye is the lens, which focuses the entering light rays on retina. A poke in the eye may dislodge the lens, blurring or changing an athlete's vision. Finally, the conjunctiva lines the inner surface of the eyelid and continues over the forepart of the eyeball.

The main structures at the posterior aspect of the eye are the retina and the optic nerve. The retina lines the back of the eye and contains the rods and cones. Rods provide vision in black and white and cones provide color vision. The retina receives the image formed by the lens and converts it into chemical and nerve signals that the optic nerve sends to the brain, where vision occurs. Damage to the optic nerve can cause blindness. Injury to the optic nerve that has resulted in blindness will also prevent the pupil from functioning.

In the upper outside (that is, superior lateral) edge of each eye is a gland that makes tears. Tears wash diagonally across to the nose and drain into it through a duct. In the rims of each eyelid are small glands that secrete lubricating fluid, allowing the eyelid to open and close smoothly.

Vision is measured by an arbitrary standard. Originally, the test consisted of reading letters on

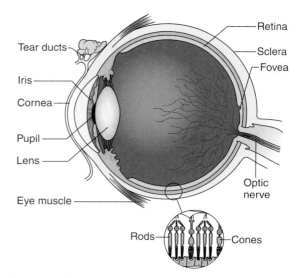

Figure 6.3	Anatomy of the eye.

Table 6.1 Muscles of the Eye

Extrinsic muscles	Attachments	Functions	
Lateral rectus Medial rectus Superior rectus Inferior rectus Superior oblique Inferior oblique	Bones of the orbit and the eyeball	Movement of the eye superiorly and inferiorly, externally and internally, and obliquely	
Intrinsic muscles	**Attachments**	**Functions**	
Iris Ciliary	Interior layer of the eye	Size of the pupil and shape of the lens	

a chart from a distance of 20 feet (6 m). A person who could read the smallest letters was said to have 20/20 vision. Today's vision tests relate to that standard. A person who can see near objects more clearly than distant ones is nearsighted, and a person who can see distant objects better than near ones is farsighted. These common vision problems are treated with corrective lenses or eye exercises.

Muscles of the eye are divided into two categories: extrinsic and intrinsic. Table 6.1 provides muscle locations and functions.

The Ear

The ear has three distinct areas: the external ear, the middle ear, and the inner ear (see figure 6.4). The external ear is composed of the pinna, the ear

What Would You Do If...

One of your friends shows you his ice hockey helmet, which has a crack in the back portion that he has glued together. He says there is no rule that prevents him from playing in a game with his repaired helmet.

canal, and the tympanic membrane. The pinna, which is the projecting portion of the external ear, is cartilage covered by skin. Its purpose is to catch sound and funnel it into the auditory canal.

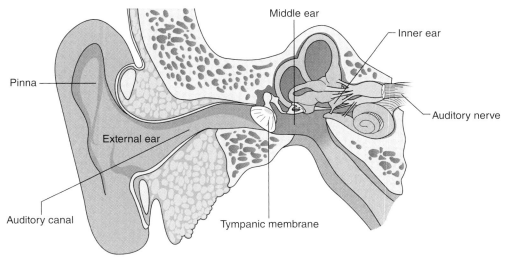

Figure 6.4 Anatomy of the ear.

The auditory canal carries sound from the pinna to the tympanic membrane, or eardrum. Earwax, which is designed to keep dirt away from the sensitive eardrum, is found in the auditory canal. Too much wax in the ear prevents or delays sound from reaching the middle ear.

> ### Understanding Diversity
>
> Some American Indians traditionally used dried raspberry leaves for an ear infection (Kennett 1976).

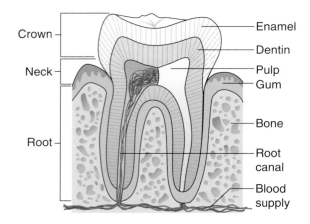

Figure 6.5 Cross section of a tooth.

The Nose

Two small bones, called the *nasal bones*, attach to the frontal bone of the skull. About an inch (2.5 cm) in length, the nasal bones make up the bridge of the nose. The rest of the nose is cartilage.

Inside the nose is the septum, which is a piece of cartilage that separates the left and right sides of the nose. Hairs inside the nose filter impurities from the air. The palate, which is the roof of the mouth, separates the mouth from the bottom of the nose.

Air that is inhaled through the nose is warmed, moisturized, and cleansed before reaching the lungs. In winter, breathing through the nose will decrease lung pain caused by inhaling cold air through the mouth. Athletes with asthma and upper-respiratory infections should breathe moist air.

The Mouth

The mouth is made up of the mandible (lower jaw), maxillae (upper jaw), temporomandibular joint, tongue, palate (roof of the mouth), and teeth.

The mandible attaches to the skull at the temporomandibular joint and is the only moveable bone in the face. The mandible moves during speaking and eating. The teeth give the face shape and are used to chew food; they are attached to both the mandible and the maxillae. An adult has 32 permanent teeth.

A tooth is composed of the crown, which is the visible portion above the gum line, and the root,

which is below the gum line (see figure 6.5). The crown is capped with a thin layer of enamel, which protects against tooth decay. The root contains pulp and dentin. Dentin is the hard, bony portion of the tooth. The pulp is the soft portion of the tooth containing the nerve and blood supply. The nerve is sensitive to pain, pressure, and temperature, and the blood supply brings oxygen and food to the tooth to keep it alive. A live tooth is white in color, whereas a dead tooth is dark gray.

The teeth, tongue, and saliva work together to prepare food to be swallowed. The salivary glands under the tongue and in the back of the mouth provide saliva to begin digestion. The saliva makes it easier for the teeth to break down food, and it binds the food together before the food is sent to the stomach.

The muscles used for chewing include the masseter, temporal, and pterygoid. Table 6.2 lists the muscles involved in chewing, including attachments and functions.

> ### Understanding Diversity
>
> Cubans are more commonly afflicted with gingivitis and periodontitis as a result of lack of dental care (Downes 1997; Erickson D'Avanzo, C., & Geissler, E. 2003; Purnell and Paulanka 2003, 2005).

Table 6.2 Muscles of the Mandible

Muscle	Attachments	Functions
Masseter	Zygomatic arch and the mandible	Closing the mouth
Temporal	Temporal bone and mandible	Closing the mouth
Pterygoids	Inferior surface of skull and mandible	Grinding the teeth

PREVENTING FACIAL INJURIES

Preventing facial injuries requires common sense. Athletes who fail to wear the proper equipment can easily become injured—a prime example is a catcher who does not wear a face mask when warming up a pitcher. Equipment is available in all sports to prevent facial injury; it includes helmets, mouth guards, face masks, goggles, protective eyewear, and headgear. Mouth guards are relatively inexpensive, but repairing injuries to the teeth and jaw is very expensive. A properly fitted athletic face mask decreases the number of eye, nose, face, and mouth injuries. The face mask should be spaced a minimum of 1 inch (2.5 cm) from the nose; if it is closer, an impact to the mask can cause it to distort inward, resulting in injury to the face or nose. When selecting a face mask, make sure that no game equipment, such as a hockey puck or stick blade, can get through the openings in the mask and hit the face. Protective eyewear is crucial in preventing blindness. All sports have the potential for eye injuries; balls, sticks, elbows, and fingers are common items that injure eyes. Because eye

What Would You Do If...

An athlete comes running into the athletic training room. She is in tears, cannot see, and has pain in her eyes. She reveals that she is wearing a friend's contact lenses because she wanted to try them out.

What Would You Do If...

You find the lost contact lens of a soccer player. It is covered with dirt and grass.

injuries are unpredictable, it is best for all athletes to wear eye protection designed for their sport. Eye guards, which are similar to glasses and generally consist of plastic frames and lenses, or goggles should be worn if face masks are not worn (see table 6.3 on page 70). Athletes with fractures of the nasal bones, skull, or jaw should wear special padding, masks, or helmets to prevent additional injuries.

TREATING EYE INJURIES AND CONDITIONS

Eyes are precious, and it is better to err on the side of caution and send the athlete to a doctor even if the eye injury doesn't seem serious than to discover later that injury was serious and treatment could have prevented permanent injury or loss of vision. The AT also should be thinking about other injuries that might have occurred along with the eye injury. For example, a head injury is a definite possibility that should be assessed.

Eyes move in coordination. Even if an eye is injured, it still tends to move in cooperation with the noninjured eye. Thus, if an eye must be patched or shielded, the AT should cover both eyes. This will reduce the movement of both eyes and thus reduce irritation of the injured eye.

Table 6.3   Recommended Eye Protectors for Selected Sports

Sport	Minimal eye protector	Comment
Baseball/softball (youth batter and base runner)	ASTM F910*	Face guard attached to helmet
Baseball/softball (fielder)	ASTM F803 for baseball*	ASTM specifies age ranges
Basketball	ASTM F803 for basketball*	ASTM specifies age ranges
Field hockey (men's and women's)	ASTM F803 for women's lacrosse;* goalie, full-face mask	Protectors that pass for women's lacrosse also pass for field hockey
Football	Polycarbonate eye shield attached to helmet-mounted wire face mask	
Ice hockey	ASTM F513 face mask on helmet;* goaltenders, ASTM F1587*	HECC or CSA certified; full-face shield
Lacrosse (men's)	Face mask attached to lacrosse helmet	
Lacrosse (women's)	ASTM F803 for women's lacrosse*	Should have option to wear helmet
Soccer	ASTM F803 for selected sport*	
Track and field	Streetwear with polycarbonate lenses/ fashion eyewear†	
Water polo/swimming	Swim goggles with polycarbonate Lenses	
Wrestling	No standard available	Custom protective eyewear can be made

ASTM = American Society for Testing and Materials, CSA = Canadian Standards Association, HECC = Hockey Equipment Certification Council.

*Sports equipment; safety and traction for footwear; amusement rides; consumer products. 2003. Annual Book of ASTM Standards. Vol. 15.07. West Conshohocken, PA: ASTM International.

†Eyewear that passes ASTM F803 is safer than street eyewear for all sport activities with impact potential.

This article was published in *Ophthalmology*, Vol. 111, American Academy of Ophthalmology, pgs. 600-603, "Joint policy statement: A Joint statement of the American Academy of Pediatrics and American Academy of Ophthalmology," Copyright Elsevier 2004.

Conjunctivitis

Conjunctivitis is more commonly known as *pink eye*. The conjunctiva turns red and the eye appears to be irritated. Conjunctivitis has a variety of causes, including bacteria, allergies, eye irritants (e.g., soap), viruses, and diseases (Vorvick 2008). Symptoms of conjunctivitis include redness of the eye, eye irritation, crusting matter along the corners and lid of the eye, blurred vision, and itching.

A physician needs to examine and assess eye fluids to determine the cause. Pink eye is usually caused by a highly contagious virus, so to prevent others from getting it, the athlete should stay at home until effectively treated and no longer contagious. Eye drops will be necessary for effective treatment.

For those who have the allergic form of conjunctivitis, an antihistamine or removal of the athlete from the allergen will work. An athlete who has a bacterial infection will need antibiotics.

Foreign Body

A foreign body in the eye causes tears, which attempt to wash the foreign body toward the nose. In some instances, tears will not clear the eye. In these cases, rinsing with water from the nose outward can flush the particle out of the eye or over to one side where it can be removed.

If the object is stuck under the eyelid, the AT or athlete should lift the lid outward over the bottom lashes. The bottom lashes can brush the object out. If this process does not remove the object, it will be necessary to invert the upper eyelid. Inversion of the lid is accomplished by grasping the lid and pulling it outward; a cotton-tipped applicator is placed in the fold of the lid, and the lid is laid over the applicator. This exposes the underside of the lid so that the object can be removed. If the inversion technique fails, the athlete should be referred to a physician for care. Both eyes must be patched to decrease eye movement and prevent scratching of the cornea.

Embedded Object

An embedded object is one that is stuck in the eye; it may have been blown into the eye, for example, or a blow from a ball may have shattered a contact lens. No matter how the object entered the eye, the care received will determine the quality of the athlete's vision in the future. The athlete will know the object is in the eye. She will reach for the eye and tears will occur, resulting in pain, visual impairment, and anxiety.

The best treatment is to place an eye shield over both eyes and send the athlete to a physician. If the object is sticking out of the eye, the AT will not remove the object but will stabilize it with bulky dressings. The physician will determine the severity of the injury, surgically remove the object, and stop any fluid release. The physician will prescribe antibiotics, and the eye will remain patched for about a week. A vision test will be necessary to determine visual acuity. Eye guards and goggles will help the athlete protect the eye from reinjury.

What Would You Do If...

A golfer comes into the training room assisted by several others. They tell you that someone yelled, "Fore," and when the golfer turned to look, the ball hit her in the eye. The athlete is in extreme pain and wants you to remove her contact lens. You can see several pieces of her contact lens sticking into her eye.

Dislodged Contact Lens

Contact lenses come in two types: hard and soft. A hard contact lens covers the pupil of the eye, whereas a soft lens covers the entire cornea. A displaced hard contact lens feels like a rock in the eye. The athlete's vision will be impaired, and the displaced lens will irritate the eye. Usually the athlete knows where the lens is located in the eye because of the initial pain. When the eye is examined, the lens can be seen because of its color in contrast to the sclera. Some people believe that the lens can be lost behind the eye, but that is impossible. The lens will be in the eye—the AT just has to keep looking. The hard lens can be moved back over the pupil, and usually the athlete can do this himself if the AT provides a mirror. If he is unable to remove it, the AT can remove it using a small suction-cup device that is placed over the lens. The athlete should then clean the lens before placing it back in the eye.

The displacement of a soft lens is less uncomfortable. The athlete will know the lens is out of place because she won't be able to see. A soft lens is more difficult to put back in place because it tends to curl up like a soggy cornflake. The athlete should wash her hands and then gently grab the lens. She must use caution, because roughly handling a soft lens will tear it. The lens should be cleaned with solution before being returned to the eye. Sometimes an athlete believes that rinsing the lens by putting it in her mouth is acceptable. The practice of placing a hard or soft contact lens in the mouth is like dipping it in garbage before reinserting it. This practice must be discouraged!

Corneal Abrasion

A **corneal abrasion** or laceration is caused by being poked in the eye with a foreign object or by wearing contact lenses too long. An abrasion is superficial, whereas a laceration is deeper and more severe. The athlete will experience pain and feel as if something is lodged in the eye. She will have tears and sensitivity to bright light. If the injury is not treated, the eye may become infected or the athlete may have permanent vision problems. The physician treats the abrasion by patching the injured eye for 24 hours and applying antibiotic ointment. The athlete will need help getting to the hospital because of limited vision. If wearing a contact lens too long caused the injury, a restriction will be placed on the athlete to keep this from recurring. Sunglasses may be worn while recovering. Corrective lenses may be necessary if the cornea becomes distorted. The athlete may have difficulty returning to competition for fear of reinjuring the eye, but using eye guards or goggles will help her overcome this fear.

Eyelid Laceration

Think of an athlete who reaches out to grab the head of the opposing wrestler to gain control for a takedown. The opponent jerks his head away from the grasp but gets poked in the eye and experiences immediate eye pain. The eye is bleeding, and the athlete refuses to pull his hand away so the AT can determine the extent of the injury. Once the athlete relaxes, the AT can see that the eyelid is lacerated, maybe all the way through to the margin of the eyelash.

The immediate procedure is to control the bleeding with direct pressure. The AT will question the athlete about his ability to see clearly in order to determine the extent of other possible consequences of the poke. An eyelid laceration is similar to most lacerations except the tear duct may also be injured, possibly resulting in permanent damage. Once the bleeding is controlled, the athlete must be referred to a physician to repair the lid.

A plastic surgeon should repair a laceration of the eyelid to prevent scarring or permanent deformity of the lid. The ophthalmologist will want to check the eye for proper vision and to ensure that there are no other complications.

Athletes should keep their fingernails cut to prevent eyelid lacerations (this is a rule in wrestling). Goggles can also prevent this type of injury.

Black Eye

A hard blow to the eye may cause a black eye. As with any contusion, a black eye is caused by bleeding and discoloration just under the skin, which affects the tissue surrounding the eye but not the eye itself. Therefore, athlete will not complain of visual impairment, but there will be swelling and pain. If the athlete complains of any other difficulty, a referral to a physician is necessary. Ice application over a black eye is an accepted treatment.

Hemorrhage Into the Anterior Chamber (Hyphema)

A blow to the eye can cause bleeding within the eye. A **hyphema** is blood pooling in the anterior portion of the eye. When looking at the athlete, the athlete will complain of both the inability to see and of pain. She should have both eyes covered with a protective shield, but the AT should not apply an ice pack. The physician needs to determine the severity of the injury. The athlete with a hyphema may suffer permanent damage, blindness, or cataracts.

Detached Retina

A blow to the eye or even a hard sneeze can cause the retina to detach. The athlete will experience pain, but the surest sign of a **detached retina** is that the athlete sees sparks, lights, and flashes that nobody else can see. The athlete may indicate that he is having difficulty seeing or that things look foggy. The athlete should be referred to a physician who can do laser surgery to repair the detached retina. When the athlete returns to activity, he must wear protective goggles to prevent reinjury. If a physician does not repair the damage promptly, blindness could result.

Subconjunctival Hemorrhage

Athletes who have a terrible cough from an upper-respiratory infection are prone to subconjunctival hemorrhage. The constant coughing may cause the small vessels in the eye to rupture, turning the conjunctiva red. An athlete may also get poked in the conjunctiva or hit by a ball, which causes the same result.

Although the eye looks painful, the athlete experiences minimal or no pain and no visual impairment. It is best to refer the athlete to a physician for an eye exam to be sure no other structures are injured. The treatment for this hemorrhage is to do nothing. The athlete is allowed to participate without restriction. Her biggest problem will be the funny looks she gets from others concerned about the appearance of her eye.

Orbital Roof Fracture

A blow to the eye or the area just above the eye can cause a fracture in the roof of the orbit. When this happens, the athlete will experience pain, a headache, signs and symptoms of a concussion, and a hematoma over the area. The nose may bleed, and cerebrospinal fluid may drain from the nose. This injury requires immediate care by a physician. Hospitalization for observation and care of the fracture and rest will most likely be required. The athlete will not be able to return to competition for about a year.

Sinus Fracture

A sinus fracture can occur when there is a sharp blow to the face, for example, from a baseball taking a bad hop or from a stick across the face. A headache, dizziness, and unsteadiness may occur. The athlete's nose may bleed on the same side as the injury. He will experience pain, but once the bleeding has stopped, the AT should do a quick assessment of the injury. With this fracture, air seeps into the skin and tissues around the eye and nose, resulting in a crackling sensation when the area is touched. The AT should apply ice and immediately refer the athlete to a physician. The physician will require special X rays to discover the exact location of the fracture.

A complication of this injury is a concussion, which could diminish the athlete's ability to give a history. In the case of a blow to the face, it is always prudent to recommend a physician's evaluation.

Blowout Fracture

A blow to the eye can force the eyeball backward into the socket. The thin bones beneath the eye absorb the sudden increase in pressure and fracture. This type of fracture is referred to as a **blowout**.

The athlete may experience double vision and may not be able to feel much pain as a result of damage to surrounding nerve endings. The athlete may also experience numbing of the lip and upper jaw on the same side as the injury. The muscles of the eye often get caught in the fractured bones. Therefore, the AT may notice that the athlete cannot control the injured eye—it will be looking in a different direction than the uninjured eye. The eye may appear to be sunken in the socket. There will be immediate swelling, and the conjunctiva will begin to discolor. The athlete may have a bloody nose on the same side as the injury, and the bleeding may fill the sinus, making it difficult to breathe. The eye may bulge when the athlete attempts to blow her nose.

The AT should call 911 and help control any bleeding. The athlete should be monitored in case her condition worsens. A physician may have to surgically repair the fracture and release the muscles.

The athlete may suffer permanent vision problems, including glaucoma and cataracts. She will remain out of competition for several months.

Boxers wear headgear to prevent such eye injuries. Although blowout fractures are rarely seen in wrestling, basketball, and racquetball, athletes in these sports should wear some form of eye protection to prevent them.

Ruptured Globe

The globe—the eyeball itself—can be ruptured by any object small enough to enter the eye, such as a squash ball or racquetball. Upon examination of the eye, the AT will notice a lack of roundness of the globe and a hemorrhage of the eye. Associated injuries may include an eyelid laceration, blood in the front of the eye, the interior contents of the eye spilling out, or the pupil out of round (figure 6.6). Any sign that the globe has been ruptured requires that the AT cover the eye with a protective eye shield

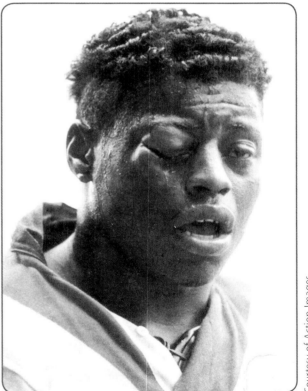

Courtesy of Action Images.

Figure 6.6 Anytime there is excessive swelling with possible leakage of fluid, a ruptured globe should be suspected. Patches must be put over both eyes and the athlete sent to the emergency room immediately.

that will not allow external pressure. The athlete must be taken to the emergency room immediately and referred to an ophthalmologist if his eyesight is going to be saved. He will not be able to return to competition for months.

TREATING EAR INJURIES

The external ear helps to funnel sound to the inner ear, and the inner ear plays a role in equilibrium. With its placement on the side of the head, the ear does not have a high incidence of injury. In high school athletics, earrings are barred from competition because of the potential for ear injury.

Swimmer's Ear (Otitis Externa)

Proper care of the ear requires that the ear and the canal be dried after swimming. There are times when a swimmer cannot remove water from her ear, such as when she is hurrying to get home or water is stuck in the ear. If water remains in the ear, an inflammation of the canal can occur, which is referred to as *otitis externa*, more commonly called **swimmer's ear**. The athlete will experience pain, itching, hearing loss, and possibly a smelly discharge from the ear. It will be easy to notice the discharge and the swollen, red canal. If the infection is not controlled, it can spread deeper into the canal. The athlete should be sent to a physician for ear drops and antibiotics. Prevention of swimmer's ear can be as simple as drying the ear after swimming by using a hair dryer on a low setting. Rubber or wax plugs are sometimes used to lessen

the flow of water into the ear, but these can actually increase the risk of infection because they irritate the ear canal. Also, when using plugs, hearing is impaired, making it difficult to hear coaches. Some athletes prefer to use alcohol-based ear drops, which dry the ear canal.

Many athletes clean their ears regularly to prevent infection, but this too can become problematic. The American Academy of Otolaryngology states that cerumen, or earwax, is an important barrier to infection, and regular cleaning that forces wax out of the canal may not only irritate the canal but also increase the risk of infection.

Foreign Body

In athletics, foreign bodies in the ear are rare, but bugs have been known to take a look in an athlete's ear. The athlete will have the sensation that something is in the ear and may experience pain.

Probing the ear with a cotton-tipped applicator may push the object farther into the ear and should be avoided. The AT could also rupture the eardrum while trying to get the object out. A physician can remove an object using mineral oil or special tweezers.

Cauliflower Ear (Hematoma Auris)

Wrestlers are the athletes who suffer the most from **cauliflower ear**. The wrestler involved usually is not wearing his headgear and gets hit hard in the ear, or his head is pushed hard into the wrestling mat. The pinna of the ear begins to bleed internally, causing swelling, redness, and pain. As the ear heals there is an excessive growth of reparative tissue, which distorts the pinna, causing it to look like a piece of cauliflower (see figure 6.7).

Treatment of cauliflower ear starts with ice and compression with moldable material, performed by the team physician. The team physician may lance, or drain, the ear to reduce the swelling and use steroid medication to keep the hemorrhage under control. In more complicated cases the physician may remove the tissue through surgery. Some athletes opt for plastic surgery to fix the

The Real World

One night while I was covering a high school football game, an athlete whose nickname was Cowboy came over to the sidelines as the defense came off the field. The team physician and I were there when the athlete stated that he was experiencing ear pain. Upon removing his helmet, I examined his ear and saw a fly at the entrance to the ear canal. I must have startled the poor insect because it retreated back into the ear. The physician asked if I had a penlight. I produced one, she aimed it at the ear, and the fly immediately came forward—drawn to the light—and buzzed away, solving Cowboy's dilemma.

Todd Keasling, ATC

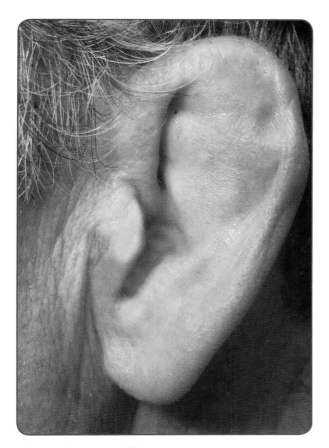

Figure 6.7   Cauliflower ear.

ear if it is permanently distorted. Wearing headgear and applying petroleum jelly to reduce friction can prevent cauliflower ear.

Pinna Laceration

Ears stick out from the head enough that they may get in the way. Athletes should never wear earrings in practices or competitions because they increase the vulnerability of an already exposed body part. An earring can be caught by another athlete's finger, tearing the ear lobe. Even in sports in which the ears are protected by a helmet, earrings may be jammed against the wearer's head if the head is struck, causing serious discomfort and even injury. A laceration of the pinna is treated the same as any other wound—by controlling the bleeding with direct pressure, which can be applied on both sides for rapid control.

When a portion of the pinna is no longer attached, the missing piece must be found so that it may be reattached. The detached part should be wrapped in sterile gauze, put in a plastic bag, and

placed in a container full of ice. (It is appropriate to place it on ice as long as the ear is not directly touching the ice.) In the case of a laceration, the athlete should be referred to a physician for stitches and a tetanus shot. The athlete can prevent lacerations and other wounds of the pinna by wearing proper protection and removing earrings.

Ruptured Eardrum

A tear of the tympanic membrane, or **ruptured eardrum**, can occur from an ear infection, a blow to the side of the head, loud noises, and atmospheric pressure. The athlete may experience loss of hearing, buzzing in the ear, and drainage from the ear. A physician will have to examine the ear and do a hearing test to determine the extent of the injury. In some cases no treatment is necessary and the membrane will heal on its own. In some cases antibiotics will be necessary to deal with the ear infection if that was the cause. For severe ruptures or ruptures that do not heal, surgery may be necessary. An athlete will need to wear headgear to protect the membrane and must not put anything in the ear, such as a cotton swab.

TREATING NOSE INJURIES

For some athletes, the nose is always in the way. In boxing it is constantly being smashed by a fist. Wrestlers can find their noses rubbed into the mat and even used as a carrying handle by opponents. And basketball players' noses seem to be attracted to the elbows of opposing players. The nose is vital: It warms incoming air and acts as a filter to catch particles.

Nosebleed (Epistaxis)

When an athlete goes up to head a soccer ball and it lands on her nose, the impact can cause an **epistaxis**, or bloody nose. An athlete may get a nosebleed from constantly blowing the nose during a cold. Athletes taking special medications, as well as those who have had a recent nosebleed, are prone to epistaxis.

The nose will bleed from one or both nostrils, and if the nosebleed is from a blow, it will be painful. The AT should instruct the athlete to lean forward while pinching the nose. Applying ice and packing the nose with gauze that has been soaked with an astringent (medication that slows bleeding) are helpful. Leaning the head backward forces the blood into the throat, obstructs the airway, and should be avoided. The athlete should lean forward to allow blood to discharge from the nose and should spit out any blood draining into the throat—swallowing blood will cause vomiting. Discourage any attempt to blow the nose, because this will start the bleeding process again. If there is excessive bleeding (gushing like a faucet) from the nose, the athlete should be treated for shock and sent to the hospital for evaluation. The physician may cauterize the bleeding vessel.

Deviated Septum

The septum is the piece of cartilage that separates the left and right sides of the nose. A deviated septum has moved to one side, causing decreased airflow through the nasal passageway. Any form of direct impact to the nose can cause a deviation.

The blow to the nose will have caused a nosebleed, so follow the instructions for epistaxis first. Then wait a day or two to test the athlete for a deviated septum by blocking off one nostril and having the athlete force air out of the nose and then repeating the procedure on the other side. If one nostril forces more air through than the other does, the septum may be deviated. If the athlete has a deviated septum, the nose may also be broken. The athlete should be referred to a physician to determine if surgery is necessary. Many athletes who have a deviated septum choose not to have surgery. Wearing a face mask will prevent further injury to the nose.

Nasal Fracture

A direct blow to the nose can fracture one or both of the nasal bones. There will be a severe nosebleed, often similar to water running from a faucet. The AT will treat the athlete by having her lean forward. Pinching the nose may not be possible. The AT uses gauze to catch the blood as it comes out of the nose and applies ice. Gauze should not be forced into the nostril to slow bleeding.

The athlete may indicate that he heard a snap, and he may have pain and difficulty breathing. The AT should observe deformity (flat on one side) and swelling. She may hear **crepitus**, or crunchiness, during palpation and observe a deviated septum.

The athlete should be referred to a physician for care. The physician may proceed with surgery to put the bones back into place. Some athletes who opt to avoid surgery suffer from a permanently deformed nose. In the days after a nasal fracture, the athlete will have black eyes from internal bleeding that pools underneath the orbits of the eyes.

TREATING MOUTH INJURIES

Although some people believe that losing teeth is no big deal because they can always get false teeth, they are wrong. False teeth are not nearly as good as real teeth at biting and chewing, making it difficult to maintain healthy nutrition. The AT should use caution when treating the mouth—some athletes may bite because of a seizure or because they are gagging.

Tooth Fracture

Direct impact to the lower jaw or the teeth can result in a tooth fracture. The athlete will experience pain and difficulty closing his mouth. A fracture can be seen if the tooth is examined closely. In some instances, a portion of the tooth will be gone. If a portion has broken off, it should be sent with the athlete to the dentist. Although the portion cannot be put back on, the dentist may find it helpful when reconstructing the tooth. The broken tooth may die and have to be removed.

Tooth Dislocation

Direct impact to a tooth can knock it out of the jaw. The athlete will experience severe pain, bleeding, and swelling. The tooth is dislodged and needs to be handled carefully. After putting on gloves, the AT should pick up the tooth with a sterile gauze pad. It must be kept moist and should be placed

What Would You Do If...

A couple of volleyball players are horsing around in the locker room. One slips and hits her mouth on the edge of the sink. She brings her two fractured front teeth into the training room and hands them to you.

in a designated saline tooth container or a glass of milk. The athlete must be seen by a dentist so that the tooth can be put back in place, assuming it is not too severely injured to be reinserted. The AT should treat the bleeding socket, placing a piece of sterile gauze where the tooth was located and having the athlete gently bite down to keep it in place with direct pressure.

Jaw Fracture

Imagine getting hit in the face by a sharply hit baseball, a scenario that is not uncommon in athletics. A direct blow to the jaw, either upper or lower, can result in a fracture. The athlete will experience pain that increases with movement. When the AT observes the area of impact, she will be able to see swelling. If the lower jaw has been fractured, she may be able to observe a space between teeth that was not there previously. The athlete will have discoloration under the tongue, and his teeth may not line up. Palpation will reveal crepitus, and the athlete will be cautious about moving the jaw. The AT should make sure all the teeth are in place and the airway is clear.

Ice should be applied to the area as tolerated by the athlete, who should be referred immediately to a physician for care. The physician will realign the jaw for proper closure and wire the mouth shut. The athlete will eat through a straw for four to six weeks. Some athletes are allowed to return to activity as long as a special face mask protects the jaw.

Improper care or neglect of a jaw fracture can result in permanent deformity. The jaw may not be able to open wide enough to allow for eating a hamburger, and malalignment of the teeth can lead to further mouth problems.

Temporomandibular Dislocation

A blow to the chin or a violent, forced opening of the mouth can cause a dislocation. The athlete will immediately grab and hold his mouth to keep it from moving. The jaw will lock itself in place by spasm of the local muscles, and the athlete will be in extreme pain. His jaw will look deformed, locked open, or to one side. The AT can feel that the condyles are out of normal position. The AT should

The Real World

I was covering a girls' soccer match. With two minutes left in the first half, the opposing team was inside the scoring circle. From where I was standing I could see a lot of bodies kicking and flailing around as our team was defending. Then our goalie was on the ground with the ball in her hands, and I knew something was wrong by the reaction of our players. The official summoned me onto the field. Our goalie had been kicked in the mouth, and there was blood everywhere. Unfortunately, she had not been wearing a mouth guard. She was conscious and spitting out blood. I did a head and neck evaluation and found no other problems. Upon examining her mouth I saw blood coming up from her gums in the molar region. She was able to move her mouth to talk, but her jaw was painful in the front. I packed sterile gauze between her gums and teeth all the way around her mandible. I had her put ice on the jaw where she had pain. Her father wanted to drive her to the emergency room because that was quicker than calling an ambulance. I felt she was stable enough and agreed he should take her. I gave her a pan to hold on her lap because she was still spitting blood.

The textbooks say to use a wrap around the patient's jaw and apply ice if there is a suspected jaw fracture. However, in this case I chose not to follow that protocol. The athlete was spitting blood that would have gone into her stomach if I had strapped her jaw the way the books say. Blood is an irritant to the stomach, and chances are she would have starting vomiting, thus complicating matters. The emergency room physician said I did the right thing. The mandible was fractured in two places in the front of the jaw. On the X ray it looked as if a triangle had been cut into the mandible. This player's soccer season was over. However, she was back in goal next year, wearing a mouth guard.

Suzy Heinzman, ATC

never try to put the jaw back in place, because the area around the jaw is filled with nerves and cartilage that can be permanently damaged. The team physician should relocate the jaw, which must be kept shut for several weeks. Some physicians wire the jaw shut to ensure this rest.

Temporomandibular Joint Dysfunction

Temporomandibular joint (TMJ) dysfunction is a condition in which the muscles surrounding the joint spasm. The spasms can be caused by stress, a blow to the mandible, or an injury to the muscles.

The dysfunction can cause misalignment of the teeth, inability to open the mouth fully, clicking of the jaw, earache, pain in the musculature of the mouth, and headaches.

Upon examination, the AT may find a lack of range of motion, holding of the jaw, poor alignment upon opening or closing, or crepitus. Treatment of TMJ dysfunction includes relaxation of the muscles of the jaw, such as from massage or trigger point techniques. In some instances the athlete may require muscle relaxants or pain medication. A dentist may choose to make a bite splint to prevent TMJ dysfunction from reoccurring.

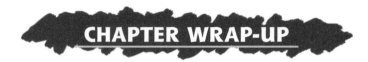

CHAPTER WRAP-UP

Summary

Any impact to the face could injure the eyes, nose, ears, or jaw and could result in permanent disfigurement. Impairment of the facial organs can be devastating to the injured athlete. To prevent facial injuries, an AT should work with the equipment staff to make sure proper equipment is provided and with coaches to make sure the athletes wear the equipment. Facial injuries should be treated conservatively and evaluated by the team physician and dentist.

Key Terms

Define the following terms found in this chapter:

blowout	epistaxis
cauliflower ear	hyphema
conjunctivitis	ruptured eardrum
corneal abrasion	subconjunctival hemorrhage
crepitus	swimmer's ear
detached retina	temporomandibular joint (TMJ) dysfunction

Questions for Review

1. How do facial injuries occur?
2. How can facial injuries be prevented?
3. If an athlete has epistaxis, what injuries may have occurred?
4. What is the treatment for a fractured tooth?
5. What injury causes an athlete to see sparks?

6. Why are both eyes covered if one eye is injured?
7. What is the best head position for epistaxis?
8. What does it mean to have 20/20 vision?
9. How can cauliflower ear be prevented?

Activities for Reinforcement

1. Have an AT demonstrate how to perform a facial injury evaluation.
2. Ask the school nurse to demonstrate a hearing test.
3. Ask the school nurse to give a vision test.
4. Invite a local dentist or dental hygienist to demonstrate proper brushing and flossing techniques.
5. Describe common eye injuries and how to care for them.
6. Invite an ophthalmologist to speak with the class.
7. Investigate various mouth guards and determine which would be best for various sports.
8. Investigate various types of eye protection and determine which would be best for various sports.

Above and Beyond

1. Collect brochures from your dentist's office and create a poster about the various types of dental injuries.
2. Write a report on a facial injury of your choice. Use the following materials for assistance.

   Behrens, D. 2006. Treatment of epistaxis in the emergency department. *Emergency Medicine Journal* 23(3): 241.

   Honsik, K. 2004. Emergency treatment of dentoalveolar trauma: Essential tips for treating active patients. *Physician and Sportsmedicine* 32(9): 23.

   Labella, C.R., B.W. Smith, and A. Sigurdsson. 2002. Effect of mouthguards on dental injuries and concussions in college basketball. *Medicine and Science in Sports and Exercise* 34(1): 41-44.

   Lahti, H., J. Sane, and P. Ylipaavalniemi. 2002. Dental injuries in ice hockey games and training. *Medicine and Science in Sports and Exercise* 34(3): 400-402.

   Leong, S.C., R.J. Roe, and A. Karkanevatos. 2005. No-frills management of epistaxis. *Emergency Medicine Journal* 22: 470-472.

   Moeller, J.L., and S.F. Rifat. 2003. Identifying and treating uncomplicated corneal abrasions. *Physician and Sportsmedicine* 31(8): 15.

   Moylan, F. 2003. Swimmer's ear mystery. *Physician and Sportsmedicine* 31(9): 48.

3. Visit the Web site of Prevent Blindness America and create a poster about how to prevent eye injuries: www.preventblindness.org/safety/prvnt_injuries.html.
4. Visit the Mayo Clinic Web site and summarize the swimmer's ear prevention tips: www.mayoclinic.com/health/swimmers-ear/DS00473/DSECTION=prevention.
5. Create a brief report on eye injuries by visiting the Coalition to Prevent Sports Eye Injuries Web site for an article summary of the policy statement by the Coalition to Prevent Sport Eye Injuries on eye injuries in sport: www.sportseyeinjuries.com/resources.aspx.

6. Visit the Web site of the Maryland Department of Health and Mental Hygiene to obtain information related to dental health:

   http://fha.maryland.gov/pdf/oralhealth/fact_sheets/Dental_complications_of_eating_disorders.pdf

   http://fha.maryland.gov/pdf/oralhealth/fact_sheets/Diabetes_and_Your_Oral_Health.pdf

   http://fha.maryland.gov/pdf/oralhealth/fact_sheets/Heart_Disease_and_Your_Oral_Health.pdf http://fha.maryland.gov/pdf/oralhealth/fact_sheets/Mouthguards_for_coaches.pdf

   http://fha.maryland.gov/pdf/oralhealth/fact_sheets/Oral_Piercing.pdf

7. Visit the Web site of the American Association for Oral and Maxillofacial Surgeons and write a summary of the information related to preventing injuries to the face: www.aaoms.org/facial_injury.php.

chapter 7

Throat and Thorax Injuries

Objectives

Upon completing this chapter, the student will be able to do the following:

- Understand the basic anatomy of the throat and thorax.
- Understand how to prevent injuries of the throat and thorax.
- Know the care necessary to treat an injury to the throat or thorax.
- Understand the implications of illness or injury related to specific organs in the thorax.

The thorax is the part of the body between the neck and the abdomen. Compromise of the organs and passageways in the throat and thorax is life threatening. Prompt care can save an athlete's life.

ANATOMY OF THE THROAT

The throat contains the carotid arteries, jugular veins, larynx, trachea, and esophagus. Because these structures are so sensitive and vital to life, the AT must understand their purpose and location (see figure 7.1).

The **esophagus** is the passageway for food going from the mouth to the stomach. It lies in front of the cervical vertebrae and behind the trachea and larynx. The **trachea** is made up of circular rings of cartilage; it is the main trunk of the system of tubes through which air passes to and from the lungs for the exchange of oxygen and carbon dioxide. The **larynx** is the modified upper part of the trachea and contains the vocal cords.

One **carotid artery** and one **jugular vein** pass on each side of the trachea. The carotid arteries carry oxygenated blood to the brain while the jugular veins carry unoxygenated blood away from the brain. Severing one of these vessels can cause death in a short time, so protection of the neck is vital in sports such as ice hockey and field hockey.

Understanding Diversity

Some sub-Saharan Africans believe that to prevent a sore throat, they must have the uvula surgically removed (Erickson D'Avanzo and Geissler 2003).

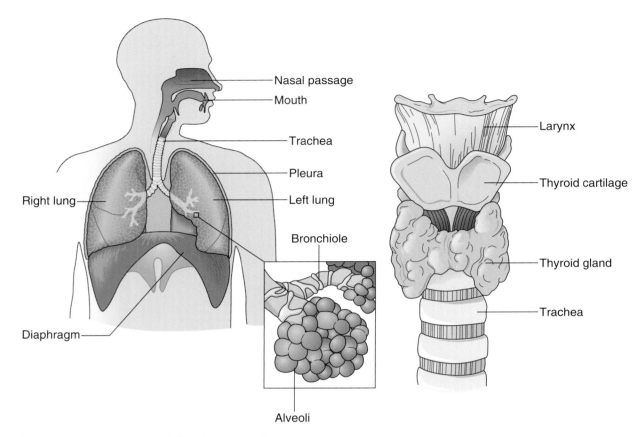

Figure 7.1 Anatomy of the thorax and throat.

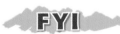

Veins

Veins carry waste products and carbon dioxide back to the heart (except for the pulmonary vein, which carries oxygenated blood to the left atrium).

Arteries

Arteries carry nutrients and oxygenated blood away from the heart and throughout the body.

Oxygenated

As blood passes through the lungs, it picks up oxygen and becomes oxygenated, or oxygen rich.

ANATOMY OF THE THORAX

The bony structure of the thorax is made up of the thoracic vertebrae posteriorly, 12 ribs on each side, and the sternum anteriorly (see figure 3.3, *a-b*, on page 34). These bones protect the sensitive organs in the thorax. The two lowest ribs do not attach to the sternum and are called *floating ribs*.

Heart and Lungs

The heart is about the size of a fist and is responsible for pumping blood to all parts of the body. The blood carries nutrients and oxygen to cells and carbon dioxide and waste products away from cells. The heart is divided into four chambers: the upper chambers, which include the left and right **atria**, and the lower chambers, which include the left and right **ventricles** (see figure 7.2). The ventricles are generally larger and have thicker walls than the atria because they pump the blood throughout the body. Exercising the heart muscle makes it larger and more efficient at pumping. However, an enlarged heart can also be a sign of heart disease.

The heart pumps blood to the lungs and around the body (see figure 7.3). The right atrium fills with blood from a vein, which is carrying waste products and carbon dioxide. The right ventricle receives blood from the right atrium and pumps it to the lungs to get rid of carbon dioxide and pick up oxygen. The left atrium fills with the oxygenated blood from the lungs. The left ventricle, which is the largest chamber of the heart, receives the

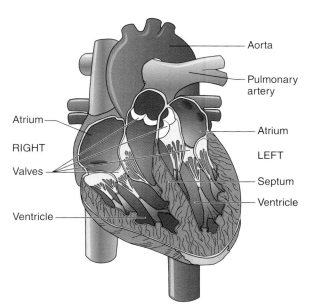

Figure 7.2 Interior of the heart.

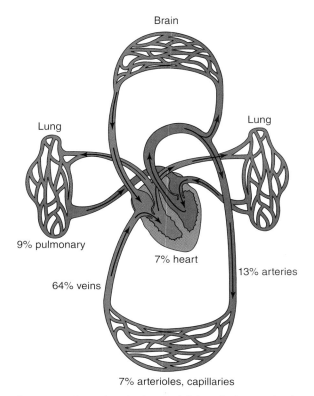

Figure 7.3 Circulation of blood through the heart and distribution to the body.

Reprinted, by permission, from J. Wilmore and D. Costill, 2007, *Physiology of sport and exercise,* 4th ed. (Champaign, IL: Human Kinetics), 138.

oxygenated blood from the left atrium and pumps it throughout the body. The main artery leaving the heart is known as the aorta. The aorta travels downward through the chest and abdomen, and other large arteries branch off to the head (carotid arteries), arms (brachial arteries), and legs (femoral arteries) (see figure 7.4). After the oxygen-rich blood has been delivered and used by the tissues, the deoxygenated blood returns to the heart through major veins (see figure 7.5).

Two electrical nodes in the right atrium begin a contraction. A slight delay in impulses conducted from the nodes through the heart allows blood to be squeezed from one chamber to another. Injured or diseased electrical nodes cause the heart to stop or to beat ineffectively.

The lungs, which are located on each side of the heart, exchange oxygen and carbon dioxide and dissipate body heat. The trachea divides into two bronchi, the bronchi further subdivide into bronchioles, and each bronchiole ends in an alveolus, an air-containing cell of the lungs (see figure 7.1). It is in the **alveoli** that the exchange of oxygen and carbon dioxide occurs. The lung tissue is divided into sections, or lobes. There are three lobes in the right lung and two lobes in the left lung. Lung capacity is hampered primarily by smoking, pollution, and lung disease. The bronchi are filled with cilia, which are small, hairlike projections that help remove foreign substances such as dust and pollen. Coughing and

sneezing help to keep the trachea and bronchi clear and remove **phlegm** and allergy-causing agents.

Lung function and breathing rate are controlled by carbon dioxide receptors. When receptors register the presence of too much carbon dioxide, inhalation occurs. Exercise increases cell metabolism and causes cells to need more oxygen and eliminate more carbon dioxide. This increased cellular need increases the number of breaths per minute. Over time, the ability of the lungs to exchange air effectively increases as the athlete exercises, and the athlete's breaths become deeper and more forceful. Moreover, a conditioned athlete will return to a normal breathing rate more quickly after exercising compared with someone who is out of shape.

A thin, lubricated tissue called the *pleura* lines each half of the thorax and is folded back over the surface of the lung on the same side. The pleurae allow smooth movement of the lungs as they encounter the wall of ribs during inhalation and exhalation. There is a small space between the pleura and the lung.

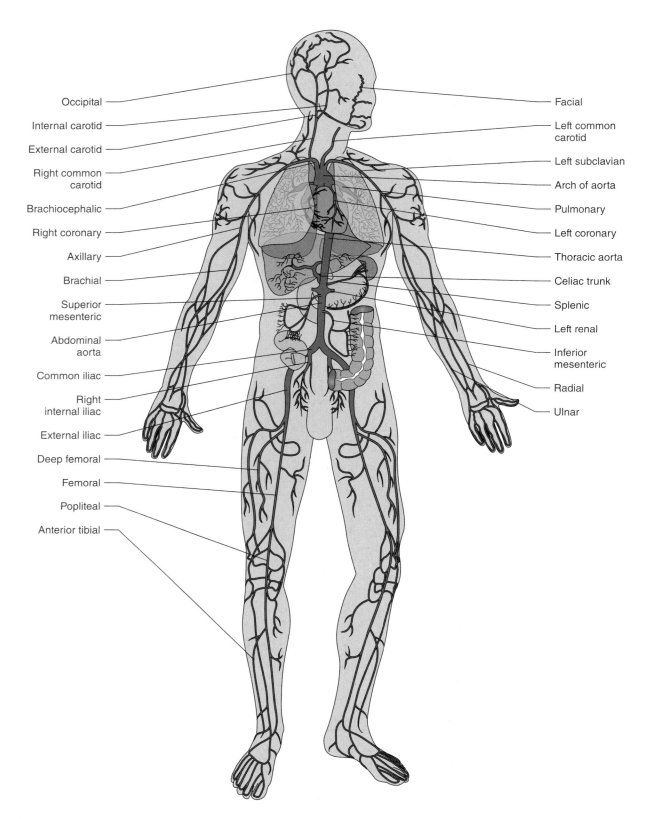

Figure 7.4 Major arteries.

Adapted, by permission, from R.S. Behnke, 2001, *Kinetic anatomy* (Champaign, IL: Human Kinetics), 17.

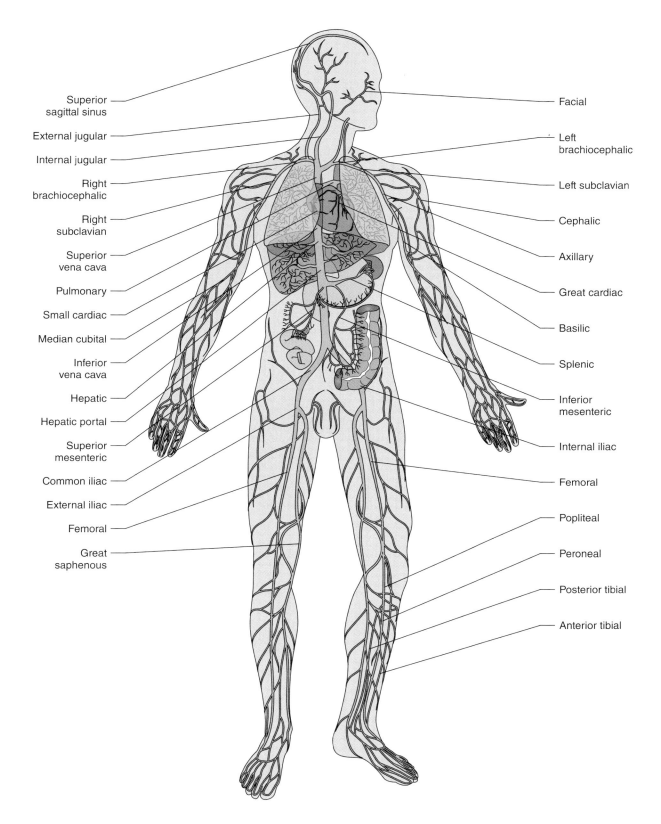

Superior sagittal sinus

External jugular

Internal jugular

Right brachiocephalic

Right subclavian

Superior vena cava

Pulmonary

Small cardiac

Median cubital

Inferior vena cava

Hepatic

Hepatic portal

Superior mesenteric

Common iliac

External iliac

Femoral

Great saphenous

Facial

Left brachiocephalic

Left subclavian

Cephalic

Axillary

Great cardiac

Basilic

Splenic

Inferior mesenteric

Internal iliac

Femoral

Popliteal

Peroneal

Posterior tibial

Anterior tibial

Figure 7.5 Major veins.

Adapted, by permission, from R.S. Behnke, 2001, *Kinetic anatomy* (Champaign, IL: Human Kinetics), 18.

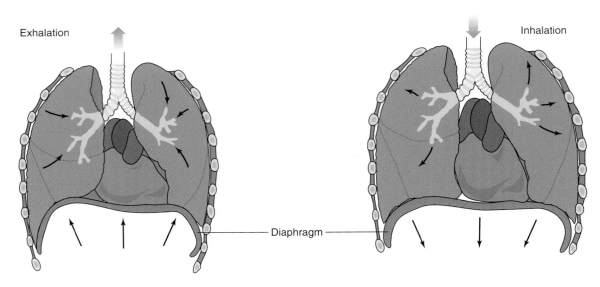

Figure 7.6 Breathing. The diaphragm moves upward during exhalation and downward during inhalation.

Diaphragm

The **diaphragm** muscle separates the thorax and the abdominal cavity. The diaphragm contracts and pulls down to assist in inhalation and moves upward to push air out of the lungs on exhalation (see figure 7.6). The diaphragm has three openings to allow passage of the esophagus, the abdominal aorta (artery), and the inferior vena cava (vein).

PREVENTING THROAT AND THORAX INJURIES

Protective equipment and rules in athletic contests are both designed to prevent injuries to the throat and thorax because these areas contain organs that are vital to life. Thus, athletes wear throat protectors in softball, baseball, lacrosse, field hockey, and ice hockey. In field hockey, lacrosse, football, ice hockey, softball, and baseball, protective equipment—shoulder pads, chest protectors, and sternal pads—is provided for the thorax, especially for goalies. A safe distance between the boundary of a playing surface and objects such as bleachers, fences, scorers' tables, and spectators is 15 feet (4.5 m). In addition, walls, tables, and fences are often padded to prevent injury to athletes who may collide with these objects.

Many Little League softball and baseball players are required to wear chest protectors when batting because of the danger of being struck in the chest with a ball. If a ball strikes the chest just before a heartbeat is initiated, it can cause the heart to beat irregularly or even stop, which could result in death.

When buying equipment to protect an athlete in a potential life-and-death situation, buy the best equipment available. Make sure the equipment is certified and will do what it claims. When a baseball hits the chest of a Little Leaguer, the chest protector is supposed to absorb the force and reduce the impact on the heart. However, some of the chest protectors used by Little Leaguers are not certified and may actually increase the chance of irregular heartbeat if a ball hits the chest because they focus the impact over the heart.

What Would You Do If...

You are proudly wearing your new student assistant's uniform of a white sweater. This is the first sweater you have received after working with the AT for two years. At the ice hockey game, the goalie suffers a lacerated vein in the neck. You are asked to assist the AT in stopping the bleeding. Blood is everywhere—it is definitely going to get on your new sweater.

TREATING THROAT INJURIES AND CONDITIONS

Throat injuries can be simple or devastating. Most of the injuries that occur to the throat are contusions caused by blows from sticks, feet, or arms. Contusions can be treated by applying ice. In any type of throat injury the general response by the athlete is coughing, spitting, difficulty breathing, and pain.

Throat Laceration

A throat laceration could occur, for example, when one player's ice skate goes across another player's throat. Lacerations that are not deep can be handled with direct pressure. Deep lacerations or those that affect a jugular vein or carotid artery are medical emergencies and require immediate treatment. Apply direct pressure over the site of the laceration and treat the athlete for shock. The vessels in the neck are large and a massive amount of blood will be lost rapidly, so the AT must respond quickly to save the athlete's life. To review procedures for treating hemorrhages, see page 234.

Cartilage Fracture

A severe blow to the throat can result in a fracture of the circular cartilaginous rings of the trachea, which can be life threatening. The athlete will have difficulty breathing and gasp for air, spit up blood, complain of pain, have difficulty talking, and be very anxious. His skin may turn a bluish color due to lack of oxygen. The AT must exercise caution when treating a cartilage fracture because the trauma also may have caused a fracture of the cervical spine. This is a medical emergency. The AT will place the athlete on a backboard for transport to the hospital and apply ice to the area to reduce swelling. Those treating the athlete must remain calm to keep the athlete calm. Keep the airway free of blood, and make sure medical care is on the way.

The Real World

At an ice hockey game, a young man was trying to stop a shot on goal with a diving headfirst slide. The slap shot hit him square in the throat. It was immediately apparent that he was in life-threatening danger. The team physician and AT jumped onto the ice before play was stopped. They quickly assessed him and found he had difficulty breathing, a blue skin tone, an inability to speak, and rapid swelling over the throat. They iced his throat and put him on a backboard. His breathing was constantly monitored, and the physician was ready to make an emergency airway. Paramedics arrived and took the young man to the hospital. He recovered—with a deeper voice and partial loss of the use of his vocal cords. He now wears a throat protector, and he slides feetfirst to stop slap shots!

Lorin Cartwright, MS, ATC

TREATING THORAX INJURIES AND CONDITIONS

Many people suffer from conditions such as asthma or experience hyperventilation. Additionally, if the thorax is not adequately protected, it is vulnerable to blunt trauma that can result in fractures of the ribs or sternum. Moreover, severe trauma may cause a lung injury.

Hyperventilation

Hyperventilation is quick, deep breathing at a rate of more than 24 breaths per minute, which leads to abnormal loss of carbon dioxide from the blood. The condition can be caused by an athlete becoming too excited and beginning to breathe rapidly or by an underlying illness such as diabetes. If the athlete does not get her breathing under control, she will experience lightheadedness; numbing of the fingers, toes, and lips; and loss of consciousness. As hyperventilation continues, muscular contractions will occur in the limbs. To treat hyperventilation, the AT should talk calmly to the athlete and encourage her to control her breathing rate.

Exercise-Induced Asthma

Asthma is a chronic inflammation of the breathing passageways to the lungs. The triggers can be many, but in this instance exercise causes the asthma attack. The bronchi spasm and narrow the breathing passageways. This narrowing causes the athlete to wheeze and struggle with taking a full breath. It has been described by some as breathing through a straw. An athlete may also experience coughing, tightness of the chest, and mucus production.

The immediate treatment is to have the athlete stop activity, sit upright, and breathe in through the nose and out through the mouth. The athlete should take the medication that has been prescribed before the attack gets worse. Breathing must be controlled even though he feels as if he is not getting enough air. Breathing in through the nose humidifies and cleans the air. Exhalations should last for a count of five. If mucus is coughed up, the athlete should lean forward and remove it. He should continue to control his breathing and to relax as much as possible. If the athlete is unable to breathe or is progressively worsening, EMS must be called and the AT must be prepared to perform CPR.

One preventative method that has been used with success is to have athletes take their medication about 20 minutes before exercise. Athletes who have a known asthma problem should be tested during their preparticipation physical using a spirometer. A spirometer is a device that measures air volume both in and out. The spirometer measurements are recorded on the athlete's physical form. The spirometer can be used to test air volume at the time of a suspected attack, and if it is less than before, an asthma attack should be the diagnosis.

Jogger's Nipple

Jogger's nipple is most commonly found among male athletes. It occurs when the shirt one is wearing rubs against the nipple repetitively. It is called *jogger's nipple* because long-distance runners are the most inclined to suffer this condition. The nipple becomes irritated, sometimes to the point where application of a lubricant or bandages becomes necessary.

Prevention involves using lubricant or applying an adhesive bandage over the nipple. If the irritation does not subside with minimal treatment, a physician may have to evaluate the athlete to determine if an infection has occurred.

What Would You Do If...

An athlete comes off the playing field where you are standing. She is having trouble catching her breath. You ask her what happened and she says, "I just got the wind knocked out of me. I'll be fine in a minute." The minute passes, and she is still struggling to catch her breath.

Blow to the Solar Plexus

The typical cause of a solar plexus injury is a blow to the area of the diaphragm that can hits the nerve in the solar plexus. When this occurs, the athlete will struggle to take a breath because the diaphragm spasms. After a short span of time, the diaphragm relaxes and the person is able to breathe normally again. The AT should reassure the athlete while he recovers.

Pulmonary Contusion

A pulmonary contusion is a bruise of the lung due to impact, such as from a baseball to the chest or a tackle. The contusion results in an accumulation of blood and other fluids within the lung tissue. Unfortunately, the accumulated fluid keeps the lung from exchanging oxygen and carbon dioxide, and the larger the contusion, the more serious the injury. The athlete will have difficulty breathing and may have a bluish skin color. Application of ice may be helpful, but EMS must be called immediately.

Myocardial Contusion

When there is an impact to the chest over the heart, the heart can become bruised. In sport, a typical impact would come from a ball or a shoulder into the chest. An athlete may experience pain in the chest, especially over the sternum, and a rapid heart rate. In this instance the injury merits calling EMS and treating the athlete for shock.

Rib Contusion

A rib contusion is caused by the same impact or compression as a rib fracture, but the force does not cause a fracture. There is pain, and signs and symptoms may be similar to those of a rib fracture. When the AT evaluates the athlete, there is pain over the site of the impact but not on compression away from the site.

Treatment involves ice application and rest. An athlete may participate as pain allows. The area may have to be padded to allow participation.

Ruptured Diaphragm

Infrequently in athletics the diaphragm can rupture as a result of a blow to the general area of the diaphragm. The athlete will present with difficulty breathing with no real trauma to the chest. The athlete may have other internal injuries, most likely in the abdominal region. If the AT auscultates the chest, bowel sounds may be heard.

Treatment is to care for the presenting signs or symptoms. If the athlete is having difficulty breathing, elevating the head will be helpful. Treat the athlete for shock and call EMS. This injury is hard to diagnose, so if difficulty with breathing continues to be a problem, call EMS.

Sternal Fracture

Sternal fractures occur because of direct impact. Impact to the sternum that causes a fracture can be expected to also cause internal injuries, so the heart and lungs may be involved. A suspected fracture of the sternum is treated with application of ice and referral to the hospital. If the sternum is only contused from the impact, the athlete could possibly return to activity with a special sternal pad.

Rib Fracture

A rib fracture is caused by direct impact or chest compression. On rare occasions, a sudden violent muscular contraction, such as throwing a baseball, will cause a rib stress fracture. Blows to the front or back of the ribs generally do not result in inward displacement of the fractured rib. Blows to the lateral aspect, however, are more likely to lead to inward penetration, causing complications such as internal bleeding or a punctured lung.

An athlete with fractured ribs experiences pain and difficulty breathing. The pain increases with inhalation, and the athlete usually holds a hand over the injured area in an effort to support the ribs. The area may be deformed due to swelling. A key to determining if a rib is fractured or severely contused is to note whether the athlete experiences increased pain with inhalation but not exhalation. If she has pain during both inhalation and exhalation, she more likely has a contusion.

Treatment for uncomplicated rib fractures involves applying ice and sending the athlete for X rays. The team physician will restrict the athlete's physical activity until inhalation is not painful. If the athlete participates in a contact sport, all activity should be stopped for six weeks. Upon return to competition, he should wear protective padding or equipment.

Flail Chest

Flail chest occurs when several consecutive ribs are fractured in two or more places (see figure 7.7). This injury occurs from an impact directly to the ribs. The entire fractured portion moves in and out when the athlete breathes; however, the portion moves opposite to the normal breathing pattern. Normally the chest expands and the ribs move outward during inhalation, and during exhalation the chest moves inward. With a flail chest the fractured

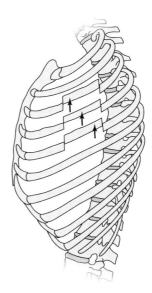

Figure 7.7 When two or more ribs are broken in two places, it makes flail chest possible—the broken section of ribs moves inward toward the heart and lungs during inhalation and outward during exhalation.

portion moves outward during exhalation and inward during inhalation. This movement creates extreme pain and difficulty breathing. Breathing will be painful and distressed, the athlete will be anxious, and skin tone will be bluish. The athlete should be checked for other internal injuries, especially lung contusions.

Treatment of a flail chest includes decreasing the movement of the fractured ribs. This can be accomplished by placing an object such as a sandbag or pillow over the fractured segment to keep it from moving. The athlete can be placed on her injured side as a way of controlling the movement of the flail chest, and she also should be treated for shock. This is a medical emergency and requires rapid advanced care.

Pneumothorax

A **pneumothorax** is the presence of air in the pleural cavity, commonly known as a collapsed lung, which can occur either as a result of trauma or without trauma. A traumatic pneumothorax can occur from a rib puncturing the lung, a gunshot wound, or a severe laceration. A nontraumatic pneumothorax occurs due to a weakness of the lung tissue. When a pneumothorax occurs, the injured lung moves toward the center of the chest, which puts pressure on the heart and the other lung. Because only one lung is functioning, the athlete will experience difficulty breathing and will gasp for air. As the athlete continues to breathe, air goes through the hole in the lung and into the chest cavity, which causes the collapsed lung to compress the heart and opposite lung even further.

Spontaneous Pneumothorax

When there is an imperfection in the tissue of the lung, it can break and cause the lung to collapse, also known as a spontaneous pneumothorax. There need not be any impact or illness associated with a spontaneous pneumothorax; the athlete may have appeared healthy in the past and had no previous signs of illness. The athlete will experience difficulty with breathing, chest pain, and possibly bluish color of the skin if breathing is poor.

The athlete should be placed so that the side with the injured lung is closest to the ground. The AT will treat the athlete for shock and get him to a hospital. In general, a spontaneous pneumothorax will heal itself without surgical intervention.

Tension Pneumothorax

An athlete with a pneumothorax may develop a more serious problem called a *tension pneumothorax*. As air leaks out of the collapsed lung and into the chest cavity, it forces the lung to press against the other lung and the heart. If the AT observes the trachea deviated to the side of the throat, she should suspect tracheal shifting. As pressure builds in the chest, the trachea moves away from the side of the pneumothorax. If the trachea moves, the athlete will experience severe respiratory distress. As more air enters the chest cavity, more pressure builds against the heart and uninjured lung. As the pressure mounts, the heart begins to labor as blood flow and breathing are impeded. Death can occur if the athlete is not treated rapidly. If the athlete has an external puncture wound, partially cover it, leaving one side unsealed. Sealing the wound entirely will prevent the inner air from escaping, worsening the tension pneumothorax.

With tension pneumothorax, the athlete will experience respiratory distress, absent breath sounds on the injured side, anxiety, and bluish skin color. His pulse will be rapid and weak, and his blood pressure will drop. As the pneumothorax worsens, tracheal deviation and neck vein distention will occur, as will bulging of the muscles between each of the ribs. The AT should place the athlete so that the side with the injured lung is closest to the ground, treat him for shock, and get him to a hospital. This injury requires a physician to insert a chest tube to allow air to escape as well as possible surgical intervention.

Sucking Chest Wound

If the wall of the chest is punctured and air from the outside is drawn noisily into the cavity, the athlete has a **sucking chest wound** (see figure 7.8). In this injury, the lung is not punctured. However, the air

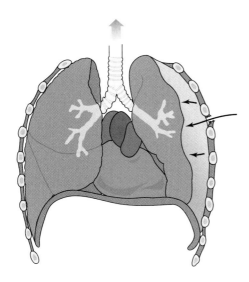

Figure 7.8 Sucking chest wound. When the chest is pierced, air can enter the chest cavity directly from the outside, which causes the lung on the same side to compress. Breathing becomes difficult.

that is being sucked into the chest cavity applies pressure on the lungs and heart, causing distress. The athlete will have difficulty breathing, and circulation may become impaired, resulting in a bluish skin color. The athlete is best treated by sealing the wound with a cellophane wrap or a piece from a plastic bag. EMS must be called immediately.

Hemothorax

A **hemothorax** is blood in the chest cavity. The bleeding can occur from an internal injury, such as a ruptured lung or blood vessel. A hemothorax may also occur from an external wound that penetrates the chest, such as a javelin into the chest.

A hemothorax is similar to a pneumothorax in that the blood puts pressure on the heart and lungs, which decreases their ability to function normally. As blood fills the chest cavity, the athlete will have difficulty breathing, may turn blue from lack of oxygen, may become unconscious, will have a rapid weak pulse, will sweat, and will go into shock. Breath sounds may be absent on the side of the bleeding.

Bleeding into the chest cavity is serious and requires immediate care to prevent death. The AT must call for immediate transportation to the hospital and control the bleeding as best she can. The athlete may require CPR if advanced help is delayed.

Cardiac Tamponade

Blows to the thorax can affect not only the lungs but also the heart. There is a thin pericardial sac around the heart. When fluid fills the sac, it places pressure on the heart to the point where it may stop beating. An injury to the heart increases fluid in the sac. In athletics the most likely cause is a blow to the chest.

Cardiac tamponade is a medical emergency that will cause death if not diagnosed and treated quickly. The athlete will be in shock, with all the signs and symptoms. The defining sign of cardiac tamponade is a narrowing pulse pressure, meaning the systolic and diastolic pressures come closer together after each repetitive taking of the blood pressure. EMS must be called and oxygen administered. Upon arrival at the emergency room, a needle will be inserted into the chest to remove the fluid.

Dorsal Aortic Rupture

The aorta can be ruptured with a severe deceleration force to the chest over the dorsal aorta. This is most commonly seen in car accidents when the strap of the seat belt tightens rapidly during a sudden deceleration. In sport, the most common deceleration is a severe blow to the chest, such as a hit in football.

In **dorsal aortic rupture**, the aorta commonly tears away from the heart and the athlete most often bleeds to death in seconds. Those who do not die may have a partial tear and can bleed to death more slowly. They will show signs of shock and will be anxious. The deceleration, or severe blow, may be the most revealing determination of this injury. If this happens, EMS must be called and the athlete must not be moved. Movement can cause the aorta to shift, resulting in immediate death.

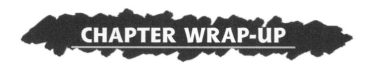

CHAPTER WRAP-UP

Summary

Injuries to the throat and thorax can cause severe, permanent damage or even death. The AT must be able to evaluate injuries to the throat and thorax because prompt treatment is crucial to an athlete's survival. The history, signs, and symptoms will define the injury. Most injuries to these areas are preventable if the athlete is wearing the proper equipment. Luckily, few injuries occur in these areas, and when they do occur, most of them are not life threatening. For serious injuries, EMS is needed immediately.

Key Terms

Define the following terms found in this chapter:

alveoli	esophagus	phlegm
atrium	flail chest	pneumothorax
cardiac tamponade	hemothorax	sucking chest wound
carotid artery	hyperventilation	trachea
diaphragm	jugular vein	ventricle
dorsal aortic rupture	larynx	

Questions for Review

1. Describe the normal breathing process.
2. Describe the normal heart and circulation process.
3. What types of throat and thorax injuries are life threatening?
4. What are the common signs and symptoms of thorax injuries?
5. How are injuries to the thorax distinguished from each other?
6. What are the common treatments for thorax injuries?

Activities for Reinforcement

1. Have an AT show the protective equipment that is available for various sports to prevent injuries of the throat and thorax.
2. Have an AT demonstrate how to evaluate throat and thorax injuries.
3. Use a stethoscope to listen to the heart and lungs.
4. Invite the local EMS to demonstrate CPR and electrical monitoring of the heart.

Above and Beyond

1. Interview a cardiologist and write a report on sudden-death syndrome.
2. Using a cow heart (available at grocery stores), label the parts of the heart. Give a classroom demonstration.
3. Visit the following Web site and examine how the heart works: http://library.med.utah.edu/kw/pharm/hyper_heart1.html.
4. Visit www.blaufuss.org to listen to various heart sounds.
5. Examine the information at the following Web site and report on common chest injuries in hockey: http://www.sportsinjuryclinic.net/sports/ice_hockey.php/
6. Visit the following Web site and listen to the various heart and lung sounds: www.med.ucla.edu/wilkes/index.htm.

8

Abdominal Injuries

Objectives

Upon completing this chapter, the student will be able to do the following:

- Understand the anatomy of the abdomen.
- Understand the implications of illness or injury related to specific organs.
- Understand how to prevent injuries of the abdomen.
- Describe the care necessary to treat an abdominal injury.

Although abdominal organs are not generally protected in sporting activity by padding, abdominal injuries occur infrequently. A serious injury of the abdomen, however, may not become apparent for days. In this chapter we discuss function of the abdominal organs, injury prevention, and treatment.

ANATOMY OF THE ABDOMEN

The abdominal cavity is bounded by the lumbar spine posteriorly, the diaphragm superiorly, the abdominal musculature anteriorly, and the pelvis inferiorly. For purposes of discussion, the abdominal cavity is divided into four quadrants by an imaginary horizontal line running across the abdomen through the navel and an imaginary vertical line running from the sternum through the navel to the area between the legs (see figure 8.1). The right upper quadrant lies just below the ribs on the athlete's right side, and it contains the liver, a portion of the pancreas, the right kidney, the gallbladder, and the large and small intestines. The left upper quadrant lies just below the ribs on the athlete's left side, and it contains the stomach, a portion of the liver, a portion of the pancreas, the left kidney, the spleen, and the large and small intestines. The right lower quadrant contains the large and small intestines, the appendix, a portion of the bladder, the uterus and right ovary (in females), and the prostate (in males). The left lower quadrant contains the large and small intestines, a portion of the bladder, the uterus and left ovary (in females), and the prostate (in males).

The abdomen contains both solid and hollow organs. Injuries to the hollow organs, such as the bladder, intestines, stomach, and appendix, rarely cause rapid death. Moreover, the hollow organs tend to move and bend away if an athlete is hit in

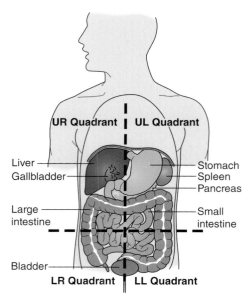

Figure 8.1   The abdominal quadrants.

Adapted, by permission, from S. Shultz et al, 2010, *Examination of musculoskeletal injuries*, 3rd ed. (Champaign, IL: Human Kinetics), 573.

the abdomen. Hollow organs are tubes that assist in transporting substances from one organ to another and are connected to one another by sheetlike membranes. Solid organs such as the liver, kidneys, and spleen aid in body chemistry. They can cause rapid death if injured because they have a large blood supply.

Abdominal organs can be divided into three categories: digestive organs, urinary organs, and reproductive organs. The organs included in the digestive system are the stomach, liver, pancreas, large and small intestines, appendix, spleen, and gallbladder. The organs of the urinary system are the kidneys, ureters, and bladder. Organs of the female reproductive system include the ovaries and uterus. Organs in the male reproductive system include the prostate and seminal vesicles.

Digestive Organs

The stomach secretes gastric juices that assist in breaking down food before it enters the intestines. The liver has several functions, including the detoxification of chemicals that the body perceives as poisons, such as alcohol. The liver also stores several vitamins, produces bile, and assists with food metabolism. The gallbladder is located at the liver and is a storage tank for **bile**, which is passed into the small intestine where it assists with the digestion of fat.

The pancreas produces insulin and enzymes for digestion. The small intestine completes the digestive process of breaking down food; from here the products of digestion are absorbed into the circulatory system. The sequential contraction and relaxation of the intestinal muscles, or peristalsis, pushes the food onward through the intestines. By the time it reaches the large intestine, the material that has not been digested or absorbed into the circulatory system is considered waste. In the large intestine water is absorbed, leaving solid waste for excretion. The appendix is part of the large intestine and has no known function. The spleen, which is covered with a thin sheath, has numerous functions: It produces and destroys red blood cells, it assists in the destruction of harmful microorganisms, and it is a storage site for blood.

Urinary Organs

The kidneys are responsible for maintaining the sensitive acid–base balance within the body. If the acid–base balance changes, the body systems begin to shut down, eventually resulting in death. The kidneys filter the blood and remove the waste products of metabolism to keep the acid–base relationship stable. If either kidney does not have adequate blood supply (whether by injury or illness), the kidney can cause hypertension from a chemical constriction of the body's blood vessels. The ureters are tubes attached to the kidneys that transport urine to the bladder, which is the holding tank for liquid waste products.

Reproductive Organs

In females, the ovaries produce eggs for possible fertilization and the hormone estrogen. Estrogen is the chemical that stimulates the development and maintenance of feminine characteristics. The uterus is the organ in which a fertilized egg develops. The lining of the uterus is released during a menstrual period if a fertilized egg is not present.

In males, the seminal vesicles and prostate gland are responsible for adding fluid and nutrients to seminal fluid. Males are particularly at risk of injuries to the reproductive organs because these organs are external to the pelvic and abdominal cavity. A common injury for males is a testicular contusion. This injury is caused by direct impact and results in severe pain and swelling. Testicular trauma can be prevented by wearing a protective cup during contact sports such as football and an athletic supporter during other sports such as basketball.

The Pelvis

The pelvis is a structure that provides a bony base and solid protection for some abdominal organs. The top edge of the pelvis is known as the iliac crest (see figure 3.3, *a* and *b*, on page 34), which is the attachment point for the abdominal muscles. The pelvis of the female has a larger opening and is wider than in the male in order to permit childbirth.

Abdominal Muscles

Although the liver and spleen are slightly covered by the inferior-most portion of the ribs, protection of the abdominal organs is mainly provided by the abdominal musculature and fat. The primary muscles of the abdomen are the rectus abdominis and the obliques. When well developed, the rectus abdominis gives the washboard-ripple effect to the abdomen. It attaches at the hip bones and extends to the lower ribs and sternum. The rectus abdominis is responsible for forward flexion or bending of the trunk. Each oblique muscle attaches to the lateral aspect of the lower ribs on one side of the body and runs diagonally to the hipbone. The obliques help compress the abdomen—for example, if someone threatens to hit you and you tighten your muscles, you are contracting the obliques. Refer to figure 3.4 on page 36 for a review of these muscles and the bones to which they are attached.

PREVENTING ABDOMINAL INJURIES

Preventing injuries of the abdominal organs is essential because abdominal trauma can quickly cause death. Sport rules that require protective equipment and limited contact are designed to prevent abdominal injuries. Ice hockey goalies, for example, generally wear protective equipment for the abdomen and reproductive organs. Other players can protect themselves by tightening their abdominal muscles. Most sports do not allow tackling or checking (physically moving an athlete) from behind so that athletes can protect themselves. Boxing has a rule that says it is illegal to hit below the belt. Before games, all athletes should be reminded to empty

their bladders because full bladders are more prone to rupture on impact than empty ones.

TREATING ABDOMINAL INJURIES AND CONDITIONS

Injuries within the abdominal cavity, especially to the hollow organs, are rare. The solid organs—the liver, spleen, and kidneys—can be injured, and internal bleeding may result. The AT should assess any athlete who has received a blow to the abdominal area, especially if he has abdominal pain, signs of shock, muscle spasms, or blood in the urine.

Side Stitch

A side stitch refers to pain just below the ribs in the upper abdominal region. There are various theories about why this pain occurs—a lack of oxygen getting to the abdominal muscles, improper breathing technique, eating food just before exercising, air trapped in the abdominal organs, and muscle spasms are a few—but in general, people who are less fit tend to get more stitches. Athletes experiencing the pain of a stitch resolve it by stopping exercise or by pressing directly over the area. If an athlete believes the stitch is a result of eating, she should change her eating patterns. A muscle-spasm stitch can be resolved by raising the arm on the same side as the pain and leaning away from the painful area. Pain that does not resolve needs to be referred to a physician for further evaluation.

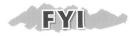

Enzymes
 An enzyme is a protein that allows a biochemical reaction to take place at normal body temperature but is itself not changed in the reaction.

Inguinal Canal
 The inguinal canal is a hole in the abdominal wall in the groin region.

Mechanism of Injury
 The *mechanism of injury* refers to the way in which an injury occurs. The mechanism can be observed if one is paying attention during a practice or game, or it can be explained by the athlete.

Hernia

A **hernia** is a lump of tissue, usually the intestine, that bulges through a weakness in the abdominal wall. Hernias can result from increased abdominal pressure, which may occur if the athlete holds his breath while weightlifting or going to the bathroom. The lump may go away when he lies down and bulge again when he stands up or exerts abdominal pressure. In males the intestine may go through the inguinal canal and stay in the scrotal sac. The athlete may or may not have pain. A hernia must be surgically repaired, although a truss, or strap, can be used temporarily to apply pressure to keep the bulge inside the abdomen. A truss does not work for inguinal hernias and cannot be used by athletes who participate in contact sports or sports such as weightlifting that require the exertion of internal abdominal pressure. If not treated, the bulge of tissue can get stuck in the abdominal wall or inguinal canal, which is called *strangulation*. Strangulation cuts off the blood supply to the tissue and eventually the tissue will die. If intestinal tissue is involved, a bowel obstruction will result. The obstruction prevents the passage of waste material from the body, causing pain and illness, and must be surgically repaired.

Pancreas Injury

The pancreas lies just behind the stomach near the liver and the spinal column. It is prone to injury during deceleration—for example, when an athlete running with the ball hits a wall. The wall does not cause the injury, but as the pancreas shifts forward when the rest of the body has stopped, it tears. The athlete will have pain in the middle of the abdomen to the back as well as nausea, vomiting, and signs of

shock. The athlete should be referred to the hospital for additional examination—a ruptured pancreas must be surgically repaired.

Liver Injury

A blow to the right upper abdomen can result in a contusion or rupture of the liver. The athlete will experience pain over the area that may radiate to the right shoulder. As the athlete loses blood she will go into shock; have a rapid, weak pulse; and experience a drop in blood pressure. She must be referred to a physician immediately. The AT should be suspicious of a liver contusion if the athlete receives any blows to the area. The athlete may die if the liver is ruptured and it goes untreated.

Kidney Injury

A direct blow over the kidney can cause a contusion, laceration, or rupture. The athlete will experience pain just under the posterior ribs to the side of the spine, and the pain may radiate to the bladder. Pain will increase with trunk extension and ease with knee or hip flexion. The athlete may feel nauseated and vomit. Urine may have visible blood, and the blood loss may cause the athlete to go into shock. Thus, the injury requires prompt emergency care and hospitalization. Generally, an athlete with a kidney injury is required to rest for several weeks before returning to competition. Possible complications are scarring of the kidney and hypertension.

Bladder Injury

A rupture of the bladder causes urine to leak into the surrounding area. The athlete may have painful urination, a contusion over the bladder, or blood in the urine. She should report any of these symptoms to the AT. In severe cases of bladder injury, athletes go into shock, causing rapid heart rate, decreased blood pressure, anxiety, and sweating. When the injury mechanism suggests a bladder injury, the athlete should be referred to a physician for immediate evaluation. The AT should instruct the athlete to look for the signs and symptoms listed previously and report problems immediately.

Spleen Rupture

A blow to the abdomen may injure the spleen. A spleen that is enlarged from an infection is more prone to rupture, so athletes recovering from

What Would You Do If...

A cross country runner reports that she has blood in her urine. She does not remember being hit over her kidney.

illnesses, especially mononucleosis, should not be allowed to play without a physician's permission. Athletes with a spleen injury will experience abdominal pain and perhaps pain in the left shoulder, which is referred to as **Kehr's sign**. The left shoulder pain is caused by internal bleeding that puts pressure on the diaphragm, which presses on a nerve, causing referred pain to the shoulder. The

athlete will often indicate that she is nauseated, experiencing cramps, and weak, and she may pass out. Upon examination, the AT may note abdominal spasms, vomiting, rapid heart rate, decreased blood pressure, and shock. The athlete must be transported by EMS to a hospital immediately—an injured spleen is a medical emergency. A ruptured spleen can bleed severely, causing rapid blood loss and a drop in blood pressure.

An athlete with less severe spleen injuries will be hospitalized overnight for observation. A ruptured spleen must be surgically removed. Athletes who have had their spleens removed are able to play sports after total recovery. The spleen can be protected from injury through the use of padding.

The Real World

While I was working a summer basketball camp, one of the athletes was accidentally kneed in the abdomen. When we got to him, he complained of high pain levels in the lower abdomen off to the left side. We determined that he could move, so we helped him walk to the sideline and finished our evaluation. He exhibited tenderness over the spleen with a positive Kehr's sign. The coach encouraged the athlete to walk it off, but because a Kehr's sign most often suggests a spleen injury, I overruled him. We removed the athlete to the training room, where he began to show signs of shock. We thought his spleen must be ruptured, and we called EMS immediately. While we waited, we monitored his vital signs and treated him for shock. He showed a decreasing level of consciousness and a significant drop in blood pressure. We recorded vital signs at five-minute intervals before EMS arrived, and that cut down on time of transfer from our care to theirs. He was taken to the local hospital and was later airlifted to a larger hospital. He did have a ruptured spleen, and he was rushed into surgery. The athlete recovered fully, and the next summer he was back at the same camp.

Alex Embry, ATC, EMT

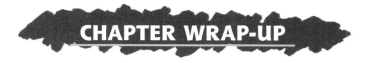

CHAPTER WRAP-UP

Summary

Most of the organs in the abdominal region are involved in the digestive process and therefore are hollow. It is difficult to injure the hollow organs, but the solid organs of the abdomen can be seriously injured. The AT must know where the organs of the abdomen are located in order to evaluate abdominal injuries. Some serious injuries will not be immediately evident because they have delayed signs and symptoms. Athletes with abdominal injuries require immediate aid from EMS. The number of serious abdominal injuries in sport has been reduced by rules restricting body contact and by required protective equipment.

Key Terms

Define the following terms found in this chapter:

bile

hernia

Kehr's sign

Questions for Review

1. List the major organs of the abdomen and their functions.
2. What measures can be taken to prevent abdominal injury?
3. What abdominal organs are easiest to injure?

Activities for Reinforcement

1. Have an AT demonstrate how to evaluate an athlete with a suspected abdominal injury.
2. Use a stethoscope to listen to the four abdominal quadrants.
3. If you could redesign the abdominal cavity, how could you provide more protection for solid organs?

Above and Beyond

1. Using one of the references that follow, draw the external abdomen. Include the pain-referral points of the abdominal organs.
2. Examine one of the following research studies and write a summary:

   Johnson, J.D., and W.W. Briner, Jr. 2005. Primary care of the sports hernia. *Physician and Sportsmedicine* 33(2): 35.

   McGuine, T. 1996. Recognizing abdominal injuries in high school athletes. *Sports Plus* Winter/Spring: 2-3.

   Meyers, W., E. Yoo, O. Devon, N. Jain, M. Horner, C. Lauencin, et al. 2007. Understanding "sports hernia" (athletic pubalgia): the anatomic and pathophysiologic basis for abdominal and groin pain in athletes. *Operative Techniques in Sports Medicine* 15(4): 165-177.

   National Safety Council. 2001. *First aid and CPR.* 4th ed. Boston: Jones and Bartlett.

3. Read one of the following case studies and write a brief report to share with your class:

   Itagaki, M., and N. Knight. 2004. Kidney trauma in martial arts: A case report of kidney contusion in jujitsu. *American Journal of Sports Medicine* 32(2): 522-524.

   Massie, J., D. Donnelly, and K. Ricker. 2009. Liver laceration sustained by a college football player. *Athletic Therapy Today* 14(2): 23-26.

   Unverzagt, C., T. Schuemann, and J. Mathisen. 2008. Differential diagnosis of a sports hernia in a high-school athlete. *Journal of Orthopaedic and Sports Physical Therapy* 38(2): 63-70.

chapter 9

Spinal Injuries

Objectives

Upon completing this chapter, the student will be able to do the following:

- Describe the basic anatomy of the spine.
- Explain common spinal injuries that occur with athletic participation.
- Identify common signs and symptoms of spinal injuries.
- Explain the treatments performed by ATs for specific spinal injuries.
- Describe common postural problems.

Similar to the other joints in the body, the joints in the spine consist of articulated bones supported by muscles and ligaments. However, the spinal column is more complex than many joints and includes other structures such as disks and nerves. Because it protects the spinal cord, injuries to the spine can be life threatening and need careful attention by the AT. Most spinal cord injuries are in the lumbar and cervical regions, so we will only consider injuries to those areas.

ANATOMY OF THE SPINE

The spine is a complex structure of bones with four segments—the **sacrum** (tailbone area), **lumbar spine** (lower spine), **thoracic spine** (middle spine), and **cervical spine** (upper spine) (figure 9.1). Normal anatomical alignment and muscular strength keep the spinal segments aligned properly. The spine should have normal curvature at each of these areas. Normal alignment is termed a **neutral spine**—this means

that the spinal curves of the lumbar, thoracic, and cervical region are curved neither too much nor too little, and the spine is comfortable. Such a position is anatomically the strongest.

Bones

The bones in the spine are separated by disks and held together by ligaments. The muscles of the spine and trunk permit many movements and also help to stabilize the spine.

The bones of the spine are called *vertebrae*. There are 7 cervical, 12 thoracic, 5 lumbar, and 5 sacral (which are fused together) vertebrae. Though there are differences among the vertebrae of each region, they also share many similarities. For example, each vertebra has a body, a spinous process, and a canal through which the spinal cord passes (see figures 9.2 and 9.3). The bony spinal column has several functions: protecting the spinal cord, holding the body upright for walking, and serving as a site for muscular attachments.

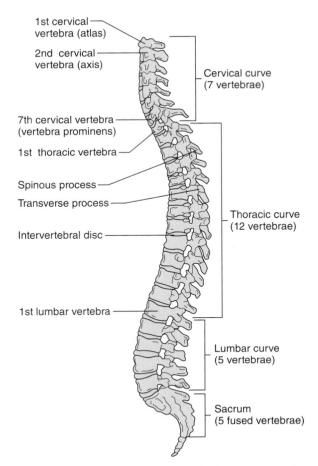

Figure 9.1 Lateral view of the spine. The natural anterior and posterior curves of the spine allow it to absorb shock. Note also the differences in size of the cervical, thoracic, and lumbar vertebrae.

Adapted, by permission, from W.C. Whiting and R.F. Zernicke, 2008, *Biomechanics of musculoskeletal injury,* 2nd ed. (Champaign, IL: Human Kinetics), 263.

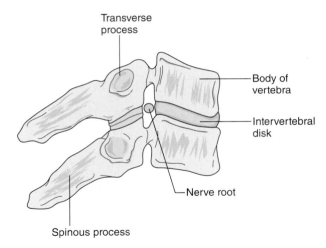

Figure 9.2 A normal vertebra. Each vertebra consists of a body, a transverse process, and a spinous process. An intervertebral disk lies between each pair of vertebrae to absorb shock.

Adapted, by permission, from W.C. Whiting and R.F. Zernicke, 2008, *Biomechanics of musculoskeletal injury,* 2nd ed. (Champaign, IL: Human Kinetics), 263.

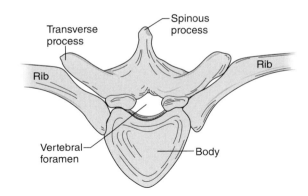

Figure 9.3 Inferior view of normal vertebra.

Disks

The **intervertebral disks** that lie between the vertebrae absorb shock and resist compression during activity. They separate the vertebrae, which allows movement and flexibility, and they provide space for nerves to exit the spinal cord and enter the rest of the body. Figure 9.4 shows a disk cross section.

A disk has two parts: a jellylike core called the **nucleus pulposus** that is surrounded by several layers of cartilage called the **annulus fibrosus**. The disks of the spine do not receive any blood supply, so they do not have the same healing potential as other tissues of the body. The disks are compressible—a person is slightly taller first thing in the morning than she will be later in the day after gravity has been compressing the disks, and in old age we become shorter.

Muscles and Tendons

The muscles of the trunk and neck attach to the spine via tendons and provide both a wide range of movement and much needed stability. Two highly respected physical therapists, James Porterfield

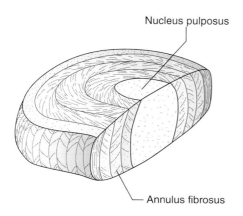

Nucleus pulposus

Annulus fibrosus

Figure 9.4 Disk cross section. The disk lies between the vertebral bodies. The nucleus pulposus, located at the center of the disk, is a jellylike substance.

Reprinted, by permission, from J. Watkins, 2010, *Structure and function of the musculoskeletal system*, 2nd ed. (Champaign, IL: Human Kinetics), 122.

and Carl DeRosa, describe the spine as a mast on a ship. A mast has many cables attached to it at various points that extend to various places on the ship. These cables keep the mast stable as the wind catches its sail. Likewise, the spine has many muscles attached at various points that extend to the pelvis, legs, and arms. These muscles keep the spine stable as the body performs tasks such as throwing, catching, and kicking. If the ship has a mast that bends and folds, the sail will not catch the wind effectively. Similarly, if the body has a spine that bends and gives because of poor stability, it will not perform athletic tasks effectively.

The abdominal muscles are crucial for supporting trunk movement, especially the rectus abdominis and the internal and external obliques (see figure 3.4a, page 36). The spinal extensors run the entire length of the spine posteriorly and attach to various structures including the pelvis, ribs, and vertebrae. These muscles work together to keep the body upright.

The upper trapezius extends the cervical spine (see figure 3.4, page 36). It attaches to the occipital bone (back of head) and fans out to each side of the neck before attaching to the acromion process of the scapula (see figure 3.3, page 34).

Cervical flexion is accomplished by the scalene muscles, which attach to the cervical vertebrae and run down to the first and second ribs. There are three muscles in all, each of which has a different attachment point. These muscles also help with the breathing process. Cervical side bending and rotation are accomplished by the sternocleidomastoid muscle, which is attached to the top of the sternum and runs up the neck, attaching to the mastoid process just behind the ear. The sternocleidomastoid rotates the head to the direction opposite the attachment.

Ligaments

Many ligaments support the vertebral segments. The anterior aspect of the spine has a thick, tough ligament called the *anterior longitudinal ligament*. This ligament prevents bony separation during extension.

The posterior aspect of the spine contains the supraspinous ligament, a thin ligament that passes from the tip of one spinous process to another. As the spine flexes, this ligament supports the vertebral segments. Also at the posterior aspect of the spine, the posterior longitudinal ligament runs from the posterior regions of the vertebral bodies. This ligament works with the supraspinous ligament to stabilize the posterior aspect of the spine, particularly during flexion.

Various other ligaments also support the vertebral segments. For example, on each side of the spine the intertransverse ligaments run from the transverse process of the vertebra above to the transverse process of the vertebra below.

POSTURAL CONSIDERATIONS

Take a look at a friend's posture. How do you know if the posture is normal? To understand postural problems, you must first understand normal postural alignment.

Normal Posture

The AT can determine if a person has normal posture by viewing him from the side (see figure 9.5). Picture a straight line dropping from the ceiling.

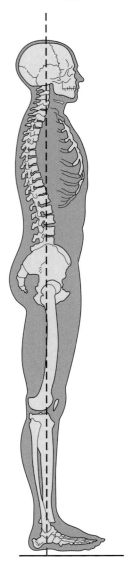

Figure 9.5 Normal posture. Note how the plumb line runs just behind the ear, through the shoulder, past the hip, and through the knee to just in front of the lateral malleolus.

Adapted, by permission, from J. Griffin, 2006, *Client-centered exercise prescription*, 2nd ed. (Champaign, IL: Human Kinetics), 106.

If an athlete were standing with proper posture beside the line, specific body segments could be observed in alignment. The line would pass just behind the ear, through the center of the shoulder, down through the middle of the greater trochanter of the hip, just behind the patella, and down to just in front of the lateral malleolus.

Abnormal Posture

Imagine a plumb line in reference to an athlete you are viewing from the side—you may identify several postural faults (see figure 9.6, *a-c*). For example, if her ear were projected in front of the line, she would have a **forward head posture**. This puts a great deal of stress at the back of the neck. If the line passed through the back of the shoulders instead of the middle, she would have rounded shoulders. The thoracic spine should be somewhat curved, but excessive roundedness is undesirable and is called **kyphosis** (figure 9.6*a*). Likewise, too much forward curve at the lumbar spine is called **lordosis** (figure 9.6*b*). If the spine is correctly aligned, the normal cervical, thoracic, and lumbar curves are ideal for flexibility and absorbing shock. When the athlete cannot maintain proper posture, the ability of the spine to absorb shock is diminished, eventually resulting in injury.

Not only can the spine be too rounded at the thoracic region and too curved forward at the lumbar region, it can also curve from side to side. When observed from behind, the spine may be crooked rather than running straight from the skull to the sacrum. This is called **scoliosis** (figure 9.6*c*). Some people have this condition in mild forms. However, occasionally ATs will find an athlete with a prominent deviation. Although doctors often screen for this during preparticipation physical examinations, it is sometimes difficult to see. If a previously undetected deviation is suspected, the athlete should be referred to an orthopedic surgeon for an assessment.

What Would You Do If...

You have been observing and assisting the AT with the rehabilitation of an athlete suffering from back pain. While in class you notice that the athlete slouches in his chair.

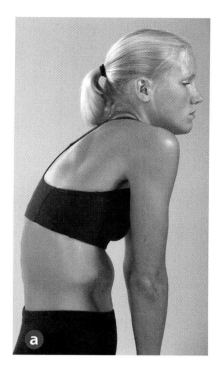
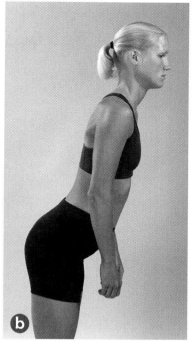
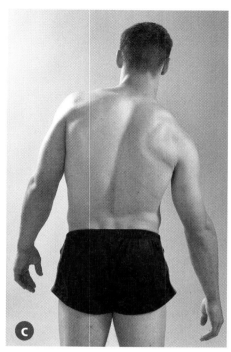

Figure 9.6   Abnormal postures: *(a)* kyphosis, *(b)* lordosis, and *(c)* scoliosis.

Reprinted, by permission, from R. Behnke, 2005, *Kinetic Anatomy,* 2nd ed. (Champaign, IL: Human Kinetics), 121.

You can take steps to prevent poor postural habits, such as imagining balloons attached to your head that are pulling you up straight. You can also alternate carrying your book bag or gym bag on opposite shoulders. Putting a heavy book bag on the same shoulder every day throughout your high school and college career can take its toll on the spine. You can stay fit and exercise regularly, too. Your body is made to move, and being a slug will cause stiffness. Be kind to your spine, and use proper posture whenever possible.

PREVENTING SPINAL INJURIES

Preventing injury to the cervical and lumbar regions of the spine is an active process. Athletes should participate in exercise and flexibility programs, maintain proper posture, learn to lift properly, use proper technique (e.g., proper tackling in football), and perhaps use back support when lifting heavy objects.

Exercise and flexibility programs are necessary for the muscles surrounding and supporting the spine, especially the abdominal muscles. A strong abdomen can help decrease stress on the lumbar

spine. The muscles around the hip should also be strengthened because the hip directly influences the spine. If the hip is tilted forward, the spine will move into extension, and if the hip is tilted backward, the spine will move into flexion. Therefore, the hip musculature should be both flexible and strong to allow proper movement and positioning in the lumbar region.

Proper lifting procedures reduce the risk of injury (see figure 9.7). Business people understand that if an employee improperly lifts a weight, she can injure her back. To prevent such injuries, businesses have begun sending employees to training called *back school*. Back schools are short-term instructional programs that teach people proper posture and lifting techniques. Proper lifting technique is maintaining a slight curve in the lumbar spine while lifting with the knees and the hips rather than the spine. It also involves keeping the head up when lifting. A lifting posture in which the spine is too rounded or flexed may cause a strain or disk injury.

Back supports have become popular recently. Go to any home repair store, lumberyard, or even some grocery stores, and you will see many of the workers wearing these belts. Back supports increase the pressure around the spine and decrease the

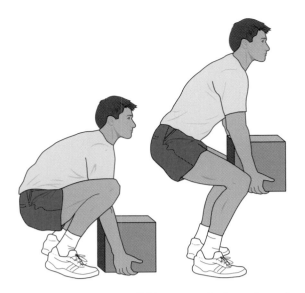

Figure 9.7 Proper lifting entails keeping the head up, the feet in a wide stance, and the spine in a neutral position. Also, keeping the load close to the body reduces stress on the back.

Adapted, by permission, from E.T. Howley and B.D. Franks, 2003, *Health fitness instructor's handbook*, 4th ed. (Champaign, IL: Human Kinetics), 467.

amount of stress to the vertebrae. A back support, however, should not take the place of other means of injury prevention—the use of the brace alone cannot prevent all injuries.

Recognizing that proper technique plays a role in preventing cervical spine injuries, NATA published a position statement regarding head-down technique in football (Heck, Clarke, Peterson, Torg, and Weis 2004). It states that initiating contact at the top of the helmet (also known as spearing) creates an axial load. An **axial load** occurs when force is applied to the head while the head is lowered into flexion that straightens the cervical spine like a drinking straw. If you take a drinking straw and push on the ends hard enough, it will eventually bend. A similar event occurs at the cervical spine, causing vertebrae fractures.

According to the NATA position statement, axial loading is the key mechanism for catastrophic injuries in football; thus, football players should tackle with the shoulders while positioning the head in an upward position. Many coaches teach athletes to see their tackling targets. This is a cue to remind players to keep the head up while tackling.

TREATING LUMBAR SPINE INJURIES AND CONDITIONS

As with other parts of the body, the spine is susceptible to ligament, muscle and tendon, and bone injuries. In addition, the disks that lie between the bodies of the vertebrae cause unique problems.

Bone Injuries

Bone fractures are possible in the lumbar spine, especially with severe mechanisms of injury such as compression; for instance, forcefully landing on the buttocks could cause a compression fracture. Fractures of the spine are hard to determine without an X ray. However, if an AT knows the mechanism of injury and finds a great deal of back pain, muscle spasm, and tenderness when touching the vertebrae, a fracture must be suspected. If the AT suspects a lumbar fracture, the athlete should be treated conservatively; that is, he should be put on a backboard with the help of appropriate emergency medical personnel and taken to the nearest hospital.

Two common bone injuries found among athletes are **spondylolysis** and **spondylolisthesis**. These bony problems are most commonly found in athletes such as gymnasts who arch their backs and subject their spines to a great deal of hyperextension. Spondylolysis is often described as a stress fracture or bone degeneration of the vertebrae, specifically at a location referred to as the *pars interarticularis*. The pars interarticularis is located on a thin portion of the vertebrae between the superior and inferior facets. The location of the bone degeneration is important because if the fracture fails to heal, it can separate, causing the spine to become unstable. The resulting instability allows a vertebra to slip forward (shunt) on the vertebra below it. This is called *spondylolisthesis* (see figure 9.8). The most common location for this injury is the fifth lumbar vertebra slipping forward on the first sacral vertebra.

Spondylolysis and spondylolisthesis are serious problems, and they require examination by a physician. In many instances the athlete is required to discontinue the aggravating activity and wear a lumbar brace to keep the vertebral segment stable. The athlete must then perform extensive reha-

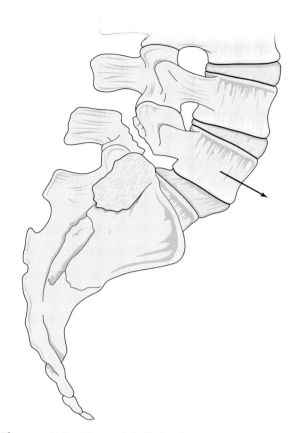

Figure 9.8 Spondylolisthesis.

bilitation that focuses on strengthening the trunk muscles in a neutral spine position.

Disk Injuries

One of the most common injuries of the lumbar spine is a disk bulge (see figure 9.9). This condition is not common in younger athletes, but older athletes seem to be susceptible to it. Although some people call it a *slipped disk*, that is not an appropriate term. The disk is attached to the body of the vertebra and rarely slips forward or backward. In a disk bulge, the jellylike nucleus pulposus at the center of the disk pushes through the rings of cartilage. For example, if you were to place the palms of your hands on the top and bottom of a jelly doughnut and squeeze, jelly would begin to ooze through the layers of dough. Similarly, when a disk is compressed, the nucleus pulposus begins to press through the layers of cartilage around it and eventually can press against the outer layer, causing it to bulge.

Disks rarely bulge toward the front of the spine for two reasons. First, the front of the spine is covered with a thick ligament called the *anterior longitudinal ligament*, and second, most people have postures that flex the spine forward most of the time. Flexion of the spine tends to put more pressure on the front of the disk, pushing the nucleus pulposus toward the posterior. Most often disks bulge posteriorly to one side or another, which may put pressure on the nerve exiting the spinal cord at that level (see figure 9.9).

Disk bulges are aggravating and can be disabling. If the disk bulge is putting pressure on a nerve, numbness, tingling, and pain can occur down the leg. Another characteristic of this condition is pain in the low back that increases with sitting.

Treating an athlete with a disk bulge requires the AT to understand the causes of this condition. Most often disk bulges are the result of poor posture and body mechanics that put the spine in a great deal of flexion over a long time. For example, a softball infielder who does not maintain a neutral posture may await a pitch with the spine flexed forward. If this same person also sits with a slouchy posture and uses poor lifting mechanics, she may eventually put herself at risk of a disk bulge.

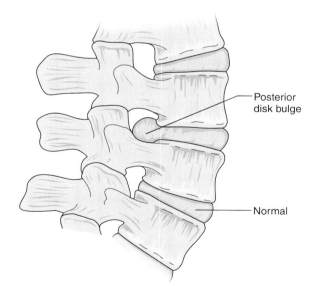

Figure 9.9 A posterior disk bulge. As the spine is flexed, pressure is put on the anterior part of the disk, which encourages the nucleus pulposus to push through layers of the annulus fibrosus.

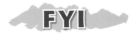

Compressing the Spine

Sitting creates a greater compressive load on the spine than standing does.

Under the direction of the team physician, an AT may initially treat a disk bulge by using active rest, as with a sprain (see the next section). Also, correcting poor posture and helping the athlete move into spinal extension can be helpful. It is thought that if proper posture and body mechanics are used, the nucleus pulposus will not bulge quite as much, which will give the athlete some relief. The AT should make certain that none of the exercises aggravates the leg pain or causes more numbness or tingling. As the athlete progresses, extension exercises, and sometimes traction (discussed in chapter 16), may help reduce the disk bulge. He should also be taught about proper sitting, standing, and lifting postures that minimize pressure on the disk, and he should avoid prolonged sitting. Strengthening the spine with lumbar stabilization techniques is also helpful.

Muscle and Tendon Injuries

An AT rarely sees a ruptured muscle at the lumbar spine, but mild and moderate strains are common. Characteristics of lumbar strain include pain to one side of the spine, spasm, and lack of movement. Also, the athlete will often present with pain on the opposite side of the direction in which she bends. For example, if she bends to the left and the pain is on the right side of the spine, the muscle to the right of the spine may be strained. The pain associated with sprains is very localized, whereas pain caused by a muscle strain usually moves up and down the length of the muscle, especially when the athlete tries to use the muscle while bending. Remember that the spine is like a mast on a ship, and the muscles are the guy wires. If the spine is bent to one side, the muscles on the opposite side will attempt to stabilize it. The AT can initially apply ice to the injury, and gentle stretching using a knees-to-chest routine often speeds healing. Once pain is decreased, flexibility and strength can be restored to normal using

strengthening and stretching routines. The AT should observe the athlete for proper posture and lifting mechanics to prevent reinjury.

Ligament Injuries

Sprains at the lumbar joints commonly occur when athletes are forced into excessive trunk flexion or attempt to flex the spine and rotate at the same time. An example of this mechanism is when a football player is tackled and forced forward. When the trunk flexion is combined with rotation, the posterior aspect of the vertebral joints can separate and stretch over the ligaments. Characteristics of a lumbar sprain include pain to one side of the spine and limited movement because of pain and muscle spasm. An AT who takes a thorough history of the injury and performs special spinal tests can determine if the ligaments are involved, although it can be difficult to differentiate from a muscle strain. During an assessment, an AT might gently perform a stress test that pushes each vertebra anteriorly. This will usually be painful if the joint is sprained, but it should not be painful if a strain is present, unless the strain is severe. Of course, an AT will not perform such a test if signs or symptoms of a fracture are present (see chapter 4).

When a sprain initially occurs, the AT should treat it the same as any other acute injury; that is, PRICES should be performed. As we discuss in chapter 20, the critical treatment in this phase is PRICES. In other words, the injured area must be protected, rested, iced, compressed, elevated, and supported. Many believe that heat should always be used for spine injuries. With an acute injury, however, this may do more harm than good because heat tends to increase swelling and pain. After 48 hours postinjury, it is typically all right to use heat.

Though rest is recommended, complete bed rest is no longer the accepted norm. Rather, the athlete should engage in active rest, maintaining a comfortable neutral spine position and gently performing strengthening exercises to stabilize the spine. (Strengthening exercises are discussed in chapter 17.) As the initial inflammation subsides, the AT can have the athlete begin some flexibility exercises as well as some advanced lumbar stabilization exercises as long as they do not aggravate the area. The spinal musculature needs to be strengthened in preparation for return to activity.

TREATING CERVICAL SPINE INJURIES AND CONDITIONS

As you might imagine, the types of injuries incurred at the cervical spine are similar to those at the lumbar spine. However, the cervical spine has more mobility than the lumbar spine, and thus the treatments differ.

Bone Injuries

Bone injuries to the cervical spine include fractures and dislocations, which can have devastating results including permanent disabilities and death. Fractures to the cervical spine are often the result of an axial load, as discussed earlier in the chapter. This occurs when a force is applied to the head while it is lowered into flexion that straightens the cervical spine, resulting in vertebrae fractures. A dislocation of the cervical vertebrae often results from a combination of excessive neck flexion and rotation.

Cervical spine fractures and dislocations have similar signs and symptoms. The athlete will often report pain around the cervical spine and weakness, numbness, and tingling down the arms. With a dislocation, there is often a visible deformity, but because of equipment or positioning, it is sometimes difficult to observe. Initial care for both injuries is identical. Emergency care procedures should be followed, and after ruling out life-threatening conditions, the neck should be immobilized and the athlete put on a backboard. If he is wearing a helmet and a cervical fracture or dislocation is suspected, the helmet should be left in place because attempting to remove it may cause excessive movement of the neck, which could lead to further damage. Appropriate emergency medical personnel should take the athlete to the nearest hospital facility.

Disk Injuries

Disk injuries in the cervical spine are not nearly as common as those in the lumbar spine, but they can occur. An athlete with a cervical disk bulge often will report more neck pain while sitting and while flexing the neck forward than while standing and walking. He may also report discomfort down the back between the shoulder blades. Treatment for disk bulges of the cervical spine includes improving the neck posture and then progressing to cervical extension exercises that do not aggravate the condition. Cervical traction can also be used by the AT under the direction of the team physician to help reduce the disk bulge. Full neck mobility and strength should gradually be regained. As with suspected fractures, if an athlete presents with severe symptoms, such as numbness, tingling, and burning of the arm, he

The Real World

After school the AT was called to assist an injured female gymnast. She had been performing a back flip in the gym when she landed shoulders and neck first. She was lying face-down, with her right arm under her body and her head turned to the side. The initial exam revealed point tenderness along her trapezius muscle and lower cervical spine. All neurological signs were fine. The athlete was laughing and wanted to get up. The AT felt extra caution was necessary based on how she fell, so EMS was summoned. The student became upset, but the AT reassured her that this was the best option. The AT knew that appearances and an athlete's attitude do not always represent an accurate picture.

Several hours later, the injured girl's father called the AT to thank him for being so cautious. The girl had suffered a fracture dislocation of C3 and fractures of C4 and C5. By insisting that she be backboarded and transported, the AT may have saved her from paralysis or death. The athlete was placed in a special neck brace for three months. The fractures healed, but the C3 dislocation remained out of alignment, so she had surgery to fuse the vertebrae. The young woman kept a positive attitude, was courageous, and had a wonderful smile throughout her ordeal. She was a definite inspiration to those around her. And although she was unable to return to gymnastics, she is now able to function normally in other aspects of her life. She even teaches gymnastics to younger athletes and has recently enrolled in a college athletic training curriculum.

Roger Kalisiak, ATC

should be put on a spine board and referred to a hospital by an AT. The AT should consult the team physician regarding the athlete's return to participation following this condition.

Muscle and Tendon Injuries

A cervical muscle strain can also occur from a whiplash injury by the mechanism described in the following section. Characteristics of cervical muscle strains include muscle spasm, restricted range of motion, weakness against resistance, pain, and tenderness of the muscle. An AT should treat cervical strains much like cervical ligament sprains. The criteria for returning to play are the same as for cervical sprains. Manual resistance works well for strengthening the neck. Not a lot of exercise equipment is designed specifically for the neck; an alternative is performing cervical stretches while a partner provides resistance with her hand.

Ligament Injuries

Despite having an excellent range of motion, the cervical spine is subject to ligament sprains when it is forcefully moved beyond its normal range. Cervical sprains are usually the result of hyperextension or hyperflexion of the neck. Take a football receiver who stops, turns toward the quarterback to catch the ball, and then gets tackled by a defender. When hit forcefully from behind, the receiver often suffers a whiplash injury—in fact, many a receiver would say that he felt as if he were hit by a car. The body is forced forward by the blow while the head moves backward, placing the cervical spine into extension and stretching the ligaments and muscles at the front of the neck. When his body stops—because he hits the ground or is tackled from the front—his head snaps forward, stretching the posterior neck ligaments and muscles.

Cervical ligament sprains have symptoms of neck and arm pain. The athlete may even complain of pain between the scapulae. Because of the possibility of a spinal cord injury, any neck trauma should be thoroughly evaluated by the AT. Provided there is no sign of nerve injury, the AT can treat the neck. As with many other ligament injuries, the neck needs to be treated with protection, rest, ice, and support. No compression with an elastic bandage

should be applied to the neck, however, because this may slow blood flow to the brain. A neck brace can be used to help the athlete hold her head up. A follow-up examination from the team physician is a must to rule out any other conditions. Further treatment for the cervical spine sprain includes strengthening exercises to regain stability, and full range of motion should be reestablished. Before the athlete is allowed to return to participation, she must have the following:

- Full strength
- Full range of motion
- Full confidence
- No symptoms
- Physician clearance

Brachial Plexus Injuries

The brachial plexus is a network of nerves that exit the cervical spine and run through the shoulder and down the arm. An athlete who falls, runs into, or attempts to tackle another player can stretch the brachial plexus. Picture a linebacker tackling an opponent. As he makes the tackle, the shoulder is pressed downward and the neck is forced into a stretch in the opposite direction. This mechanism of injury often stretches the brachial plexus, resulting in burning, tingling, numbness, and stinging sensa-

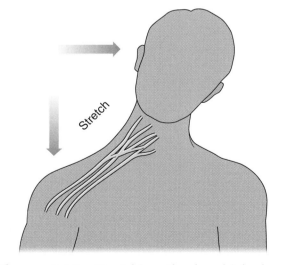

Figure 9.10 Stretching the brachial plexus causes burning, tingling, numbness, and stinging sensations of the arm and shoulder.

tions of the arm and shoulder (figure 9.10). For this reason, this condition is often called a **burner** or **stinger**. Depending on the severity of the injury, the burner may last for a matter of seconds or minutes. More severe cases can last much longer, even weeks. Treatment often consists of neck-strengthening exercises and range-of-motion stretching of the area. A football player is usually fitted with a neck roll that limits lateral flexion. Before returning to play following a burner, an athlete must have the following:

- No symptoms
- Full strength
- Full range of motion of the neck and shoulder
- A problem-free neck and shoulder evaluation by the AT and the team physician

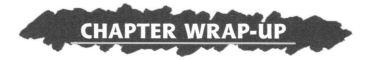

CHAPTER WRAP-UP

Summary

The spine is an articulated series of vertebrae that protect the spinal cord, and numerous muscles attach to it. A neutral spine, promoted by proper posture, is stable and absorbs shock. The spine may receive sprains and strains in the lumbar and cervical regions, but because of the spinal cord, nerve roots, and disks, other injuries to the spine may be more serious, even life threatening. After any injury to the spinal area, an athlete must learn proper bending and lifting techniques and perform muscle-strengthening exercises to reduce the risk of further injury.

Key Terms

Define the following terms found in this chapter:

annulus fibrosus	kyphosis	scoliosis
axial load	lordosis	spondylolisthesis
burner	lumbar spine	spondylolysis
cervical spine	neutral spine	stinger
forward head posture	nucleus pulposus	thoracic spine
intervertebral disk	sacrum	

Questions for Review

1. List the spinal segments, and discuss which of the segments is most commonly injured and why.
2. Describe the types of spinal injuries and how they occur.
3. If an AT were working with an athlete who reported burning sensations down the arm that lasted only about 15 seconds, what might have happened?
4. Why is proper posture important, and why do you think it is hard for some people to use proper posture?
5. What is the difference between spondylolysis and spondylolisthesis?
6. With the supervision of an AT, try wearing several lumbar supports. Why do you think these are recommended for lifting?
7. Observe the lifting mechanics of a partner in class. Are the mechanics appropriate for preventing a back injury?

Activities for Reinforcement

1. Check each other's posture—who has lordosis, kyphosis, or forward head?

2. Have an AT demonstrate how to evaluate the lumbar and cervical spine.

3. Watch the NATA's heads-up video that is designed to teach athlete's how to prevent head-down contact: www.nata.org/Heads-Up

Above and Beyond

1. What types of spine injuries do you think are most common in football? Why? What types of spine injuries are most common in gymnastics? Why? What about sports such as tennis and racquetball?

2. Select one or more of the following suggested readings and write a report on spine injuries.

   Beattie, P. 2008. Current understanding of lumbar intervertebral disc degeneration: a review with emphasis upon etiology, pathophysiology, and lumbar magnetic resonance imaging findings. *Journal of Orthopaedic and Sports Physical Therapy* 38(6): 329-340.

   Boden, B., and C. Jarvis. 2009. Spinal injuries in sports. *Physical Medicine and Rehabilitation Clinics of North America* 20(1): 55-68.

   Cassidy, R., W. Shaffer, and D. Johnson. 2005. Sports medicine update: spondylolysis and spondylolisthesis in the athlete. *Orthopedics* 28(11): 1331-1333.

   Moeller, J.L., and S.F. Rifat. 2001. Spondylolysis in active adolescents: Expediting return to play. *Physician and Sportsmedicine* 29(12): 27-32.

   Oakley, J.C. 2003. An update on the treatment of chronic low back pain. *Critical Reviews in Physical and Rehabilitation Medicine* 15(2): 113-140.

   Standaert, C.J. 2002. Practice management: spondylolysis in the adolescent athlete. *Clinical Journal of Sport Medicine* 12(2): 119-122.

   Watkins, R.C. 2002. Lumbar disc injury in the athlete. *Clinics in Sports Medicine* 21(1): 147-165.

3. Write a back-strengthening program for one of your school teams. Keep in mind the level of conditioning required as well as the amount of training time that the team can devote to your program. Share your program with your AT and get some feedback.

4. Examine the information at the following Web sites and make a poster about the causes of spine injuries:

   www.back.com/causes-trauma-musculoskeletal.html

   www.hughston.com/hha/a_14_1_1.htm

   www.cndpa.com/spine_condition_C.asp

5. Visit the Southern California Orthopedic Institute Web site and review the anatomy of the spine: www.scoi.com/spinanat.htm

6. Visit the following Web site and watch the narrated video related to spinal anatomy and movement: www.spine-health.com/video/spine-anatomy-interactive-video.

7. Visit www.spineuniverse.com for resources relating to spine health.

UNIT IV

Understanding Athletics-Related Injuries to the Upper Extremity

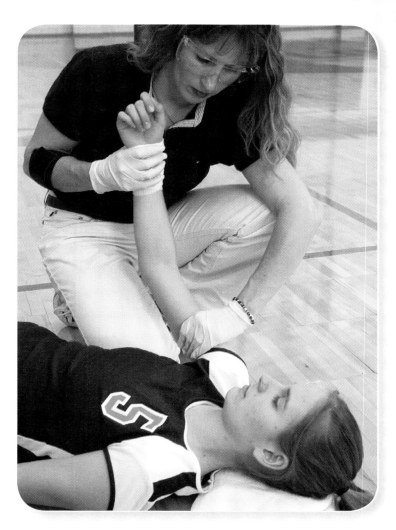

chapter 10

Shoulder Injuries

Objectives

Upon completing this chapter, the student will be able to do the following:

- Understand the basic anatomy of the shoulder.
- Explain how shoulder injuries occur.
- Describe the types of injuries to the shoulder.
- Explain treatment procedures for common shoulder injuries.

The shoulder is an amazing structure with a great deal of movement capability. Many athletics-related injuries to the shoulder are the result of overhead movement such as throwing a softball or serving a tennis ball.

ANATOMY OF THE SHOULDER

The shoulder is a ball-and-socket joint similar to the hip but much shallower. Therefore, it relies on muscular strength for its stability. Several bones link up at the shoulder, combining possibilities for movement across a wide range. The entire bony linkage of the shoulder is often referred to as the *shoulder girdle*.

Bones

The shoulder joint has three bony components, the humerus, the clavicle, and the scapula, which are held together by ligaments (see figures 10.1 and 10.2). The head of the humerus, which is the bone

of the upper arm, is round and smooth and fits into the glenoid fossa of the scapula. The humerus has a groove near the top, referred to as the *bicipital groove*, where the biceps tendon moves up and down during flexion and extension of the elbow. The clavicle, or collarbone, articulates at the tip of the shoulder and at the sternum near the throat. The scapula, or shoulder blade, has two forward projections that are located on the anterior aspect of the shoulder: the acromion process and the coracoid process. The rotator cuff muscles attach to the scapula.

Muscles and Tendons

The **rotator cuff** consists of four muscles—the subscapularis, infraspinatus, teres minor, and supraspinatus (see figure 10.3)—and their associated tendons that insert onto the humerus. These muscles are responsible for rotating the arm internally and externally as well as abducting the shoulder. The rotator cuff muscles are easy to remember if you use the acronym **SITS** (**s**ubscapularis, **i**nfraspinatus, **t**eres minor, and **s**upraspinatus).

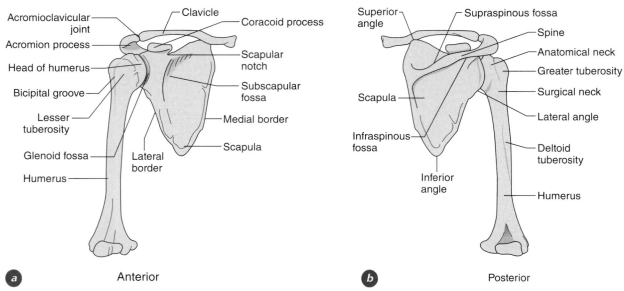

Figure 10.1   The bones of the shoulder girdle: *(a)* anterior view, *(b)* posterior view.

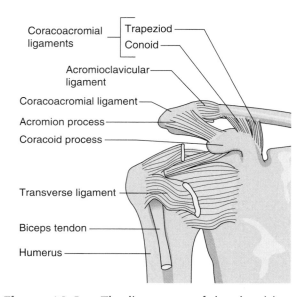

Figure 10.2   The ligaments of the shoulder.

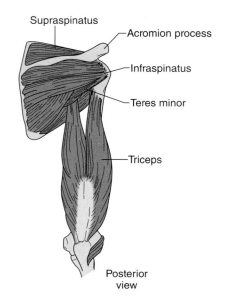

Figure 10.3   Rotator cuff muscles. The three posterior muscles are depicted. The subscapularis is found at the anterior aspect of the scapula and runs a course to the anterior aspect of the superior humerus.

Adapted, by permission, from W.C. Whiting and R.F. Zernicke, 1998, *Biomechanics of musculoskeletal injury* (Champaign, IL: Human Kinetics), 179.

The deltoid muscle lies over the head of the humerus. It attaches to the acromion process and the lateral aspect of the humerus. The deltoid abducts, flexes, and extends the shoulder.

The muscles in the anterior portion of the shoulder are the pectoralis major and minor. The pectoralis muscles attach at the sternum and the anterior portion of the humerus.

The biceps muscle flexes the elbow. It attaches to the humerus and coracoid process on one end and to the radius on the other. The biceps tendon runs through the bicipital groove and is kept in the groove by a ligament. The triceps muscles oppose the biceps. They extend the forearm and shoulder. The triceps muscles attach to the posterior of the humeral head and the scapula. (See figure 3.3*b*, page 34.)

Ligaments and Joints

The shoulder girdle is composed of several joints that are held together by ligaments, but the most commonly injured ones include the acromioclavicular joint and the glenohumeral joint. The acromioclavicular joint is made up of the acromion process of the scapula and the distal end of the clavicle. It is held together by the acromioclavicular ligament. The muscles that hold the scapula to the thorax allow movement in the scapulothoracic joint. This may be the most forgotten joint in the shoulder, but it is essential to its motion and strength.

The glenohumeral joint is the articulation, or point of contact, of the head of the humerus and the glenoid fossa, the saucerlike portion of the scapula. The glenoid fossa is shallow, making the joint susceptible to injury. The end of the humerus is covered with a hard articular cartilage that moves against the glenoid fossa. A capsular ligament, also known as the glenohumeral ligament, surrounds the entire glenohumeral joint from the scapula to the humerus, maintaining the scapula and humeral head in proper relationship and giving the joint stability. Muscles hold the scapula close to the thoracic ribs.

PREVENTING SHOULDER INJURIES

The AT and the athlete must know what kinds of shoulder injuries occur and how to prevent them. Shoulder injuries are often caused by muscle weaknesses, postural problems, and the nature of the sport.

Addressing Muscular Weakness

The saying "Out of sight, out of mind" applies to weight training in that people often lift weights only for those muscles they can see in the mirror (i.e., mirror muscles). As a result they experience weaknesses in the opposing muscles, most often the muscles on the posterior side.

Athletes who have rounded shoulders, tight pectoral muscles, or weak posterior shoulder muscles may predispose themselves to injury. The supraspinatus muscle, nerve, and blood vessel run through a narrow space between the acromion process and the head of the humerus, and a narrowing of that space can pinch those tissues. The moral of the story is that when your mother tells you to stand up straight and stick your chest out, she is not only improving your posture, she is also preventing you from getting a shoulder injury. Mom always knows best!

When an athlete uses her arm repeatedly in the same way, such as in freestyle swimming or overhand throwing, she is prone to injury. She needs to strengthen the muscles opposing the motion to prevent injury. A swimmer who swims 300 strokes of freestyle must swim 300 strokes of backstroke to balance the strength of the muscles on both sides of the body. Athletes involved in throwing sports need to learn proper techniques. If an athlete does not throw with the body, she will be more prone to shoulder injury.

During the physical examination, the physician must determine muscular weaknesses of an athlete so that they can be remedied with properly prescribed exercises. Some athletes have one shoulder that sits higher than the other shoulder. Relaxation techniques and stretching can level the shoulders and prevent spasms.

Many throwing athletes use a shoulder-strengthening program referred to as the *Thrower's Ten*. This exercise regimen consists of 10 movements that strengthen key muscles of the shoulder to prevent injuries.

Using Protective Padding

Games that have a tremendous amount of shoulder impact allow the use of shoulder pads—the heavier the impact, the thicker the padding. Ice hockey, football, and men's lacrosse are examples of sports where shoulder pads are used.

Modifying Activity

Many sports require a great deal of overhead activity with high levels of stress placed on the shoulder joint and surrounding soft tissues. Consider that a throwing athlete can accelerate his limb more

What Would You Do If...

While walking through the locker room to help the AT check on some injured athletes, you notice that an athlete's football shoulder pads are too narrow and do not cover the acromioclavicular joint.

than 6,000° a second when throwing, and you can understand how overuse injuries can occur. One study published in the *American Journal of Sports Medicine* (Lyman, Fleisig, Andrews, and Osinski 2002) found that throwing a curveball was associated with more than a 50% increase in risk of shoulder pain. High numbers of pitches thrown can increase upper-extremity pain as well. To lessen the extent of injury, it is advisable to modify the type of activity that an athlete engages in. For example, young athletes aged 9 to 14 should not throw curveballs. In addition, they should be limited to 75 pitches in a game and 600 pitches in a season.

TREATING SHOULDER INJURIES

The shoulder is often overworked through throwing, striking, and catching. This makes it vulnerable to a variety of musculoskeletal injuries.

Bone Injuries

As you might imagine, given the range of motion at the shoulder and amount of use it gets, a lot of stress is put on the bones. Epiphyses injuries must be considered, especially with younger athletes.

The shoulder is covered by heavy musculature and ligaments. The layers of tissue can make a fracture difficult to determine. Keen awareness of the mechanism of injury will tell the AT when to suspect a fracture.

Clavicular Fractures

The clavicle is most often fractured at its weakest point, the distal third. As you feel the clavicle, notice that it curves as it gets closer to the tip of the shoulder. An athlete can receive a direct blow or fall on the tip of the shoulder, causing a fracture. The athlete will experience pain and hold the arm close to the body to prevent movement. Because the clavicle moves, arm movement must be restricted with a sling. The use of ice to decrease swelling and pain is important. The team physician can set the clavicle in place using a harness. The fracture takes six weeks to heal, during which time many injured athletes wear a clavicle harness (see figure 10.4).

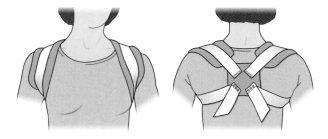

Figure 10.4   Clavicle harness.

Humeral Fractures

Fractures of the humerus are not difficult to find if they are located midshaft, but the shoulder musculature can sometimes hide a fracture of the humeral head. A shoulder sprain can mimic a fracture, so care must be taken to ensure proper assessment. The athlete will be unable to move the arm and will experience pain. He may report hearing or feeling a pop, and he will be holding the arm against the body. The easiest way to determine a humeral fracture is to palpate the circumference of the bone. If it is painful on all sides, it is likely a fracture. The AT should refer the athlete to the team physician for immediate care. AT will place the athlete in a splint from the shoulder to the fingertips. Checking the pulse before and after splinting is critical to determining the extent of the injury. If the pulse has decreased, the fracture has a serious complication. The nature of the fracture will determine the athlete's treatment. In some instances a sling can be used, and in others surgery and a long arm cast are necessary. The humerus will take at least six weeks to heal.

Epiphysis Injuries

The growth plate in a young athlete's shoulder is susceptible to direct and indirect blows. A blow to the head of the humerus can cause an epiphyseal fracture. Falling on the elbow and driving the humerus into the glenoid fossa can also cause an epiphyseal fracture. Epiphyseal fractures have the same signs and symptoms as humeral fractures: pain, inability to use the arm, desire to hold the arm still, and feeling a pop. Injuries to the epiphyses can cause permanent growth impairment. Application of ice, splinting, and a sling are the best courses of action the AT can take. The physician will determine the severity of the epiphyseal injury and the treatment. Some epiphyseal injuries require surgery to hold the humerus head to the shaft. These cases are obviously more serious. Teenage pitchers are prone to epiphyseal injury from excessive throwing. Because of this, pitchers should be limited in the number of games they are allowed to play as well as the number of pitches they throw. With this injury, the athlete has pain around the circumference of the humerus. Pain will be exaggerated with flexion, as during the throwing motion. Caution must be exercised when dealing with this injury or else the loss in range of motion could be permanent. The team physician must see the athlete, and immobilization is essential.

Avulsion Fractures

Avulsion fractures can occur in the shoulder. Avulsions may accompany a glenohumeral or acromioclavicular sprain. Recall that avulsion fractures are those in which a ligament or tendon pulls away a small portion of the bone as it is stressed during an injury. When the humerus is dislocating from the glenoid fossa, the capsular ligament is stressed and can sometimes pull on the scapula, resulting in an avulsion fracture. The athlete will experience pain associated with the dislocation and the avulsion fracture. It is difficult, if not impossible, for the AT to know if an avulsion fracture exists. She must assume an avulsion fracture until an X ray reveals otherwise. Splinting and ice are appropriate care for sprains.

Glenohumeral Dislocations and Subluxations

Glenohumeral dislocation means that the head of the humerus is out of its socket (see figure 10.5). Subluxation means that the head of the humerus came out of its socket and then went back in. The cause for both injuries is usually the same—excessive abduction and external rotation—but the results are completely different. Dislocations and subluxations require attention by the AT and team physician.

A dislocation will sometimes cause the head of the humerus to tear the capsular ligament anteriorly.

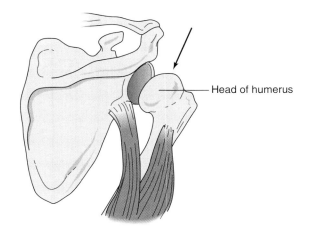

Figure 10.5   Shoulder dislocation occurs at the glenohumeral joint. The head of the humerus drops out of the socket, injuring the capsular ligament. The most common direction for a shoulder dislocation is anterior.

The instability of the capsular ligament allows the head of the humerus to shift forward, which is the most common type of shoulder dislocation. The athlete will experience pain and inability to use the shoulder. When the AT looks at the dislocated shoulder, he will see a deformity at the deltoid muscle; the shoulder will not be round but flat. The team physician must put a dislocation back into place. In the case of a subluxation the athlete may indicate that she felt the shoulder go out of its socket but then pop back in. An X ray is necessary to determine the extent of the dislocation or the subluxation—there may be associated fractures, a tear in the cartilage of the glenoid fossa, or nerve or blood vessel injury.

An athlete may not indicate to the AT that he has experienced a shoulder subluxation. Eventually, he will notice some changes as more subluxations occur. There can be permanent injury to the nerves, cartilage, and blood vessels. The athlete who has a dislocation or subluxation should strengthen the muscles of adduction and internal rotation. He may also wear a harness that restricts external rotation and abduction. An athlete who experiences recurrent subluxations or dislocations will require surgery to repair the capsular ligaments.

Muscle and Tendon Injuries

Most shoulder muscle and tendon injuries are caused by overuse. Athletes who throw, shoot, or repeat a swim stroke are prone to overuse injuries in the shoulder. Overuse injuries require rest, ice application, immobilization, and referrals to physicians for care. Common muscle and tendon injuries occur to the rotator cuff. Injury to the rotator cuff can also lead to impingement syndrome and bicipital tendon problems.

Rotator Cuff Strain

Similar to other strains, a strain of the rotator cuff is categorized as a first-, second-, or third-degree strain. As noted in chapter 4, first-degree strains are indicated by pain with no loss of stability or range of motion. Second-degree strains will have pain with some loss of stability and range of motion. Third-degree strains will have pain with partial or complete loss of stability and range of motion.

Strains of the rotator cuff occur from excessive motion beyond the normal range. Most often the supraspinatus muscle is injured. The athlete will have pain with motion and sometimes when the shoulder is not moving. The pain generally occurs with abduction of the shoulder. If the athlete is unable to abduct, a complete tear, or third-degree strain, is suspected. Strains caused by repetitive movements can also result in crepitus and impingement syndrome. A complete tear must be surgically repaired, whereas a first- or second-degree tear can be treated initially with PRICES and then with gentle strengthening and flexibility exercises.

Impingement Syndrome

An athlete develops **impingement syndrome** from repetitive overhead movements. Freestyle swimmers, throwers, and tennis players are prone to impingement syndrome. The supraspinatus and biceps muscles run together through a space beneath the acromion process. If the space narrows—from swelling, tendinitis, weak posterior muscles, or poor posture—the two muscles are impinged in the space. This creates pain and discomfort with overhead movements. Treatment of impingement syndrome includes modifying activity, strengthening the posterior muscles of the shoulder, and improving flexibility of tight pectoral muscles.

Bicipital Tendinitis

Bicipital tendinitis is common among athletes such as tennis players who are constantly raising their arms above their heads. The repetitive nature of the movement will cause irritation of the tendon in the bicipital groove. The AT may be able to palpate the tendon and feel crepitus. The athlete must stop the repetitive action causing the tendinitis. Pain is common, especially when repeating the motion that caused the tendinitis. Immobilization in a sling will make the athlete more comfortable. The team physician may prescribe ultrasound therapy and anti-inflammatory medication.

Biceps Tendon Rupture

The biceps tendon can rupture from either a direct blow or severe contractional forces. When the tendon ruptures, the athlete will be unable to flex the elbow. There will be a noticeable change in the appearance of the muscle as the tendon rolls up on itself—it will look like a golf ball under the skin (see figure 10.6). The arm must be iced and immobilized, and the athlete should be referred to a physician.

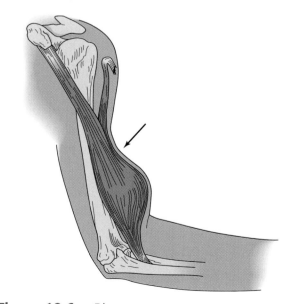

Figure 10.6　Biceps rupture.

The physician will surgically repair the tendon so that the muscle can return to full function.

Ligament and Joint Injuries

Several joints of the shoulder girdle are prone to sprains. The joints that are most commonly sprained include the acromioclavicular and glenohumeral joints.

Acromioclavicular Ligament Sprain

A sprain of the acromioclavicular ligament is referred to as a **shoulder separation** (see figure 10.7) so as not to confuse it with a glenohumeral ligament sprain. Although these joints are in close proximity, they involve different structures. The acromioclavicular joint can be injured by impact to the top of the shoulder or by falling on an outstretched arm. Falling on the elbow forces the humerus up and into the acromioclavicular joint. The athlete will indicate pain with movement whether it is a first-, second-, or third-degree sprain. The more serious sprains cause the clavicle to move superiorly. In a third-degree separation there will be a large abnormal bump caused by excessive upward displacement of the clavicle. The athlete is usually unable to move the arm and will hold it tightly against the body. To treat a first-degree sprain, the AT must use the PRICES method. A second- or third-degree sprain can be treated with PRICES initially, but the athlete

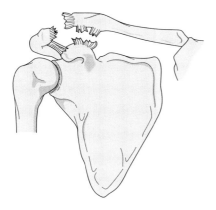

Figure 10.7 A shoulder separation occurs at the acromioclavicular joint. It is a sprain of the acromioclavicular ligament.

must be referred to an orthopedist to rule out a fracture.

A physician can take two courses of action to treat a third-degree tear: surgery or harness. During surgery the acromioclavicular joint is wired or screwed together. A harness straps the clavicle down in an attempt to hold the joint together long enough to allow the ligament to heal.

Glenohumeral Ligament Sprain

The glenohumeral joint is especially vulnerable to sprains when it is placed in abduction and external rotation. If there is a third-degree sprain, a more serious problem such as subluxation or dislocation is likely. The athlete with a glenohumeral ligament sprain will have pain with motion. The athlete is treated using PRICES and is referred to a physician.

A shoulder dislocation or repetitive subluxations are the most likely causes of a **glenoid labrum** tear. The labrum is the disk of cartilage in the glenohumeral joint. When the labrum tears it can obstruct the range of motion or allow excessive movement within the joint.

Initial care for a tear is to immobilize the shoulder. The physician will have to evaluate the shoulder to determine the extent of the injury. Conservative treatment would be to immobilize the shoulder with the hope that the labrum would reattach without surgical intervention. In many cases the labrum must be surgically reattached or removed.

Steroclavicular Joint Dislocation

A blow to the clavicle that causes a rupture of the sternoclavicular joint ligaments can cause a posterior dislocation. A posterior dislocation of the clavicle can press on the trachea, causing difficulty breathing. An athlete who is in the midst of this injury will become anxious, and the AT must act to resolve this situation quickly. The treatment is to place the athlete on a backboard with the side of the affected shoulder off the board. With the shoulder below the board, the proximal end of the clavicle moves anteriorly away from the trachea. The athlete will have to see a physician for additional treatment.

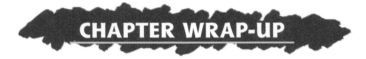

CHAPTER WRAP-UP

Summary

The shoulder girdle has many ligaments; consequently, it is vulnerable to sprains. The glenohumeral joint relies on the strength of the rotator cuff for stability, but a dislocation can occur, usually by forceful abduction and external rotation. The acromioclavicular joint can be sprained as well, resulting in a shoulder separation. A rotator cuff strain can be debilitating, and proper recovery is imperative before the athlete returns to competition. A strong rotator cuff and a well-conditioned shoulder will prevent many shoulder injuries.

Key Terms

Define the following terms found in this chapter:

glenoid labrum   shoulder separation
impingement syndrome   SITS
rotator cuff

Questions for Review

1. Describe the rotator cuff.
2. Why do you think athletes who perform many overhead motions, such as tennis players, pitchers, and swimmers, often have shoulder problems?
3. How can shoulder injuries be prevented?
4. Various sports require a lot from the shoulder. Make a list of sports and the types of shoulder injuries that occur with each.
5. What is meant by *impingement syndrome?*

Activities for Reinforcement

1. Have an AT demonstrate how to assess a shoulder injury.
2. Interview several athletes who have had shoulder dislocations. Determine what position the arms were in when the injury occurred.
3. With a partner, name and point to each of the bones in the shoulder girdle.
4. With a partner, locate each joint in the shoulder girdle.
5. Examine the following Web site and view the various exercises to strengthen the rotator cuff: http://familydoctor.org/265.xml.
6. Visit the Web site of the American Academy of Orthopaedic Surgeons and examine many exercises for the shoulder girdle: http://orthoinfo.aaos.org/topic.cfm?topic=A00067.

Above and Beyond

1. Write a brief one-page essay about the shoulder. Talk about redesigning the shoulder to make it less prone to the injuries listed in this chapter.
2. Examine the American Sports Medicine Institute's position statement regarding pitching by young athletes and write a summary: www.asmi.org/asmiweb/position_statement.htm.
3. Visit the following source to examine how to perform some shoulder-strengthening exercises: www.asmi.org/SportsMed/throwing/thrower10.html
4. Go online and find a source that explains how to rehabilitate a shoulder injury.
5. Examine one of the following sources and write a brief report:

   Bonza, J., S. Fields, E. Yard, and R. Comstock. 2009. Shoulder injuries among United States high school athletes during the 2005-2006 and 2006-2007 school years. *Journal of Athletic Training* 44(1): 76-83.

   Housner, J.A., and J.E. Kuhn. 2003. Clavicle fractures: individualizing treatment for fracture type. *Physician and Sportsmedicine* 31(12): 30-36.

   Kibler, W.B. 2003. Rehabilitation of rotator cuff tendinopathy. *Clinics in Sports Medicine* 22(4): 837-847.

   Kibler, W., and A. Sciascia. 2008. Rehabilitation of the athlete's shoulder. *Clinics in Sports Medicine* 27(4): 821-831.

   Olsen, S.J., G.S. Fleisig, S. Dun, J. Loftice, and J.R. Andrews. 2006. Risk factors for shoulder and elbow injuries in adolescent baseball pitchers. *American Journal of Sports Medicine* 34: 905-912.

   Park, M.C., T.A. Blaine, and W.N. Levine. 2002. Shoulder dislocation in young athletes: Current concepts in management. *Physician and Sportsmedicine* 30(12): 41-48, 55-56.

11

Elbow Injuries

Objectives

Upon completing this chapter, the student will be able to do the following:

- Describe the basic anatomy of the arm and elbow.
- Explain common arm and elbow injuries that occur with athletic participation.
- Identify signs and symptoms of arm and elbow injuries.
- Explain treatment parameters performed by ATs for elbow injuries.

The elbow functions with any upper-extremity movement. It is prone to muscle and tendon injuries because it is the site of many muscle attachments.

ANATOMY OF THE ELBOW

The elbow is a hinge joint involving three major bones: the humerus, radius, and ulna (see figure 11.1). The radius and ulna are the bones between the elbow and wrist. The distal end of the humerus becomes wider, similar to the distal end of the femur, and forms the medial and lateral epicondyles. The ulna is hooked to the end of the humerus and forms a tight joint. The radius is the bone on the thumb side of the forearm. It rests against the humerus and is able to rotate, allowing the forearm to pronate and supinate.

Muscles

As noted in chapter 10, the triceps muscle primarily performs elbow extension whereas the biceps accomplishes elbow flexion. The wrist flexors

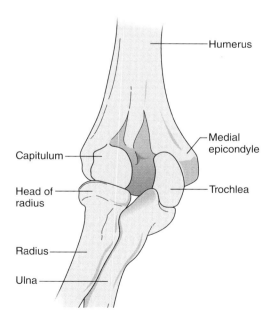

Figure 11.1 Anterior view of elbow. The elbow is a tight joint held together by many ligaments.

Adapted, by permission, from W.C. Whiting and R.F. Zernicke, 1998, *Biomechanics of musculoskeletal injury* (Champaign, IL: Human Kinetics), 190.

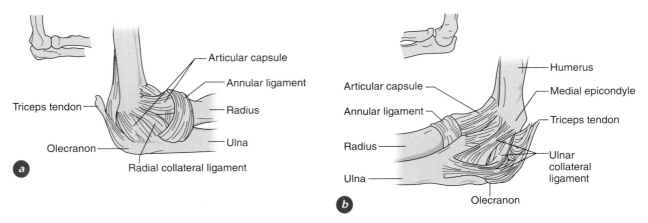

Figure 11.2 *(a)* Lateral and *(b)* medial views of elbow. The ulna hooks on to the end of the humerus, whereas the radius rests against it.

Adapted, by permission, from W.C. Whiting and R.F. Zernicke, 1998, *Biomechanics of musculoskeletal injury* (Champaign, IL: Human Kinetics), 190.

attach at the medial epicondyle of the humerus and then run toward the hand. The wrist extensors attach to the lateral epicondyle of the humerus (figure 11.2, *a-b*). These muscles help stabilize the elbow.

Several nerves and blood vessels pass through the small spaces and grooves around the elbow en route to the lower arm. Therefore, an injury occurring at the elbow must be assessed to determine if any of these blood vessels or nerves have been damaged. Checking for a pulse and ascertaining if an athlete is able to feel her hand is a helpful procedure.

Ligaments

The joint capsule is a ligament that surrounds the elbow. It provides some general stability to the elbow joint, but the elbow also relies on several major ligaments for stability, particularly the ulnar collateral, radial collateral, and annular ligaments.

The ulnar collateral ligament helps to stabilize the inside, or medial, aspect of the elbow, whereas the radial collateral ligament helps to stabilize the outside, or lateral, aspect. These ligaments are also known as the medial and lateral collateral ligaments (figure 11.3, *a-b*). The **bursa** is a fluid-filled sac located between the olecranon and the skin.

The annular ligament helps to hold the radius and ulna together near the elbow joint. The radius and ulna are also supported by the interosseus membrane. This tissue joins the radius and the ulna from the elbow to the wrist and keeps the two bones from separating.

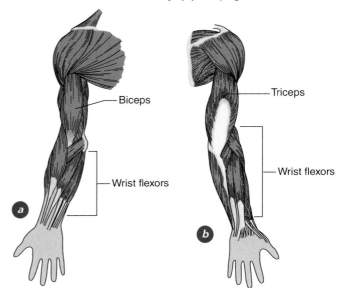

Figure 11.3 *(a)* Anterior and *(b)* posterior view of elbow and wrist musculature. Many muscles make up the wrist flexors and extensors that attach to the medial and lateral epicondyles of the humerus.

Adapted, by permission, from W.C. Whiting and R.F. Zernicke, 1998, *Biomechanics of musculoskeletal injury* (Champaign, IL: Human Kinetics), 190.

PREVENTING ELBOW INJURIES

The elbow is not injured frequently. Many of the injuries that ATs see at the elbow joint are caused by overuse—the repetitive movements and stresses delivered to the wrist and elbow over time eventually break down the tissue, causing chronic inflammation and pain. This is especially true in racket sports such as tennis and racquetball where injuries to the lateral aspect of the elbow are most common. Many athletes pay a great deal of attention to strengthening the biceps and triceps muscles, but they fail to properly condition some of the smaller muscles such as the wrist flexors and extensors. Stretching and strengthening these structures is recommended to prevent overuse injuries. We describe some stretches in chapter 17.

It is imperative for the AT to work with the coach to detect any improper techniques athletes are using, because these can eventually lead to overuse injuries. Equipment is also a factor in the prevention of elbow injuries, especially in racket sports. For example, excessive stress on the elbow musculature can result from using a racket with a grip that is too small. The AT and the coach can work together to identify these problems and prevent such injuries.

Many athletes who throw (such as baseball and softball players) should alter their activity and rest after long days of throwing. The rules limiting young pitchers' activity also help keep overuse problems of the elbow (and shoulder) to a minimum. ATs at industrial sites have reduced overuse injuries by instituting job-rotation programs whereby workers do a variety of jobs rather than the same job day after day.

TREATING ELBOW INJURIES AND CONDITIONS

The medial and lateral aspects of the elbow joint can suffer ligament sprains. Also, muscle and tendon injuries occur because the elbow and wrist are involved in repetitive stress during athletics. Fractures of the elbow can be extremely serious.

Bone Injuries

Bone fractures to the distal end of the humerus are not common in athletics. If they do occur, it is often due to powerful mechanisms of injury, such as the hand being planted on the ground and someone forcing the arm into excessive side bending. Fractures between the condyles of the humerus are also

rare in sport, but if direct impact is the mechanism of injury and pain is located at the medial aspect of the elbow about 2 inches (5 cm) above the joint, a fracture should be suspected. If either type of fracture occurs, it is an absolute emergency because it can result in compression of an artery or nerve.

Epiphyseal and Avulsion Fractures

Epiphyseal and avulsion fractures are more common on the medial epicondyle or olecranon of the elbow (the olecranon is the process of the ulna projecting behind the elbow joint). An epiphyseal injury should be suspected whenever an athlete presents with swelling, pain, and loss of movement. Remember that a growing athlete is more likely to injure the growth plate than suffer a bone fracture or ligament injury. Severe pain and deformity indicate an avulsion fracture. If either of these injuries is suspected by the AT, she should refer the athlete to a physician.

Ulnar Dislocations

The elbow is one of the most commonly dislocated joints in the body (see figure 11.4). As mentioned previously, the ulna hooks onto the end of the humerus, making the elbow a fairly tight joint. Therefore, it takes a very traumatic injury to dislocate the ulna from the humerus. Usually, a violent hyperextension injury or a severe blow to the lateral aspect of the elbow will dislodge the ulna from the humerus; most often it moves posteriorly. When a dislocation occurs, an obvious deformity will be

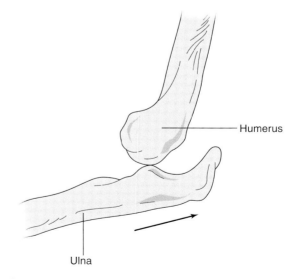

Figure 11.4 Elbow dislocations typically occur in a posterior direction.

noticed. The arm must be immediately splinted in the position it is found in, and the athlete must be seen in the emergency room by a physician so that the dislocation can be treated.

Muscle and Tendon Injuries

Strains of the elbow musculature are most often caused by either excessive resistive forces or overuse. Elbow strains can occur in the elbow flexor and extensor musculature as well as the wrist flexor and extensor musculature. As with strains discussed in previous chapters, they can be mild, moderate, or severe. A complete strain or rupture of a muscular structure, such as the biceps, is usually evident by the deformity caused when the muscle balls up due to the elasticity of the muscle.

Elbow Flexor Strains

Strains to the flexor muscles often are caused by a loaded movement that includes both the elbow and shoulder. The body's two-joint muscles—the muscles involved with creating movement at more than one joint—seem to be prone to strains. The biceps muscle is a perfect example of a two-joint muscle; it flexes the elbow joint and the shoulder joint. Minor elbow flexor strains are characterized by discomfort at the anterior aspect of the elbow and minimal swelling. The athlete will also demonstrate some weakness and extra discomfort when elbow flexion is resisted. A moderate elbow flexor strain will have mild to moderate amounts of swelling and marked weakness when tested for strength. The initial treatment an AT may give for an elbow flexor strain is PRICES. When the initial inflammation has subsided, the athlete can then perform mild stretching and strengthening exercises as indicated. A moderate strain can be treated in the same way, but the AT must keep in mind that with more tissue damage, progress will often be slower. Complete muscle or tendon ruptures or suspected avulsion injuries should be referred to the team physician.

Elbow Extensor Strains

Excessive resistance to the triceps muscle often causes tissue damage to the elbow extensors. This can happen if the athlete attempts to break a fall with an outstretched arm. The injury needs to be assessed carefully because the triceps tendon can often pull a bit of bone away from the ulna at the point where the tendon attaches. The characteristics of an extensor strain are the same as for a flexor injury, except of course the pain will be at the posterior aspect of the upper arm, and the athlete will often experience more pain when the AT resists elbow extension. Treatment with PRICES is recommended, and after inflammation has subsided, the elbow extensor should be stretched mildly and strengthened as tolerated.

Wrist Flexor Strains

Wrist flexor strains at the elbow often result in pain over the medial epicondyle of the humerus or the front of the forearm. These strains can result from excessive resistance during wrist flexion movements or, more commonly, from overuse. Initially this condition should be treated with PRICES and activity should be modified. Mild stretching can be performed by the athlete, and wrist curls and grip strengthening are helpful.

Wrist Extensor Strains

Wrist extensor strains at the elbow frequently result in pain over the lateral epicondyle of the humerus. These strains can result from excessive resistance during wrist extension movements but more commonly are caused by overuse. Initially this condition should be treated with PRICES, and activity should be modified. The athlete can also perform mild stretching, and doing reverse wrist curls can be helpful as well.

Medial and Lateral Epicondylitis

As noted previously, the elbow is prone to overuse conditions that create chronic inflammation, which frequently occurs at the medial and lateral epicondyles of the humerus. These conditions are called *medial epicondylitis* and *lateral epicondylitis*, the latter being the more frequent type of chronic inflammatory injury.

As a result of poor mechanics and continual use over a long period of time, the wrist extensor

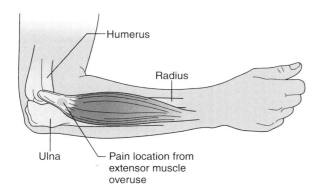

Humerus

Radius

Ulna

Pain location from extensor muscle overuse

Figure 11.5 Pain from lateral epicondylitis.

tendons at the lateral epicondyle of the humerus can become chronically inflamed (figure 11.5). Because racket sports are a common cause, this condition is also called **tennis elbow**. In the industrial setting, daily use of equipment such as a hammer and any gripping and lifting activities can cause lateral elbow inflammation.

Lateral epicondylitis is characterized by pain over the lateral epicondyle of the humerus. Minimal swelling is sometimes present.

Initially, the AT should treat the injury by attempting to reduce pain and inflammation. Therefore, the use of PRICES and a support, usually in the form of a tennis elbow strap that is wrapped around the elbow, is indicated. Limiting the amount of activity that aggravates the condition is also wise. Mild stretching of the extensor tendons is helpful, and muscle strength and endurance should be improved as tolerated. The athlete should gradually be allowed to participate in further activity. The AT may reduce the number of repetitions performed by the athlete and may also suggest the use of a two-handed backhand in racket sports. The team physician may choose to use medication to help resolve the condition.

Although not as common as lateral epicondylitis, many athletes get medial epicondylitis, often as a result of repetitive throwing. This condition involves inflammation of the wrist flexor tendons where they attach to the humerus. Some people refer to medial epicondylitis as **Little League elbow**. Little League elbow is also suggested to be a separation of the epiphysis at the medial aspect of the humerus in younger athletes (usually between the ages of 9 and 12) as a result of throwing (see figure 11.6).

Treatment for medial epicondylitis is similar to that of lateral epicondylitis—rest, ice application, and support. The athlete needs to decrease the amount of throwing and strengthen the wrist flexor muscles. The AT will monitor either condition. She will also perform a thorough evaluation because compression of the ulnar nerve is possible at the elbow joint, especially when a medial elbow injury has occurred. The AT will refer the athlete to a physician if a fracture is suspected or if the athlete is complaining of numbness, tingling, or excessive pain.

The Real World

While pitching during a college baseball game, our school's pitcher heard a pop. In obvious pain, he grabbed his elbow, fell off the pitcher's mound into the grass, and rolled around screaming that he had broken his elbow. With all that screaming, it was obvious the athlete was breathing and had a pulse. After calming him down, I determined that there were no obvious fractures around the elbow and that it would be okay for him to walk into the dugout for further examination. The athlete was very apprehensive about moving the elbow during examination because it was painful, and he continued to insist that his elbow was broken. He had extreme tenderness throughout the medial side of the elbow, especially just distal to the medial epicondyle. I took his distal pulse, checked capillary refill, and performed sensory tests. Grip strength was good, and the arm was neurovascularly normal. On valgus stress to the elbow, the athlete had a great deal of instability, which indicated an injury to the ulnar collateral ligament. We decided to ice the athlete's elbow, place it in a sling, and refer him to his family orthopedist. It turned out that he had an ulnar collateral ligament rupture that required reconstructive surgery and extensive rehabilitation. Although he never pitched again, he was able to play competitive baseball as a first baseman.

Greg Ehlers, EdD, ATC

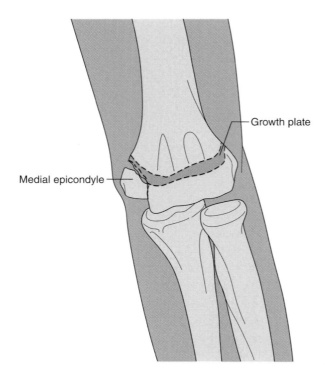

Figure 11.6   Little league elbow.

Ligament Injuries

Sprains of the elbow, as with all sprains, are classified as first, second, and third degree. Any of the elbow ligaments can be sprained, including the ulnar collateral ligament and the radial collateral ligament.

Ulnar Collateral Ligament Sprains

The ulnar collateral ligaments seem to be more prone to sprains than the other ligaments of the elbow, especially for athletes who throw. This is due in part to the amount of stress placed on the inner aspect of the elbow. Every time an athlete throws a baseball or hits a tennis ball (forehand), the medial aspect of the elbow is stretched. Over time, this repetitive trauma may result in a ligament injury. This mechanism can also cause injury to the muscles that cross the elbow joint. In addition, a direct blow may cause a disruption of the ulnar collateral ligament. Picture a wrestler supporting his weight on one arm as his opponent rolls into the lateral aspect of his elbow. This would cause valgus stress (forcing the medial aspect of the joint to separate) and would put excessive stress on the ulnar collateral ligament.

A sprain of the ulnar collateral ligament is characterized by medial elbow pain and swelling, especially if the ligament has been partially torn. When the AT tests the elbow, joint laxity may also be present. Sprains need to be treated using PRICES; an elastic bandage works well for elbow swelling and support. A moderate or severe injury may need to be splinted, and the AT will often refer the athlete to a physician for further diagnostic tests to rule out fractures. The elbow should be observed for any ulnar nerve damage when the medial collateral ligament is injured. To test this nerve, the AT can simply tap on it just behind the medial epicondyle. If the nerve is irritated, it will result in a flash of pain down to the hand. Tapping on the nerve is called *Tinel's test*.

When rehabilitating injuries to the ulnar collateral ligaments, it is essential to strengthen the wrist flexor muscles because they cross the medial aspect of the elbow and provide stability to the joint. Exercises such as wrist curls and grip strengthening are helpful. In severe cases when the ligament is ruptured, reconstructive surgery may be necessary. Reconstruction of the ulnar collateral ligament is performed by an orthopedic surgeon. The surgery involves using a length of tendon, often harvested from the palmaris longis muscle, and routing it through the distal humerus and proximal ulna. Athletes who undergo this surgical procedure can expect a long recovery before returning to sports such as baseball and tennis.

Radial Collateral Ligament Sprains

Radial collateral ligament injuries to the elbow are rare. The characteristics of a radial collateral injury are the same as for an ulnar collateral injury except that the pain is on the lateral aspect. Rehabilitation considerations for this ligament sprain include focusing on the wrist extension musculature. These muscles cross the joint line at the lateral elbow and can provide dynamic stability to an elbow that has suffered a sprain of the lateral collateral ligament.

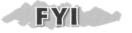

Valgus Stress

Valgus stress at the elbow means the medial part of the joint will separate or spread apart as the forearm moves laterally.

Combined Hyperextension Injuries

An athlete will often fall on an outstretched arm or receive a blow that causes the elbow to be hyperextended. This particular mechanism can result in a ligament sprain or muscle strain, although bony compression of the olecranon process as it impacts the humerus may occur.

In many instances a hyperextension injury causes each of these problems (sprain, strain, bony compression). This type of injury initially needs to be treated with PRICES. More severe conditions are referred to a physician. As the condition improves, range of motion should be reestablished and strength of the elbow flexor muscles should be improved. The athlete may need to wear an elbow hyperextension tape application upon initial return to play.

The elbow is a bony joint with little natural padding. Contusions, therefore, are fairly common, and they can typically be treated with PRICES. A variety of protective pads offer further protection to the elbow.

If the olecranon process is contused, the olecranon bursa may become irritated. This causes fluid to build up at the tip of the elbow. Although this is seldom a disabling condition, the fluid buildup can become the size of a golf ball (see figure 11.7). Compression wraps must be applied by the AT, and if the condition persists, the team physician may want to drain the fluid from the area. In any event, the elbow needs to be adequately protected with padding to avoid further contusions.

Nerve Injuries

Various nerve injuries can occur at the elbow joint. A common injury to the ulnar nerve is a contusion.

What Would You Do If...

As a student assistant, you are walking by tennis practice and you notice one of the players rubbing the lateral aspect of her elbow. She is in obvious pain.

Because the nerve is superficial and runs just behind the medial epicondyle, it is easily bumped or hit. Compression results in a shooting pain and tingling that is often said to be caused by hitting the funny bone. With severe ulnar nerve contusions, the pain and discomfort can last longer. The area will need to be protected with a pad.

The radial nerve can also be injured, usually by becoming entrapped by a bone if a fracture occurs or by a muscle after an injury such as a strain. An injury to the radial nerve can palsy, meaning the nerve does not transmit electrical signals to muscles that are necessary for them to contract. See figure 11.8 for the neural anatomy of the elbow.

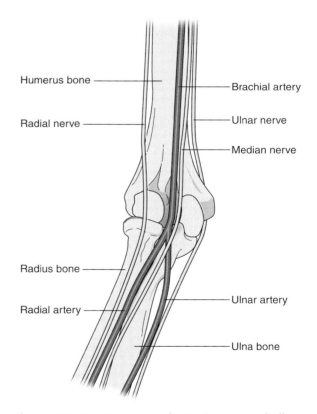

Figure 11.8 Nerves and arteries around elbow joint.

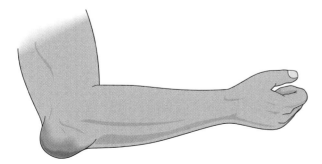

Figure 11.7 Olecranon bursitis.

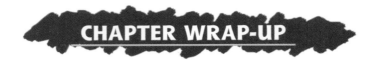

CHAPTER WRAP-UP

Summary

The elbow is a hinge joint composed of the humerus of the upper arm and the radius and ulna of the lower arm. The biceps and triceps muscles flex and extend the elbow, respectively. The wrist flexor and extensor muscles extend across the elbow and attach to the humerus. The elbow is also stabilized by the radial collateral ligament at the lateral aspect of the joint and the ulnar collateral ligament at the medial aspect of the joint. These ligaments are sometimes sprained in much the same way that the medial and lateral collateral ligaments of the knee are sprained. The elbow is also subject to overuse injuries, such as tennis elbow.

Key Terms

Define the following terms found in this chapter:

bursa
Little League elbow
tennis elbow

Questions for Review

1. Describe the bony structures of the elbow and the motions that are produced by the muscles around the elbow.
2. Describe tennis elbow. How should an AT treat this condition?
3. Explain what types of injuries may occur if the elbow is hyperextended.
4. What mechanism would cause stretching or tearing of the ulnar collateral ligament?

Activities for Reinforcement

1. Have an AT demonstrate an elbow evaluation.
2. Visit the Web site of the American Sports Medicine Institute (ASMI) and learn more about medial, lateral, and posterior shoulder injuries: www.asmi.org/SportsMed/injury/injury_elbow.html.
3. Visit the following Web site from the Stone Clinic and examine information related to medial and lateral epicondylitis basic protocol for elbow rehabilitation: www.stoneclinic.com/tenniselbow.

Above and Beyond

1. Read the following article related to reconstruction of the medial collateral ligament and write a summary: Erne, H., I. Zouzias, and M. Rosenwasser. 2009. Medial collateral ligament reconstruction in the baseball pitcher's elbow. *Hand Clinics* 25(3): 339-346
2. Read the following article related to activity modification to prevent elbow injuries and write a summary: Brockenbrough, G. 2009. Prescribe less play to prevent elbow injuries in pediatric/adolescent athletes. *Orthopedics Today* 29(6): 28.
3. Examine the following article related to designing a strength and conditioning program for pitchers in order to prevent elbow injuries, and then write a summary: Borelli, A. 2009. Engineering a strong pitching elbow: an off-season training plan. *Journal of Strength and Conditioning* 31(2): 64-73

chapter 12

Wrist and Hand Injuries

Objectives

Upon completing this chapter, the student will be able to do the following:

- Understand the basic anatomy of the wrist and hand.
- Explain the various types of wrist and hand injuries.
- Understand common mechanisms that cause the injuries.
- Understand the signs and symptoms of wrist and hand fractures.

Injuries to the wrist account for up to 9% of all sport-related injuries. Catching a ball, holding a club, and grasping an opponent are essential tasks. An injury to a wrist and hand can be exceedingly limiting and demoralizing for an athlete. Recognizing the type and extent of injury will help determine appropriate care and speed return to competition.

ANATOMY OF THE WRIST AND HAND

The wrist and hand contain many bones, muscles, ligaments, nerves, and blood vessels. All are necessary for the total functioning of the hand—one of the most active body parts—and if any anatomical part is injured, it will decrease an athlete's functional ability.

Bones and Joints

The wrist is the joint between the arm and the hand. It is made up of seven irregularly shaped carpal bones that articulate between the radius and ulna of the arm and the metacarpals of the hand to allow wrist movement (see figure 12.1). The scaphoid bone is of particular importance. It has a blood supply on only one end and therefore has difficulty healing when fractured. When the fingers are spread, the scaphoid sits in a depression at the wrist that is referred to as the *anatomical snuffbox*.

At the distal end, each of the five metacarpals joins with the proximal phalanx of one of the fingers. The metacarpals are numbered 1 through 5 beginning at the thumb side of the hand. The fingers have a total of 14 phalanges.

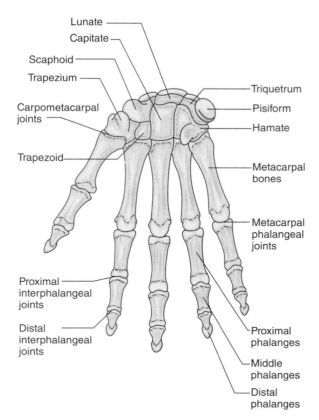

Figure 12.1 Bones and joints of the hand.

Reprinted, by permission, from W.C. Whiting and R.F. Zernicke, 1998, *Biomechanics of musculoskeletal injury* (Champaign, IL: Human Kinetics), 200.

Joints in the hand are named for the bones that compose them and whether they are distal or proximal. For example, the thumb has two joints: the metacarpophalangeal joint and the interphalangeal joint. Each of the second through fifth fingers has a metacarpophalangeal (MCP) joint, a proximal interphalangeal (PIP) joint, and a distal interphalangeal (DIP) joint.

Muscles

Wrist and hand movements are controlled by many muscles, which are categorized into extensor and flexor groups. The flexor muscle groups are found

▶ Understanding Diversity

The palmaris longus muscle is absent in 12% to 20% of Caucasians (Schrefer 1994). The lack of palmaris longus means that an athlete may be unable to forcefully flex the wrist.

on the anterior surface of the forearm, and the extensor muscles are located on the posterior aspect of the forearm.

Ligaments

The ligaments of the wrist and hand are intricate because of the many bones that must be connected. The wrist is stabilized by collateral ligaments medially and laterally. The ulnar collateral ligament attaches the distal end of the ulna to the triquetral and pisiform bones. The radial collateral ligament attaches the distal end of the radius to the trapezium and scaphoid bones.

Of particular importance to ATs is the flexor retinaculum, also known as the transverse carpal ligament. This structure is located on the anterior aspect of the carpal bones and lies over the wrist flexor tendons and median nerve. The retinaculum not only stabilizes the carpal bones but also provides a protective covering over the flexor tendons and median nerve that pass beneath it.

The thumb has several important ligaments. In particular, the ulnar collateral ligament of the thumb (also known as the medial collateral ligament) is located on the medial aspect, and the radial collateral ligament (also known as the lateral collateral ligament) is located on the lateral aspect (figure 12.2). These ligaments provide medial and lateral stability to the joint.

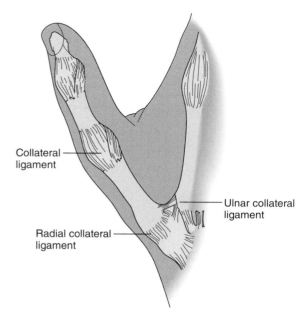

Figure 12.2 Thumb ligaments.

PREVENTING WRIST AND HAND INJURIES

Commonly used protective equipment for the wrist and hand includes braces, tape, gloves, and padding. Wearing gloves or tape can protect the area from wounds of all types, and padding can prevent contusions of the dorsal hand. Many football players wear thumb braces to protect against sprains. ATs can use plastic splints and braces to prevent injury for athletes who may be susceptible. In some sports, however, rules prohibit the use of protective equipment made of hard materials or allow the equipment only with a physician's note.

TREATING WRIST AND HAND INJURIES AND CONDITIONS

With a hand, one can manipulate objects and perform feats of astounding complexity. The slightest injury can change a movement or make it difficult for the athlete to participate in sport.

Bone Injuries

Any bone within the wrist and hand can fracture. Hands are used in all sports and are often put in harm's way. Direct impacts are the most frequent cause of the fractures. Swelling, pain, deformity, and disability are common with fractures. Two complications are associated with fractures: nonunion and death of the bone, which is also called **avascular necrosis** (death due to lack of blood flow). In the wrist, the scaphoid bone is the bone most often associated with nonunion and avascular necrosis. All fractures should be cared for with splinting and should be evaluated by a physician.

Another common fracture occurs to the metacarpal region, specifically to the fourth or fifth metacarpal. A fracture to this area is called a **boxer's fracture** because it often occurs due to punching or hitting a hard object.

A **Colles' fracture** occurs to the distal forearm. When both the radius and ulna are fractured when an athlete reaches a hand out to catch a fall, the arm often bends into extension at the fracture site.

Muscle and Tendon Injuries

Any of the numerous muscles of the wrist and hand can be strained by repetitive stress and stretching. Pain, swelling, weakness, and inability to move are common signs and symptoms. The AT will use range-of-motion testing to determine which muscle has been affected. Analysis of the athlete's movements can help determine the cause when repetitive stress is suspected. The AT should use the PRICES method and assign exercises to strengthen a weak muscle to prepare the athlete to return to competition. Taping the muscle for additional support can also be helpful.

Tendinitis

Tendinitis is defined as inflammation of the tendon. The cause of the inflammation can be overuse, stretching, or an impact. Because it is difficult to overcome, the AT's goal is to prevent tendinitis by increasing strength and flexibility, using padding, and avoiding repetitive injuries.

The thumb is vulnerable to **de Quervain's tendinitis**, which affects the abductor pollicis longus and extensor pollicis brevis. Shot-putters who hold the shot while the wrist is in radial deviation are prone to de Quervain's tendinitis. The athlete will have difficulty with abduction of the thumb, and he may experience swelling and crepitus. He needs to discontinue the repetitive movements. The PRICES method of care is appropriate in this case.

Mallet Finger

Mallet finger (see figure 12.3) is the result of the fingertip receiving an impact. The impact causes the extensor tendon to tear from the bone. The distinguishing feature of this injury is that the fingertip is in flexion. The athlete cannot lift the tip of the finger to straighten the bone because the tendon is

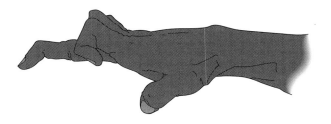

Figure 12.3   An avulsion fracture of the distal phalanx of the fingers results in a mallet finger. A mallet finger cannot be extended at the DIP joint.

no longer attached. She will experience pain and some swelling. The finger will be splinted into extension and the athlete referred to a physician for care. The physician has two courses of action: Treat the injury surgically or keep the finger splinted. The tendon can heal back to the bone if it is kept still and extended. If the tendon is retracted too far from its attachment, surgery is required to reattach the tendon. In many instances an athlete will not consider this injury to be important and may fail to report it. This negligence will result in a permanent flexion of the DIP joint.

Jersey Finger

Jersey finger is similar to mallet finger except that the flexor tendon tears from the fingertip. The athlete will not be able to flex the DIP joint of the finger. Injury occurs when the DIP joint is forcibly flexed, such as when the athlete is holding an opponent's jersey in his fist and his finger is forced to extend, tearing the tendon. He will experience pain and swelling. Splinting and ice are good initial treatments by the AT. The finger will require an X ray to determine the extent of the injury, and a physician will decide if the athlete needs surgery.

Boutonniere Deformity

A **boutonniere deformity** occurs at the PIP joint (see figure 12.4). A hard impact over the PIP joint can cause a tear in the joint capsule, which allows the extensor tendons to fall laterally. When the tendons are in the lateral position, they contract and force flexion of the DIP joint. The athlete will not be able to extend the PIP joint, and she will experience

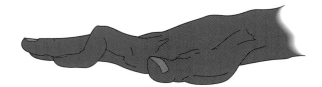

Figure 12.4   Boutonniere deformity. If the sheath that holds the extensor tendon on top of the finger is torn, causing the tendons to slide to the sides of the finger, the PIP joint flexes and the DIP joint hyperextends.

pain and swelling. The AT should splint the finger and refer the athlete to a physician for treatment. In many instances the finger can be splinted, allowing the healing of the connective tissue that keeps the extensor tendons in place. Otherwise surgical intervention is necessary.

Ligament Injuries

Many sprains are not serious and can be treated with PRICES. One common misconception about sprains is that they must be pulled back into place. This is not true! Sprains are injured ligaments, and pulling on an injured ligament can only cause more injury.

Wrist Sprain

Wrist sprains commonly occur from overuse, falls, and forceful twisting motion. Which ligament is injured depends on the stress. An excessive amount of ulnar deviation at the wrist, for example, will injure the ligament on the radial side due to too much tension or overstretching, and excessive radial deviation at the wrist will injure the ligament on the medial side. The athlete will experience pain, possibly decreased range of motion, decreased grip strength, and some swelling. The AT should recommend PRICES. When the athlete returns to activity, taping for support may prevent further injury. Rehabilitation for wrist sprains focuses on reestablishing normal range of motion and strength.

Triangular Fibrocartilage Complex Injury

The **triangular fibrocartilage complex (TFCC)** injury has been identified as a problem among athletes who sprain their wrist. The TFCC is a piece of cartilage located between the ulna and the carpal bones, and it plays a role in cushion-

What Would You Do If...

A male gymnast was putting on his gymnastics pants. His hand slipped, and he noticed he could no longer lift the end of his finger. You explain this could be a mallet finger and should be seen by the AT and team physician. The athlete refuses. You tell him that it could result in a permanent injury. The athlete responds by saying, "That's why we have insurance."

ing these structures. The TFCC is injured with forceful rotation or hyperextension of the wrist. Treatment of this injury often involves immobilization followed by a rehabilitation plan to restore wrist range of motion and strength. In some instances the TFCC must be surgically repaired.

Dislocation of the Lunate

When an athlete falls on her hand, it can be in flexion or extension at the time of impact. Either motion can result in a dislocation of a carpal bone, most commonly the lunate. This dislocation will cause deformity, pain, swelling, and decreased range of motion. The dislocation of any carpal bone should be splinted and referred to a physician, who must relocate the bone.

Ganglion Cyst

Sometimes a pocket of fluid develops within the sheath in the wrist. This is known as a **ganglion cyst** (see figure 12.5). Treatment often includes ice application and activity modification. The injury should be evaluated by a physician if symptoms persist.

Gamekeeper's Thumb

An injury to the medial collateral ligament of the thumb is known as **gamekeeper's thumb** (see figure 12.6) and sometimes as skier's thumb. The term *gamekeeper's thumb* is an old one that was first used to describe farmers who injured the ligament when breaking the necks of birds intended for the cooking pot. This injury is also known as skier's thumb because the ski pole sometimes gets stuck and forces the thumb into abduction. In general, the ligament on the medial aspect of the thumb is injured when the thumb is forcefully abducted, such as when catching a basketball. The athlete

The Real World

A male gymnast asked me to take a look at his hand. He said he had somehow cut his palm during a workout a couple of days earlier. He had cared for the injury himself but was unhappy that he was still having some problems. When I removed the bandages it became apparent why he was having a problem—he had used his mother's needle and black thread to stitch his own hand. Luckily, it did not appear to be infected. I sent the student to his family physician, who removed the stitches and placed him on antibiotics.

Lorin Cartwright, MS, ATC

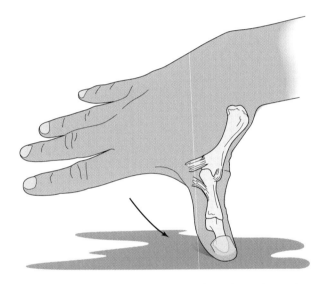

Figure 12.6   Gamekeeper's thumb and mechanism. When the thumb is pulled away from the finger, the ulnar collateral ligament can rupture.

Adapted, by permission, from W.C. Whiting and R.F. Zernicke, 1998, *Biomechanics of musculoskeletal injury* (Champaign, IL: Human Kinetics), 203.

will complain of pain over the joint, and the area may be swollen.

Treatment of the injury involves splinting the medial aspect of the thumb and icing. An X ray will be necessary to determine if an avulsion fracture is associated with the ligament tear.

Interphalangeal Collateral Ligament Sprain

A collateral ligament is located on the side of each interphalangeal joint. The ligaments provide stability when the phalanges are stressed,

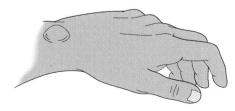

Figure 12.5   Ganglion cyst.

What Would You Do If...

A softball player slid headfirst into second base, and afterward her index finger did not look right. She tells you that she had another player pull her finger, and she felt it pop.

but they can be sprained when a joint is stressed beyond normal—for example, if the finger is hit by a ball, if the athlete lands with fingers curled or extended, or if he accidentally catches a finger on an opponent's jersey. Injury to the collateral ligament is painful and disabling. The joint can swell and become discolored. The AT will confer with the team physician to determine if an X ray is necessary to rule out a fracture. Ice application will keep the swelling to a minimum; if the finger swells too much, the athlete will be unable to bend it. When he returns to competition, it is common to tape the injured finger to an uninjured neighbor (i.e., buddy taping). Padding may be helpful in preventing additional injuries.

Dislocation of the Interphalangeal or Metacarpophalangeal Joint

When a dislocation of the interphalangeal or MCP joint occurs, one bone usually moves dorsal and one moves volar. The team physician should relocate all dislocated fingers and thumbs because tiny tendons, nerves, and blood vessels make their way through joint spaces. If the relocation is done incorrectly, there can be permanent damage to that finger. In the case of a dislocation the ligament may tear, with

possible fractures also occurring. We know of a softball player who dived for a ball and dislocated her finger. Her teammate pulled on the finger in an attempt to help, driving the splintered bone pieces into the tendon and severing it. Four pins and one surgery later the softball player has a straight finger that she will not let anyone touch.

Nerve Injury

As with the elbow, nerve injuries can occur in the wrist and hand. **Carpal tunnel syndrome** is a common injury to the median nerve that runs anterior to the carpal bones. In this area, the carpal bones form a tunnel along with the overlying ligamentous tissue. The median nerve travels through the tunnel into the hand. If this tunnel narrows due to overuse from gripping, typing, or any other repetitive movements, the nerve will be compressed. Compression of the median nerve causes pain, tingling, numbness, and weakness in the thumb, index finger, and third digit of the hand.

Treatment involves using a wrist splint, stretching the flexor muscles of the wrist, and medication. If this fails to work, a physician may inject the area with a steroid, or surgical procedures may be performed to open the space.

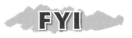

Volar
    The palm side of the hand.

Dorsal
    The back or posterior portion of the body in the anatomical position.

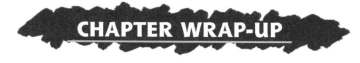

Summary

The wrist and hand are involved in every athletic activity and thus are susceptible to numerous injuries, which can range from minor to permanently disabling. An athlete who is trying to be helpful can increase the severity of an injury, such as by pulling on an injured finger. Because of the intricate structure of the wrist and hand, the signs and symptoms of many injuries are identical. To ensure the best possible outcome, the AT, coach, or team physician should be the first one to provide care. The physician should evaluate most sprains to rule out fractures.

Key Terms

Define the following terms found in this chapter:

avascular necrosis

boutonniere deformity

boxer's fracture

carpal tunnel syndrome

Colles' fracture

de Quervain's tendinitis

gamekeeper's thumb

ganglion cyst

jersey finger

mallet finger

triangular fibrocartilage complex (TFCC)

Questions for Review

1. What bone is located beneath the anatomical snuffbox?

2. Describe the mechanism of injury for mallet finger. How should it be splinted?

3. Describe the mechanism of injury for gamekeeper's thumb. Why is it also known as skier's thumb?

4. How should jersey finger be splinted?

5. What are common methods of caring for wrist, hand, and finger injuries?

Activities for Reinforcement

1. Find an anatomy text and review the location of the various carpal bones.

2. Have an AT demonstrate how to perform a wrist and hand evaluation.

3. Visit the following Web sites to explore pictures and detailed anatomy of the hand and wrist:

    www.eorthopod.com/public/patient_education/6606/hand_anatomy.html

    www.eatonhand.com/hom/hom33.htm

Above and Beyond

1. Write a report on the proper management of a specific hand injury.

2. Examine the following article and write a report related to carpal fractures in athletes:

    Marchessault, J., Conti, and M. Baratz. 2009. Carpal fractures in athletes excluding the scaphoid. *Hand Clinics* 25(3): 371-388.

3. Read the following article and summarize the key points related to the rare but problematic issue of neural and vascular injuries that occur among athletes:

    Ruchelsman, D.E., and S.K. Lee. 2009. Neurovascular injuries of the hand in athletes. *Current Orthopaedic Practice* 20(4): 409-415.

4. Read the following article related to forearm and wrist injury rates of football players and summarize the findings:

    Carlisle, J.C, C.A. Goldfarb, N. Mall, J.W. Powell, and M.J. Matava. 2008. Upper extremity injuries in the National Football League, part II: elbow, forearm, and wrist injuries. *American Journal of Sports Medicine* 36(10): 1945-1952.

5. Read the following articles related to forearm and wrist injury and summarize the findings:

Altizer, L. 2003a. Hand and wrist fractures, part I. *Orthopaedic Nursing* 22(2): 131-138.

Altizer, L. 2003b. Hand and wrist fractures, part II. *Orthopaedic Nursing* 22(3): 232-239.

Goitz, R.J., and M.M. Tomaino. 2002. Traumatic hand injuries evaluation and management: Understanding of the complex anatomy is the key to diagnosis. *Journal of Musculoskeletal Medicine* 19(5): 204-206, 208-210.

Rettig, A.C. 2003. Athletic injuries of the wrist and hand, part I: Traumatic injuries of the wrist. *American Journal of Sports Medicine* 31(6): 1038-1048.

6. Visit some sports medicine equipment Web sites and compare and contrast the types of wrist splints available to treat and prevent injuries.

7. Visit www.ubsportsmed.buffalo.edu/education/triangle.html to learn more about injuries to the TFCC.

8. Visit http://sportsmedicine.about.com/cs/wrist_hand/ and then give a presentation about common hand injuries and how to take care of them.

UNIT V

Understanding Athletics-Related Injuries to the Lower Extremity

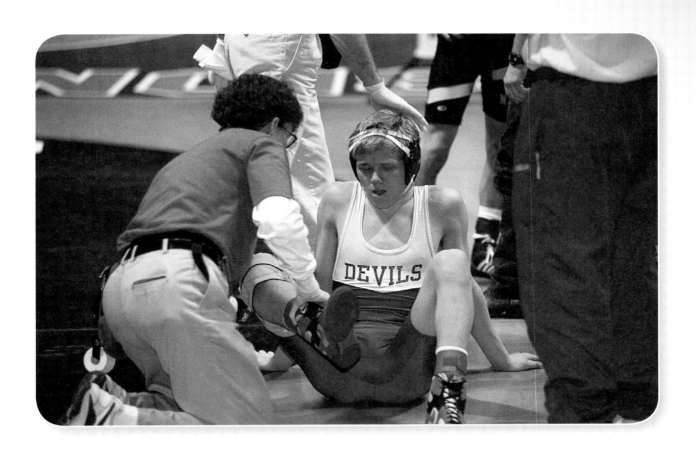

13

Hip, Pelvis, and Thigh Injuries

Objectives

Upon completing this chapter, the student will be able to do the following:

- Describe the basic anatomy of the hip.
- Explain common hip, pelvis, and thigh injuries that occur with athletic participation.
- Identify common signs and symptoms of hip, pelvis, and thigh injuries.
- Explain the treatments performed by an AT for specific hip, pelvis, and thigh injuries.

The hip, pelvis, and thigh contain some of the strongest muscles in the body, but they are also subjected to tremendous demands. Thus, they are vulnerable to injuries that can sideline a player for a long time. Both their importance in sport and their vulnerability make it particularly important to know how to prevent and treat injuries to these areas.

ANATOMY OF THE HIP, PELVIS, AND THIGH

The hip joint, which is a synovial ball-and-socket joint, is the articulation, or point of contact, between the femur and the pelvis—the head of the femur fits into the cup-shaped acetabulum. The **acetabulum** is also called the *hip socket*. It is deep and covered by thick ligamentous structures that provide stability. Figure 13.1 shows the lateral view of the hip and pelvis.

The **labrum** is attached to the edge of the acetabulum. It is a tough, fibrotic tissue that extends the edge of the acetabulum to help secure the femur in its place. It also helps to cushion the femur against the edge of the joint.

The femur, which is the longest bone in the body, and the pelvis are connected by thick, strong ligaments. Two of the muscle groups of the femur are the quadriceps and hamstrings.

The hip muscles include the most powerful muscles in the body. The hip flexor group, which includes the rectus femoris, sartorius, and

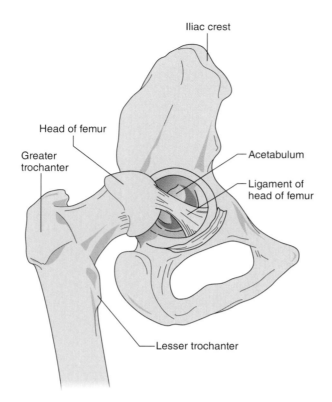

Figure 13.1   Lateral view of the hip and pelvis.

Adapted, by permission, from W.C. Whiting and R.F. Zernicke, 1998, *Biomechanics of musculoskeletal injury* (Champaign, IL: Human Kinetics), 138.

iliopsoas, flexes the thigh. The hamstrings and gluteus maximus extend the thigh (see figure 13.2). Abduction of the hip is predominantly the result of contracting the lateral muscles, which include the gluteus medius and minimus and the tensor fasciae latae. Adduction of the hip is performed primarily by contracting the groin muscles, which originate and mesh into the symphysis pubis region and run a course down the medial aspect of the femur. Some of the primary groin muscles include the gracilis, adductor magnus, adductor longus, and pectineus.

▶ *Understanding Diversity*

Hip measurements are 4 centimeters smaller in Chinese females and 7 centimeters smaller in Chinese males compared with Westerners (Purnell and Paulanka, 2003, 2005).

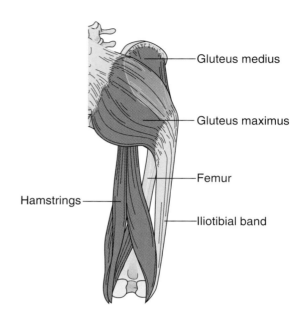

Figure 13.2   Posterior hip musculature. Along with the hamstrings, the gluteus maximus and gluteus medius extend the thigh.

PREVENTING HIP, PELVIS, AND THIGH INJURIES

Because the hip is a stable joint, ATs will not see many sprained ligaments or dislocations in this area. They will, however, see many injuries related to muscular strains. Therefore, proper flexibility training and stretching before vigorous exercise or activity is warranted. Moreover, because many sports expose the thigh to contact, athletes must wear proper equipment—for example, in football, athletes should wear a secure thigh pad that covers a significant portion of the quadriceps. Contact-type injuries also can occur at the iliac crest (the point of the hip) because this area has little natural protection. In sports such as football, players are required to wear a hip pad to cover this area. Proper strength training for any portion of the body can never be too strongly emphasized, and because the muscles around the hip and lower torso are considered the core region, strength in these muscles is necessary for balance and stability.

TREATING HIP, PELVIS, AND THIGH INJURIES AND CONDITIONS

Most injuries to the hip, pelvis, and thigh are strains and contusions. However, the area is not exempt from other injuries, such as fractures and dislocations.

Bone Injuries

Although pelvic fractures are not common, they can occur when excessive stress is placed on the bone tissue. Athletics-related fractures of the hip, pelvis, and femur often occur as a result of an avulsion (the tendon pulling away the bone), disruption of the epiphysis (damage to the growth plate), stress, or trauma to the femur.

Hip Pointers

A **hip pointer** is a contusion of the iliac crest. The iliac crest is superficial and has little soft tissue covering it; however, many muscles attach near the crest so when a serious force impacts the bone, it can be debilitating. The area must be protected from further contact by a protective pad.

Labral Tears

Although not a common injury, the labrum can tear if an acute injury occurs, though in the majority of patients the occurrence is insidious, meaning it occurs slowly with no specific mechanism of injury. A torn labrum can flip into the joint and result in catching, groin pain, and restricted range of motion at the hip. A labral tear will often need to be surgically repaired, but in some instances the athlete can learn to manage the condition so the tear does not aggravate the joint.

Avulsions

Avulsion fractures occur as a result of forceful muscle contractions that pull the bone away at the site where the tendon attaches. This may happen, for example, when a football player continues to run aggressively forward while a defender is holding his leg. The hip flexor may forcefully contract, causing a fracture.

Growth Plate Fractures

Epiphyseal fractures occur at the growth plates of bones, especially at the **capital femoral epiphysis**, where the neck of the femur joins the head. The head of the femur slips off the neck, causing pain in the groin, hip, and knee. According to some experts, this injury is the most common hip disorder in active children between the ages of 10 and 15. When an AT suspects this condition, the athlete should be referred to a physician because treatment includes stopping the slippage and closing the growth plate with a surgical procedure.

Stress Fractures

Although uncommon, femoral stress fractures do occur in athletes who do a great deal of running. Stress fractures are caused by repetitive stress, typically as a result of the pounding of the lower extremity while running. This pounding can cause the femur to bend slightly. Just as if a pencil were bending, one side of the bone is compressed while the other side is stretched. When bone tissue is repeatedly stretched, small hairline fractures can develop, causing a great deal of pain and discomfort. Rest and an alternative activity such as aquatic therapy are indicated to reduce the stress on the fracture site so it can heal.

Femur Fractures

Because the femur is the largest bone in the body, the stress required to fracture it is often extreme. A femur fracture is characterized by severe pain and loss of function as well as internal bleeding, swelling, or tearing of muscles, tendons, nerves, and arteries. Typically, the athlete is unable to move the leg. A femur fracture often causes the leg to externally rotate. Initial treatment for a femur fracture includes immobilization and transportation to the hospital by EMS personnel. They will often use a traction

What Would You Do If...

While at football practice, the AT and a student assistant are helping an injured player off the field. You see that another athlete seems to have injured his leg during a play—it appears to be externally rotated, and he is in a lot of pain. As you approach the athlete, another player starts to grab his teammate's injured leg, saying that it needs to be straightened out.

splint that gently pulls the femur, reducing leg pain and spasm.

Hip Dislocations

Extreme stress can cause a dislocation. Most hip dislocations occur posteriorly and accompany other trauma such as fractures. Severe damage can occur in this area because of the nerve and vascular structures. An athlete with a dislocated hip is likely to be in extreme pain, and the leg is often internally rotated (see figure 13.3). With such an injury, EMS should be called to transport the athlete to the hospital as soon as possible. Only a physician should reduce a hip dislocation. Significant follow-up treatment is required before the athlete can return to activity. Rehabilitation for a hip dislocation often begins with establishing normal range of motion and strength. Gait training, or relearning how to walk normally, will be necessary. As you can imagine, this is a long process.

Legg-Calvé-Perthes Disease

In some children and teens who are still growing, a disruption of blood flow to the head of the femur causes the tissue at the head of the femur to die, a condition known as **Legg-Calvé-Perthes disease**. Typical signs and symptoms of this problem include groin or knee pain and walking with a limp. If this condition is suspected,

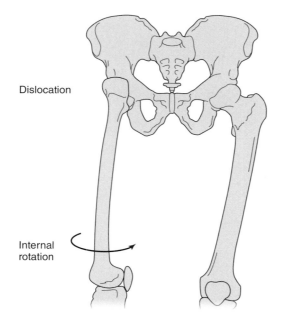

Dislocation

Internal rotation

Figure 13.3 A hip dislocation. Note that the leg is internally rotated.

the athlete should be referred to a physician immediately.

Muscle and Tendon Injuries

Thigh strains are common athletic injuries, especially to the hip flexor, extensor, and groin musculature. Many muscles in the leg cross two joints—for example, the hamstrings cross the back of the hip joint to help with extension and the knee joint to help with knee flexion—and some people see this as the cause of strains in the region. Another theory is that when a strength imbalance occurs, the stronger muscle group puts excessive tension on the opposing muscle group. For example, if an athlete has a great deal of strength in her quadriceps but her hamstrings are weak, the hamstrings are prone to strains.

Strains should initially be treated with PRICES and wrapped with a supportive elastic bandage. Moderate and severe strains may need to be referred to a physician. Rehabilitation will focus on regaining strength and range of motion and enhancing flexibility before returning to play.

Hip and Thigh Muscle Contusions

Deep thigh contusions are common, especially in collision sports. In many contact sports such as rugby or football, opponents collide with the athlete's thigh and compress the tissue. Thigh contusions can result in a lack of knee flexion due to tightness. Although many bruises suffered in athletics are minor, thigh contusions can cause disability. The more severe contusions can actually cause tissue tearing and extensive bleeding. If not managed appropriately, serious thigh contusions can cause a condition known as **myositis ossificans**, which is the formation of bone tissue within the muscle (see figure 13.4). Because bone tissue is not as extensible as muscle tissue, disability and loss of function are typical consequences.

When treating a thigh contusion it is important to proceed with PRICES, but the knee should be flexed during the ice application. An AT may put an athlete with this type of injury in a hinged knee immobilizer with the knee locked into flexion, limiting the total loss of flexibility due to the injury. With a moderate to severe contusion, the athlete should be placed on crutches to minimize stress to the area and then referred to the team physician. Active

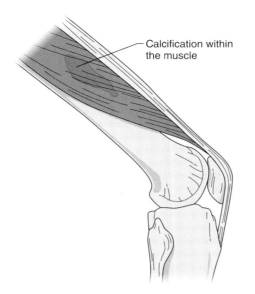

Figure 13.4 Myositis ossificans.

Calcification within the muscle

Hip Bursitis

The lateral hip, specifically over the greater trochanter of the femur, can create pressure over the bursa. The bursa is a fluid-filled sac that reduces friction of tendons that cross this bony prominence. When the bursa is irritated from too much pressure from the tendons, it becomes inflamed. Athletes with **hip bursitis** will report snapping of the hip when they climb stairs.

Ligament Injuries

The hip is a ball-and-socket joint that is extremely stable, mostly because the head of the femur sits so deeply in the pelvis. Thick ligamentous structures and strong muscles also surround the hip.

rest and the use of ice and gentle stretching routines are effective in restoring mobility. Ultrasound (discussed in chapter 16) is often used to help reabsorb the blood that collects internally and to break up the bony tissue deposits. The AT must make certain that a protective pad is placed over the contusion to prevent repeated contusions to the area, because this also can create myositis ossificans.

The Real World

I always look forward to the first football scrimmage of the year in anticipation of the season. I was watching as a defensive back came near the sideline to make a play on the wide receiver just as a blocker for the wide receiver hit the defensive back in the hip with his shoulder pad in an attempt to block. The defensive back did the splits while being blocked and tackling the receiver. He was in severe pain, supine with hip and knee flexion, and unable to get up. After I assessed him, I determined he had dislocated his hip and I called for emergency medical assistance. We placed him on a backboard with padding beneath his knee to maintain flexion. At the hospital, his hip was relocated. Unfortunately, a dislocated hip needs several months of rest and rehabilitation for proper healing—he never played in a game that year.

Lorin Cartwright, MS, ATC

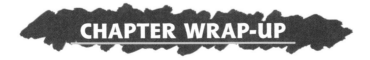

CHAPTER WRAP-UP

Summary

The hip is a stable joint not only because of its bony structure but also because it has strong muscles and ligaments surrounding it. The thigh has strong musculature but can receive deep contusions, especially to the quadriceps, if not properly protected. These injuries can be debilitating for the athlete and require immediate care. The AT must be aware that an adolescent athlete may develop Legg-Calvé-Perthes disease or growth plate fractures at the capital femoral epiphysis. She should take care to get a thorough history and observe the athlete's hip for joint position because this can help detect a fracture of the growth areas around the hip. Rehabilitation of the hip often involves reestablishing flexibility and muscle strength around the joint.

Key Terms

Define the following terms found in this chapter:

acetabulum   labrum
capital femoral epiphysis   Legg-Calvé-Perthes disease
hip bursitis   myositis ossificans
hip pointer

Questions for Review

1. What aspects of its anatomy make the hip an extremely stable joint?
2. What injuries discussed in this chapter typically occur to younger athletes?
3. How should an AT treat an athlete who has received a severe thigh contusion?
4. Describe how an AT might treat a strain to the thigh musculature.
5. Why is the thigh musculature vulnerable to muscle strains?

Activities for Reinforcement

1. Have an AT review injury assessment techniques for the hip, thigh, and pelvis.
2. Have an AT demonstrate common exercises used in hip rehabilitation.
3. Review one of the following Web sites containing information about hip injuries:

   www.human-anatomy.net/anatomy-hip-pictures.html

   www.innerbody.com/image/skel15.html

   www.uihealthcare.com/topics/sportsmedicine/spor3340.html

Above and Beyond

1. Read the following case report related to a torn labrum in an elite athlete and present a summary: Binningsley, D. 2003. Tear of the acetabular labrum in an elite athlete. *British Journal of Sports Medicine* 37(1): 84-88.

2. Read one of the following articles and explain common signs, symptoms, and treatment of the conditions described:

   Diaz, J.A., D.A. Fischer, A.C. Rettig, T.J. Davis, and K.D. Shelbourne. 2003. Severe quadriceps muscle contusions in athletes: A report of three cases. *American Journal of Sports Medicine* 31(2): 289-293.

   Larson, C.M., L.C. Almekinders, S.G. Karas, and W.E. Garrett. 2002. Evaluating and managing muscle contusions and myositis ossificans. *Physician and Sportsmedicine* 30(2): 41-44, 49-50.

   Rosenthal, M.D., and D.J. McMillan. 2004. Injury management update. Hamstring-strain rehabilitation: a functional stepwise approach for return to sports, part II. *Athletic Therapy Today* 9(1): 44-45.

   Rosenthal, M.D., and D.J. McMillan. 2003. Injury management update. Hamstring-strain rehabilitation: a functional stepwise approach for return to sports, part I. *Athletic Therapy Today* 8(6): 34-35.

3. Read the following article related to stength imbalances and the occurrence of hamstring strains, and summarize your findings: Croisier, J., S. Ganteaume, J. Binet, M. Genty, and J. Ferret. 2008. Strength imbalances and prevention of hamstring injury in professional soccer players: a prospective study. *American Journal of Sports Medicine* 36(8): 1469-1475.

4. Read this literature review related to causes of hamstring strain reoccurrence and articulate what you believe to be the strongest argument as to why hamstring strains reoccur: Croisier, J. 2004. Factors associated with recurrent hamstring injuries. *Sports Medicine* 34(10): 681-695.

5. Examine the following Web site, which contains information about hamstring strains, and create a poster presentation about how these injuries occur and how they should be treated:

   http://orthoinfo.aaos.org/fact/thr_report.cfm?thread_id=137&topcategory=wellness.

14

Knee Injuries

Objectives

Upon completing this chapter, the student will be able to do the following:

- Describe the basic anatomy of the knee.
- Explain common knee injuries that occur with athletic participation.
- Identify signs and symptoms of knee injuries.
- Explain treatment parameters performed by an AT for specific knee injuries.

The knee is vulnerable to ligament sprains, tendon strains, and cartilage damage. In this chapter, we describe the basic anatomy of the knee and injuries common to athletes.

ANATOMY OF THE KNEE

The knee is a hinge joint at the articulation, or point of contact, of three bones. The joint is stabilized by four major ligaments, cartilage, and strong musculature. The knee is also able to rotate.

Bones

The bones that form the knee joint are the femur, tibia, and patella (see figure 14.1). The primary movement of the knee occurs at the articulation of the tibia and femur, which is called the *tibiofemoral joint*. The patella is a sesamoid, or floating bone, which is embedded in the patellar tendon that attaches the quadriceps muscles to the front of

the tibia and protects the front of the joint. As the knee flexes and extends, the patella glides up and down on the front of the femur. This is called the *patellofemoral joint*.

Muscles

The muscles of the knee provide both movement and stability. The primary muscles spanning the knee include the quadriceps and the hamstrings. Knee extension is primarily performed by the four quadriceps muscles: the vastus medialis, vastus lateralis, vastus intermedius, and rectus femoris (see figure 14.2). The vastus muscles of the quadriceps originate on the femur, whereas the rectus femoris originates at the anterior aspect of the pelvis. All of the quadriceps muscles run toward the patella and attach to the patellar tendon at the anterior knee. The patellar tendon crosses the anterior aspect of the knee joint and inserts on the superior aspect of the tibia.

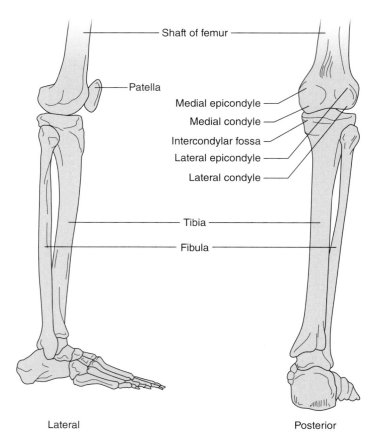

Lateral   Posterior

Figure 14.1 Lateral and posterior views of the knee.

Adapted, by permission, from W.C. Whiting and R.F. Zernicke, 1998, *Biomechanics of musculoskeletal injury* (Champaign, IL: Human Kinetics), 150.

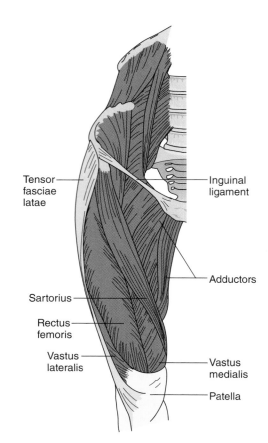

Figure 14.2 The quadriceps muscles.

Adapted, by permission, from W.C. Whiting and R.F. Zernicke, 1998, *Biomechanics of musculoskeletal injury* (Champaign, IL: Human Kinetics), 144.

Flexion of the knee is predominantly the result of contracting the hamstring muscles. The term **hamstrings** refers collectively to the biceps femoris, semimembranosus, and semitendinosus muscles (see figure 14.3). The three hamstring muscles attach on the posterior aspect of the lower pelvis and run down the back of the thigh and across the knee to their attachment on the tibia. The location of their attachments helps prevent forward movement of the tibia on the femur.

Besides the quadriceps and hamstrings, other important muscles around the knee joint allow movement and provide stability. Posteriorly, the gastrocnemius muscle crosses the knee joint, originating at the posterior aspect of the femur. The gastrocnemius is known mainly as a muscle that allows us to point our toes (plantar flexion), but it also functions with the popliteus muscle to flex the knee.

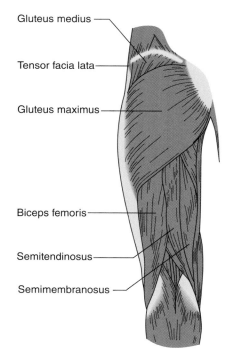

Figure 14.3 The hamstring muscles.

What Would You Do If...

An athlete has been treated in the athletic training room for jumper's knee. While you are getting the water coolers set up for practice, you notice that the athlete is starting to play one on one with a teammate before warming up and stretching.

At the medial aspect of the knee, the gracilis muscle crosses the knee joint. This muscle originates near the groin and inserts on the medial tibia; its function is to adduct the femur. On the lateral aspect of the knee, the iliotibial band crosses the knee joint. The iliotibial band is a tough connective tissue that the tensor fasciae latae and gluteus maximus of the hip mesh into. These muscles help to abduct the hip.

Ligaments

There are four primary knee ligaments (see figure 14.4). The **medial collateral ligament (MCL)** helps stabilize the inside or medial aspect of the knee, and the **lateral collateral ligament (LCL)** helps stabilize the outside or lateral aspect of the knee. The **anterior cruciate ligament (ACL)** keeps the tibia from moving forward on the femur, and the **posterior cruciate ligament (PCL)** prevents the tibia from moving backward on the femur. The ACL and PCL pass through the middle of the knee joint and cross each other; hence the name *cruciate*, which means "cross-shaped."

Cartilage

The ends of the tibia and the femur are covered and cushioned by pieces of tough cartilage tissue called the **menisci** (see figure 14.5). Without the menisci,

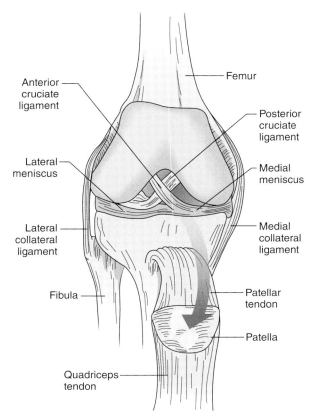

Figure 14.4 Major ligaments of the knee. Note how the cruciate ligaments cross in the center of the knee.

Adapted, by permission, from W.C. Whiting and R.F. Zernicke, 1998, *Biomechanics of musculoskeletal injury* (Champaign, IL: Human Kinetics), 150.

the tibia and femur would rub against each other, which would cause the bone to wear down quickly. The menisci also help stabilize the knee joint. The top of the tibia is flat, like a tabletop. The end of the femur, specifically the condyles, is rounded, like an orange. Without something to stabilize the

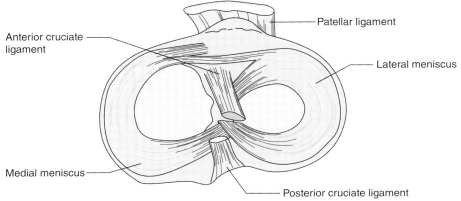

Figure 14.5 A top view of the medial and lateral menisci.

Adapted, by permission, from R.S. Behnke, 2001, *Kinetic anatomy* (Champaign, IL: Human Kinetics), 207.

joint, the femur would move a great deal on the tibia—in other words, the orange would roll around on the tabletop. The menisci are thicker on the sides and thinner in the middle, forming a dish-shaped hollow. They are also attached to the top of the tibia, which provides a seat for the femoral condyles to sit in on top of the tibia—like putting the orange in a bowl on the table. The femur can move, but it will not roll off the tibia.

PREVENTING KNEE INJURIES

Ligament sprains are among the most common injuries to the knee. Remembering that the muscles in this area provide stability to the knee and help resist abnormal bony movement, athletes should develop strength in these muscles (i.e., the quadriceps, hamstrings, gastrocnemius, and hip abductors and adductors). For instance, heel raises are a good way to strengthen the gastrocnemius, which is located at the back of the lower leg and helps to point the toes. Some ATs and athletes use preventive knee braces that are designed to protect the MCL (see figure 14.6); however, the American Academy of

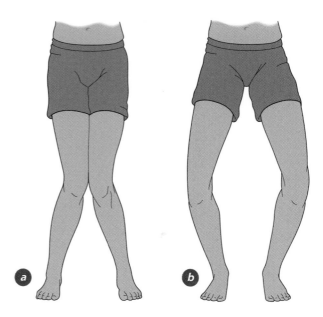

Figure 14.7 *(a)* Knock-knees and *(b)* bowlegs.

Pediatrics states that there is insufficient research to warrant the use of braces to prevent ligament injury.

If an athlete has problems with her knees, the AT should examine her leg structure to determine if she has genu valgus, also known as knock-knees, or genu varus, also known as bowlegs (figure 14.7, *a-b*). These conditions may provide insight into the type of knee problem the athlete is suffering. Also, knowing if one of these conditions is present will help in selecting appropriate equipment such as knee braces or athletic shoes.

Current research has identified neuromuscular training as an effective way to prevent knee injuries, particularly injuries to the ACL. Neuromuscular training involves teaching athletes how to land from a jump, how to change directions while maintaining appropriate lower-extremity alignment (keep the knee over the foot), and how to flex the knee and hip during movements. It also involves balance training and proper deceleration of activities involving knee flexion.

TREATING KNEE INJURIES AND CONDITIONS

The knee is exposed to many forces. This makes it vulnerable to injuries, especially to the ligaments, but tendon and bone injuries also occur. The patella and menisci are subject to unique athletics-related injuries.

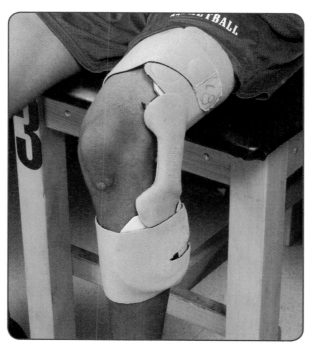

Figure 14.6 A protective knee brace is applied to an athlete's knee to prevent tearing of the MCL, which can result from a blow to the lateral side.

Bone Injuries

Although the patella is not immune to fracture, other bone injuries are more common. These include chondromalacia and patellar dislocations.

Patellofemoral Syndrome

Patellofemoral syndrome involves a set of symptoms that include pain and discomfort around the patella, often caused by patellar tracking problems. As the knee bends, the patella is grated across the femur instead of riding smoothly, causing the cartilage on the back of the patella to soften or wear away. This is known as **chondromalacia**, which is characterized by achiness around the patella, especially with prolonged sitting in the same position. The athlete will often report a grinding sensation with flexion and extension. If the AT places a hand over the patella as the athlete flexes and extends the knee, the grinding can even be felt. Treatment for chondromalacia involves correcting any problems with patellar tracking, strengthening the vastus medialis muscle, and improving flexibility of the quadriceps and hamstrings. Bent-leg activities should be avoided because they tend to aggravate the condition. Treatment for patellofemoral pain syndrome should also address any weakness around the hip joint since this has been identified as an effective intervention.

Patellar Dislocation

Occasionally an athlete's patella will be forced to the lateral aspect of the knee, usually while the knee is bent and forced to twist inward. This deformity is hard to overlook. The athlete is often in distress, and EMS must be called unless the team physician is present. Only a physician should reduce a dislocated patella; otherwise complications may result and the posterior aspect of the patella may be injured further. Treatment involves immobilizing the knee for a short time, and then the athlete should begin exercising to regain mobility and strength around the knee joint. Sometimes athletes are advised to wear a knee sleeve with a patellar hole to help keep the patella in place during activity.

The Real World

As an AT working at a large high school, I was summoned to the track and field area because an athlete had fallen over the hurdles. When I arrived at the track, the athlete was in obvious pain and moaning that his knees were injured. I gently pulled up his pant legs to see what was wrong. There were obvious deformities at the anterior aspects of both knees. Where the patellae should have been were two large depressions, and the patellae themselves were sitting several inches above the knee joints, where the quadriceps had pulled them. We called EMS immediately. I acted calm and reassuring, knowing that if the young man panicked, things would only get worse. We immobilized his legs and treated him for shock. Once he was at the hospital, the surgeons determined that he had ruptured one patellar tendon and fractured his other patella in half. Although I had limited contact with this athlete afterward, his recovery looked positive because he received quick advanced care by physicians and he was in good health.

Lisa V. Pitney, MSEd, Former ATC

Muscle and Tendon Injuries

Many of the muscle and tendon injuries at the knee are chronic and are caused by overuse. The patellar tendon in particular is commonly involved.

Patellar Tendinitis

Patellar tendinitis is an overuse disorder characterized by quadriceps weakness, tenderness over the patellar tendon, and minimal swelling. The condition is also called *jumper's knee* because athletes who perform a lot of jumping (e.g., basketball and volleyball players) often get this condition. In the early stages, the athlete typically has pain after activity, but in the later stages the condition can result in pain during activity as well as loss of strength. The AT will attempt to control inflammation by applying ice and modifying the athlete's activity level, usually restricting running and jumping. The rehabilitation program should address any flexibility problems of the quadriceps and weakness of the leg.

Although the term *tendinitis* is often used, the term *tendinosis* is often more appropriate. Tendinosis denotes a condition of the tendon, meaning it is degenerated, painful, and weak, but there is an absence of inflammation.

If a tendon is already weak but the athlete continues to participate, a rupture can occur. A patellar tendon rupture means that the amount of stress applied to the tendon exceeded the ability of the tendon to withstand the force, ripping apart the fibers. With an injury such as this, the elasticity of the quadriceps muscles will retract the patella upward; thus, a deformity at the anterior knee will be present.

Osgood-Schlatter Disorder

Younger athletes who perform a great deal of running and jumping sometimes develop an irritation at the site of the patellar tendon attachment to the front of the tibia, or the tibial tuberosity. The bones of an adolescent are still somewhat soft, and repeated stressful activity can sometimes cause the patellar tendon to partially pull away from the bone, an injury called **Osgood-Schlatter disorder**. It typically causes discomfort of the knee, swelling, tenderness, and pain during activity. Athletes with this condition should restrict their activity until it is resolved. This does not mean they should stop all activity, however. For example, although a basketball player should stop aggressive running and jumping, an alternative activity that may not irritate the injury is stationary bicycling. The athlete can maintain her fitness level without causing additional problems. As a general rule of thumb, pain should be used as a guide; that is, activity should be modified based on the athlete's pain level. If she does not modify her activity appropriately, she may experience prolonged periods of pain. Ice application before and after activity is also helpful. A special pad may need to be made to fit over the front of the tibia because this area becomes extremely tender. Osgood-Schlatter disorder often improves by age 16 or 17, but a bony growth may develop at the top of the tibia. Unfortunately, the bump remains even after the symptoms of the condition have disappeared.

Ligament Injuries

In common with other joints, ligament sprains of the knee can be mild (first degree), moderate (second degree), or severe (third degree). The four primary ligaments are the most commonly sprained.

Understanding Diversity

Female athletes are more prone to ACL injuries compared with male athletes. The reasons for this are varied. One theory is that female athletes have a higher Q-angle, which is the angle created by the femur and the tibia. Because females tend to have wider hips than males, the Q-angle is greater, resulting in the knee collapsing inward and forward during function. Another theory is that during the female menstrual cycle hormones are released that create joint laxity, or looseness in the joints. If the joint is lax, it is more unstable and the tibia may shift more on the femur. Lastly, it is thought that the landing mechanics of females are the cause—more stress is applied to the ACL instead of the surrounding muscles to absorb the impact forces.

Anterior Cruciate Ligament Injuries

The ACL keeps the tibia from moving forward on the femur. If this ligament is injured (see figure 14.8), the athlete is often disabled, complaining of the knee giving way, collapsing, and popping. Injuries to the ACL are often the most serious of all knee ligament injuries, and the ACL is the ligament that is most frequently surgically reconstructed.

The ACL is often injured as the athlete attempts to change directions quickly and twists the lower leg; he may hear a popping sound during the twisting mechanism. However, it can also be injured because of excessive hyperextension. A torn ACL

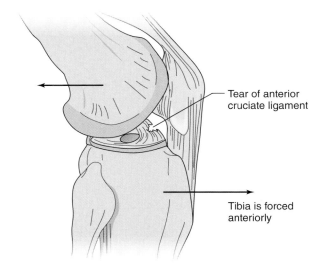

Tear of anterior cruciate ligament

Tibia is forced anteriorly

Figure 14.8 An ACL tear results from the tibia moving forward forcefully on the femur.

causes rapid swelling and loss of knee function. Immediate treatment includes PRICES, and a knee immobilizer, and crutches provide additional knee protection. Follow-up with an orthopedist is necessary if a torn ACL is suspected.

An athlete rarely functions well with a torn ACL, and the injury often needs to be surgically reconstructed. This, however, is a decision that must be made by the athlete, the surgeon, and the athlete's family. The decision may depend on the amount of instability that exists, the level of function desired by the athlete, and the age of the athlete.

Surgical reconstruction of the ACL can involve two types of tissues, autografts or allografts. An autograph involves a piece of tissue from the athlete's body. The tissues used in these instances will include either a portion (about one-third) of the patellar tendon or a hamstring tendon (usually the semitendinosus). The tissue used for an allograft involves a portion of the athlete's patellar tendon, the athlete's Achilles tendon, or a cadaver's patellar tendon.

Rehabilitation of an ACL injury focuses on restoring range of motion and strengthening the hamstrings to help stabilize the tibia as well as to regain full function. Even with an aggressive ACL rehabilitation program, it may be six months before the athlete can return to participation.

Posterior Cruciate Ligament Injuries

The PCL prevents posterior tibial movement on the femur. It is frequently injured when an athlete falls and a bent knee bears her full weight, when the knee is forcefully hyperflexed, or when a blow is delivered to the front of the tibia.

After determining the mechanism of the injury, the AT may suspect a PCL injury if the athlete reports having heard a pop. Surprisingly, there tends to be little swelling with PCL injuries. Initial treatment should include PRICES and referral to a physician. A rehabilitation program for mild or moderate PCL sprains will focus on strengthening the quadriceps and regaining full function. Although some physicians disagree about whether or not surgery should be performed on a severe PCL injury, even complete PCL tears can be rehabilitated without surgical intervention—many athletes can become functional again after the initial pain and swelling are controlled and the knee is strengthened.

Medial Collateral Ligament Sprains

The MCL is frequently injured when an athlete receives a blow to the outside of the knee. This causes the knee to bend inward (valgus stress) and stresses the MCL. A mild MCL sprain usually results in medial joint line pain, little if any swelling, no joint laxity when stressed by the AT, and full knee flexion and extension. A moderate MCL sprain often results in mild swelling, discomfort, and some joint laxity when stressed by the AT during the injury assessment. A moderate or severe amount of swelling, loss of function, and a great deal of joint laxity often characterize a severe MCL injury.

Regardless of the severity of the injury, the athlete's knee should be treated with PRICES. A mild injury may only require an elastic wrap for compression and support. However, with a moderate or severe MCL injury, the knee should be put in an immobilizer. Rehabilitation considerations include strengthening the muscles that cross the medial aspect of the knee. If the knee has moderate or severe MCL damage, the AT should consider the possibility of damage to the menisci or an ACL injury.

Lateral Collateral Ligament Injuries

LCL injuries occur less frequently than MCL injuries. The signs and symptoms are similar except the discomfort is at the lateral aspect of the knee. Treatment for an LCL injury is the same as for an MCL injury. In terms of regaining joint stability, strengthening exercises should focus on the lateral thigh muscles and hamstrings.

Cartilage Injuries

Each large piece of fibrous cartilage in the knee joint is a meniscus. The function of the menisci is shock absorption and stability. Unfortunately, the menisci are vulnerable to significant injury, specifically tears.

The most common injury to the meniscus is a tear, which can be on the outer edge, middle, inside edge, or ends (horns) of the meniscus. Tears of the meniscus typically happen with a twisting movement of the knee or with hyperflexion and hyperextension injuries. An athlete with a torn meniscus will often complain of pain at the joint line; have problems putting weight on the limb; complain of clicking, catching, or locking; and walk with a limp.

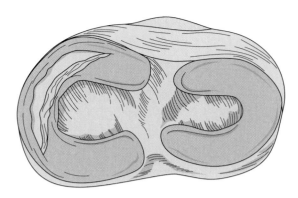

Figure 14.9   Bucket-handle tear of the meniscus.

He will be unable to fully extend and flex the knee and may have some swelling.

Tears of the meniscus used to be treated by surgically removing the entire meniscus (called a **meniscectomy**). See figure 14.9, which shows a bucket-handle tear, a type of meniscus injury. However, due in part to the prevalence of **arthroscopic surgery**, where small surgical instruments are inserted into the knee through tiny holes, treatment of a torn meniscus often involves taking out only the small piece of tissue that has been torn. Depending on where the meniscus is torn, sometimes surgeons are able to suture (sew) it back together.

During rehabilitation after an injury to or surgery on the meniscus, an athlete initially will use exercises that do not involve placing weight on the injured leg. Aquatic therapy programs are ideal for helping to reestablish range of motion and strength. Then the athlete will progress slowly to more weight-bearing exercises as tolerated.

Fat Pad Syndrome

The infrapatellar fat pad lies behind and just beneath the patella and acts as a barrier and cushion between the patella and femur. When an athlete extends her knee, the fat pad can become trapped between these bones. **Fat pad syndrome** is sometimes referred to as **Hoffa's syndrome**. The signs and symptoms of this condition include tenderness beneath the knee, swelling, and pain with extension. The area should be rested and treated with ice and possibly ultrasound.

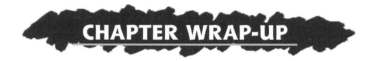

CHAPTER WRAP-UP

Summary

The knee is the joint between the femur, tibia, and patella. The quadriceps extend the knee and the hamstrings flex it. The cartilage, or menisci, of the knee provides a cushion between the tibia and femur. Four primary ligaments aid in the stability of the knee: the MCL, LCL, ACL, and PCL. A complete tear to the ACL needs to be surgically repaired by an orthopedic surgeon.

Key Terms

Define the following terms found in this chapter:

anterior cruciate ligament (ACL)	medial collateral ligament (MCL)
arthroscopic surgery	meniscectomy
chondromalacia	meniscus
fat pad syndrome	Osgood-Schlatter disorder
hamstrings	patellar tendinitis
Hoffa's syndrome	posterior cruciate ligament (PCL)
lateral collateral ligament (LCL)	

Questions for Review

1. Name the three bones that compose the knee joint.

2. Identify the four primary ligaments that stabilize the knee.

3. Name the four muscles of the quadriceps.

4. What three muscles compose the hamstrings? What movements can they produce?

5. If an injury caused the tibia to move forward on the femur, what ligament would most likely become overstretched or torn?

6. Name the ligament that would be most likely to stretch or tear if an opponent fell on the outside of an athlete's knee and it bent inward.

7. Describe how an AT should care for a second-degree, or moderate, MCL sprain.

Activities for Reinforcement

1. Invite an AT to class to demonstrate how she evaluates a knee injury.

2. Invite an orthopedic surgeon to class to discuss common knee surgeries.

3. Visit the following site to review the anatomy of the knee: www.eorthopod.com/public/patient_education/6507/knee_anatomy.html.

Above and Beyond

1. Find a text dedicated to athletic injury assessment and develop a checklist of how to assess a knee injury.

2. Visit the following site on ehealthMD and investigate the information on ACL reconstructive surgery: www.ehealthmd.com/library/acltears/ACL_whatis.html.

3. Review the following Web sites and write a report on knee injuries among female athletes:

    www.nismat.org/ptcor/female_knee/

    www.athleticscholarships.net/sports-medicine-knee-injury-girls.htm

    www.pponline.co.uk/encyc/female-athletes-strength-training-exercises-for-knee-injuries-158

    www.arthroscopy.com/sp05041.htm

4. Examine one of the following articles and write a summary:

    Adams, N. 2004. Knee injuries. *Emergency Nurse* 11(10): 19-27.

    Kozanek, M., E. Fu, S.K. Van de Velde, T. Gill, and G. Li. 2009. Posterolateral structures of the knee in posterior cruciate ligament deficiency. *American Journal of Sports Medicine* 37(3): 534-541.

    Maitland, M.E. 2003. Best of the literature: Neuromuscular training helps prevent ACL injuries. *Physician and Sportsmedicine* 31(12): 8-9.

    Myer, G.D., K.R. Ford, and T.E. Hewett. 2004. Rationale and clinical techniques for anterior cruciate ligament injury prevention among female athletes. *Journal of Athletic Training* 39(4): 352-364.

    Sandrey, M.A. 2003. Acute and chronic tendon injuries: Factors affecting the healing response and treatment. *Journal of Sport Rehabilitation* 12(1): 70-91.

    Shea, K.G., P.J. Apel, and R.P. Pfeiffer. 2003. Anterior cruciate ligament injury in paediatric and adolescent patients: a review of basic science and clinical research. *Sports Medicine* 33(6): 455-471.

    Swart, J., R. Tucker, R.P. Lamberts, Y. Albertus-Kajee, and M.I. Lambert. 2008. Potential causes of chronic knee pain in a former winner of the Tour de France. *International SportMed Journal* 9(4): 162-171.

    Whittle, R., and B. Crow. 2009. Prevention of ACL injuries in female athletes through early intervention. *Sport Journal* 12(3).

chapter 15

Foot, Ankle, and Lower-Leg Injuries

Objectives

Upon completing this chapter, the student will be able to do the following:

- Describe the basic anatomy of the foot, ankle, and lower leg.
- Explain common injuries that occur to the foot.
- Identify common injuries that occur to the ankle.
- Describe signs and symptoms of lower-leg injuries.
- Identify strategies to prevent injuries to the ankle and lower leg.

The foot, ankle, and lower leg support the body weight and transfer force as a person walks and runs. The feet and lower legs work to maintain balance and adapt to various surfaces. Ankle injuries are among the most common injuries seen by team physicians and ATs; in fact, the ankle may be the most frequently injured joint.

ANATOMY OF THE FOOT, ANKLE, AND LOWER LEG

The lower leg, foot, and ankle play a critical role in balance, shock absorption, and movement. The bones provide structure and protection, while the muscles and tendons produce movement.

Bones and Joints

There are 28 bones in the foot (see figure 15.1). The bones in the toes are called **phalanges**. The toes are numbered 1 to 5, the great toe being number 1. Except for the great toe, each toe has three bones: the distal, middle, and proximal phalanges. (The great toe has only distal and proximal phalanges.) The toe joints are referred to as *interphalangeal joints*. Under the great toe are two small bones, the sesamoids, which assist with flexion of the toe. The **metatarsals** are the long bones of the foot; similar to the toes, they are numbered 1 to 5. The joints between the phalanges and the metatarsals are the metatarsophalangeal joints. The midfoot, which lies between the metatarsals and the **talus**

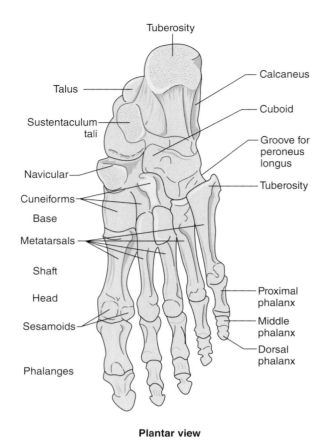

Figure 15.1 Bones of the foot.

Adapted, by permission, from R.S. Behnke, 2001, *Kinetic anatomy* (Champaign, IL: Human Kinetics), 227.

and **calcaneus**, contains several small bones that articulate (join together at a joint) with one another, producing subtle movements.

The ankle is the joint between the talus and calcaneus of the foot and the fibula and tibia of the lower leg. The calcaneus, also known as the heel bone, is below the talus. The posterior portion of the calcaneus is the attachment point of the Achilles tendon. The tibia and fibula articulate at both distal and proximal ends while muscles and ligaments between the two bones hold them together from one end to the other. The **medial malleolus** is the end of the tibia on the medial side, and the end of the fibula at the lateral aspect is known as the **lateral malleolus**. The ankle, which is the joint between the foot and the lower leg, is held together by ligaments. The fibula extends past the ankle joint and stops severe eversion.

> ## Understanding Diversity
>
> A longer second tarsal is found in 8% to 24% of Caucasians (Schrefer 1994). A long second tarsal means that an athlete may be more prone to ankle sprains.

Arches of the Foot

There are three arches on the **plantar surface** (bottom) of the foot that function as shock absorbers—the transverse, longitudinal, and metatarsal arches (see figure 15.2, *a-b*). The transverse arch is located in front of the heel and goes from the fifth metatarsal to the navicular bone of the foot. The

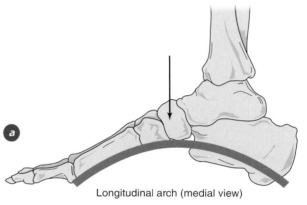

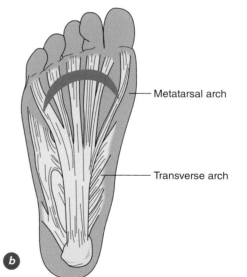

Figure 15.2 *(a)* Longitudinal and *(b)* metatarsal and transverse arches of the foot.

Adapted, by permission, from W.C. Whiting and R.F. Zernicke, 1998, *Biomechanics of musculoskeletal injury* (Champaign, IL: Human Kinetics), 170.

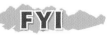

Sesamoids

Sesamoids are bones or cartilage located within a tendon, especially at a joint, that ease muscular movement over a bony surface.

longitudinal arch runs from the calcaneus to the metatarsal heads. The metatarsal arch runs along the metatarsal heads.

Muscles and Tendons

The muscles of the lower leg and ankle control movement of the foot and leg (see figure 15.3). The peroneal muscles, including the peroneus brevis and peroneus longus, attach to the lateral aspect of the lower leg and run a course to the lateral aspect and underside of the foot. This muscle group helps

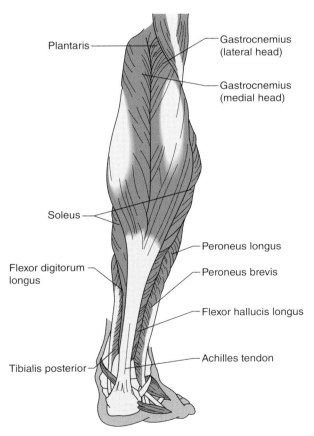

Figure 15.3 Major muscles of the lower leg.

Adapted, by permission, from W.C. Whiting and R.F. Zernicke, 1998, *Biomechanics of musculoskeletal injury* (Champaign, IL: Human Kinetics), 162.

stabilize the lateral aspect of the ankle. The **gastrocnemius** is a powerful muscle in the calf that attaches by the **Achilles tendon** at the posterior aspect of the calcaneous bone. The gastrocnemius is not the only muscle that merges into the Achilles tendon; the **soleus** muscle also meshes into the Achilles. Together the gastrocnemius and soleus act to flex the foot downward (plantar flexion) and allow athletes to propel themselves when running.

The Achilles tendon is extremely strong. It can withstand a tension force of several times the athlete's body weight while running.

Understanding Diversity

The peroneus tertius muscle is missing in approximately 13% of African Americans (Schrefer 1994). The absence of the peroneus tertius means that the athlete may have difficulty dorsiflexing and everting the ankles.

Ligaments

Strong ligaments of the foot are located laterally, medially, and on the plantar surface. Many of the ligament names give the attachment points, making it easier to identify their locations. The lateral aspect of the ankle has numerous ligaments, including the anterior talofibular, posterior talofibular, and calcaneofibular ligaments (see figure 15.4a). The lateral ligaments hold the bony structures together on the lateral side but are not as strong as the medial ligament. The medial ligament is called the *deltoid* (see figure 15.4b). The deltoid covers the entire surface of the medial side of the ankle and maintains stability, especially during eversion. The deltoid ligament is stronger than all of the lateral ligaments combined.

PREVENTING FOOT, ANKLE, AND LOWER-LEG INJURIES

Taking care of the foot, ankle, and lower leg is essential to injury prevention and continuous athletic participation. Many athletes take protective measures such as wearing shoes that provide

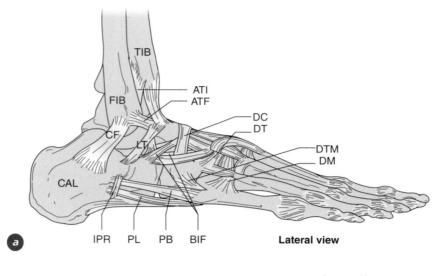

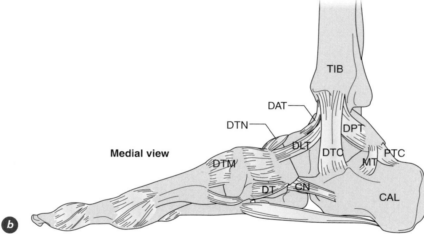

ATF	Anterior talofibular ligament
ATI	Anterior tibiofibular ligament
BIF	Bifurcated
CF	Calcaneofibular ligament
CN	Calcaneonavicular
CAL	Calcaneus
DAT	Deltoid ligament - Anterior talotibial
DPT	Deltoid ligament - Posterior talotibial
DTC	Deltoid ligament - Tibiocalcaneal
DLT	Deltoid ligament - Tibionavicular
DC	Dorsal cuboideonavicular
DM	Dorsal metatarsal
DTN	Dorsal talonavicular
DT	Dorsal tarsal
DTM	Dorsal tarsometatarsal
FIB	Fibula
IPR	Inferior peroneal retinaculum
LT	Lateral talocalcaneal
MT	Medial talocalcaneal
PB	Peroneus brevis
PL	Peroneus longus
PTC	Posterior talocalcaneal
TIB	Tibia

Figure 15.4 Ligaments of the foot: *(a)* lateral view, *(b)* medial view.

Adapted, by permission, from R.S. Behnke, 2001, *Kinetic anatomy* (Champaign, IL: Human Kinetics), 230.

ankle and arch support, using supportive ankle taping (to prevent ankle inversion), and wearing shin guards (to prevent contusions of the lower leg). Strengthening and conditioning programs can also help to prevent injuries. If the team physician finds a weakness in the athlete's foot, ankle, or lower leg, the athlete should be placed on a rehabilitation program that emphasizes strengthening. In some instances, muscles that are very tight will need to be stretched.

Conditioning under the guidance of a coach may prevent stress fractures. Proper footwear that is able to absorb shock has also been shown to reduce metatarsal stress fractures.

Balance training can reduce the onset of ankle sprains. As such, balance exercises should be incorporated into strength and conditioning programs for athletes.

What Would You Do If...

The AT has been caring for an athlete who has lower-leg pain. In gym class you note that this athlete plays without shoes. He constantly limps during class and at practices.

TREATING FOOT, ANKLE, AND LOWER-LEG INJURIES AND CONDITIONS

The feet and legs form the foundation on which an athlete walks and runs. Injuries to ligaments, muscles, tendons, and bones in this area can be disabling.

Bone Injuries

Direct impacts to an area and repetitive use can cause fractures. Common symptoms include pain, pressure, and an inability to move the body part. The AT will discover crepitus, swelling, and possible bone displacement. After splinting, the athlete must be referred to a physician for X rays and a cast. The base of the fifth metatarsal and the epiphyses of the distal tibia and fibula are common fracture sites. Stress fractures, which are caused by repetitive use, are often seen in several areas around the foot, ankle, and lower leg.

Jones Fracture (Fifth-Metatarsal Avulsion Fracture)

The most common avulsion fracture is of the fifth metatarsal—a **Jones fracture** (figure 15.5). When an ankle is forced into inversion, the muscles contract so forcefully to stabilize the lateral aspect of the ankle that the peroneus brevis tendon pulls part of the bone away at its attachment. The AT will treat the injury using the PRICES technique and refer the athlete to a physician. Many physicians will cast the ankle to allow the bone to heal.

Epiphyseal Injury of Distal Tibia and Fibula

The distal tibia and fibula epiphyses, or growth plates, can become injured when the ankle is forced

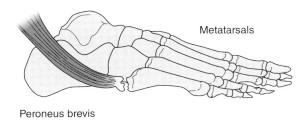

Figure 15.5 Jones fracture.

into plantar flexion and inversion. The athlete will experience pain and swelling over the epiphysis, and she will have difficulty walking or running because of the pain. The AT will splint the injury and refer the athlete to a physician for X rays. This is a potentially serious injury because it is possible for the epiphysis to close prematurely, stunting bone growth at the site.

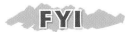

Bone Scan

A bone scan is a diagnostic test performed with a radioactive substance that allows physicians to see small disruptions in the bone.

Stress Fracture

Stress fractures of the lower leg and foot most commonly occur to the tibia, fibula, and metatarsals, and repetitive stress due to running is usually the cause. The athlete will present with pain that becomes more intense at night and following activity. Pain and swelling will be located over the bone. Some physicians believe that a stress fracture can be distinguished by using a tuning fork—the vibrations from the tuning fork vibrate the bone but do not irritate muscles. The edge of one tine of the fork is struck against the assessor's knee, and the base of the tuning fork is placed on the injured site. If the athlete indicates pain, he most likely has a fracture. A bone scan can verify the diagnosis of a stress fracture. An X ray will not show a stress fracture until two weeks after the initial injury, when a callus begins to form at the site. Stress fractures require four to six weeks of rest, and the athlete must see a physician. Although stress fractures are rarely casted, the athlete will be issued crutches to eliminate pressure on the limb. If the injury is not detected early or the athlete fails to report it, a complete fracture may result, which could create serious complications.

Muscle and Tendon Injuries

Strains occur as a result of overstretching or putting a muscle or tendon under excessive tension. **Tendinitis**, which is the inflammation of a tendon, typically results from a repetitive stress such as running or jumping. Common tendon injuries and strains in this region involve the tendons of the medial aspect of the tibia as well as the Achilles tendon.

Shin Splints
(Medial Tibial Stress Syndrome)

Shin splints is a common term for pain in the lower leg. Some people use it to refer to muscle strains, stress fractures, and even tendinitis. However, to doctors, shin splints are known as medial tibial stress syndrome. The muscle fibers on the medial side of the tibia become torn and irritated. The athlete will complain of pain and the inability to run or walk properly. The pain will be located over the distal medial side of the tibia, although there may be swelling on the lateral side as well. The athlete will generally have tight calf muscles, wear older shoes, and be out of shape for the running she is currently doing. There are several successful methods of relieving shin splints, but PRICES is first and foremost. If the athlete limps, she must take a break from running and rest or at least change her training to something else such as biking. When the athlete has permission to return to participation, the AT may wrap the medial side of the leg, pulling the soft tissue toward the bone, and recommend new shoes, stretching, and arch supports.

Achilles Tendinitis

The Achilles tendon is the strong tendon joining the gastrocnemius muscle to the heel. Any sport involving repeated running, jumping, and landing may cause cells in the tendon to break down prematurely, and this irritation or inflammation is referred to as *tendinitis*. During an evaluation, the AT will note swelling, tenderness, crepitus, and an expression of pain on the athlete's face when he palpates the Achilles tendon, especially with dorsiflexion. The athlete will also be weak when plantar flexion is resisted. She must rest the tendon and apply ice, and she may need a referral to a physician for medication. As healing progresses, gentle stretching and strengthening exercises are helpful. If the athlete does not follow instructions or resumes activity too soon, the tendon may thicken, which is the body's protective response. Unfortunately, a thickened tendon will limit the athlete's range of motion and decrease her running and jumping ability. With severe damage, the AT will feel crepitus over the tendon, and in the worst case, the tendon may completely rupture.

Achilles Tendon Rupture

An athlete falls to the court or field clutching her leg in pain, and she reports that she feels as if someone shot her in the back of the lower leg—a typical symptom of an Achilles tendon rupture. The rupture occurs when there is forced dorsiflexion of the foot, a blow over the Achilles tendon, or a sudden forceful contraction of the gastrocnemius muscle. The athlete will feel the tearing, and she will have difficulty walking. Weakness or complete loss of plantar flexion will be noticed. The AT will observe swelling and an obvious depression where the Achilles tendon used to be attached. The athlete will be in obvious pain and should be referred to the team physician immediately after she has been placed in a splint, iced, and given crutches. The Achilles tendon must be repaired surgically by reattaching it to the calcaneus.

Ligament Injuries

A sprain is a stretching or tearing of ligaments and usually occurs as a result of trauma to a joint that is forced to an extreme of its range of movement. In this region of the body, sprains commonly occur at the great toe, arch, lateral ankle joint, and medial ankle joint.

Great-Toe Sprain

The great toe helps an athlete kick a ball, push off when walking or running, and maintain balance. When excessive force is applied to the great toe, such as forced flexion or extension, the ligaments can be sprained. Some sports medicine specialists believe that artificial turf causes more great-toe sprains than real grass does. Regardless of the cause, the athlete will experience pain, swelling, discoloration, and the inability to walk or run normally. The AT will recommend rest, ice, compression, and elevation. (See chapter 16 for more information about treating acute injuries.) When the athlete returns to action, the great toe can be taped and padded to provide support and decrease pain.

Arch Sprain (Metatarsal and Longitudinal)

An arch sprain can be caused by running on a hard surface, wearing improper footwear, or subjecting the foot to repetitive stress. The athlete will report significant pain over the involved arch and will experience difficulty walking or running. An injury to the longitudinal arch will result in pain at the medial aspect of the foot. An injury to the metatarsal arch, on the other hand, will result in pain at the ball of the foot, just proximal to the toes (see figure 15.2). During the assessment the AT will notice swelling and possibly some discoloration over the plantar surface. PRICES is the best way to handle an arch sprain. The application of an arch pad may relieve some of the pain because the foot flattens somewhat during walking or running. The athlete should strengthen the arch by exercising the muscles of the foot and by stretching the Achilles tendon.

The arches of the foot are created by the contour of the bony structure and supported by thick connective tissue called *fascia*. The fascia itself can also become inflamed; this is called *plantar fasciitis*.

Plantar Fasciitis

The plantar aspect of the foot has a thick, tough layer of fascia that can become injured with chronic stress. **Plantar fasciitis** begins with tenderness at the bottom of the calcaneus and progresses toward the toes. A heel cup is often used along with stretching of the gastrocnemius and soleus muscles; stretching of the plantar muscles of the foot is also helpful. Rest is an important intervention, as is arch support, or orthotics if the condition doesn't resolve. Another treatment option is using a night splint. A night splint keeps the foot dorsiflexed so the plantar fascia stays in a slightly stretched position.

In some instances the plantar fascia can pull on the calcaneous and cause a **heel spur**. When the plantar fascia pulls on the calcaneus, it causes a small disruption in the bone that the body attempts to repair. The body repairs the bone where it is stressed, and the bony repair is shaped like a thorn on a plant. The heel spur may start to dig into existing soft tissue and cause more pain and tenderness. A heel cup or pad can distribute the pressure around the spur, but in some instances the area may need to be injected with an anti-inflammatory medication by a physician.

Lateral and Medial Ankle Sprains

One of the enemies of athletic participation is the ankle sprain. About 85% of ankle sprains are caused by excessive inversion. Only about 15% of ankle sprains occur because the ankle is excessively everted. The reason for this difference is twofold—

The Real World

A football player complained of feeling a pop in his right lower leg during the first half of a football game. We examined him and found he had full range of motion and strength of the right lower extremity, so he completed the game. In the training room after the game we examined him again. He complained of pain in the lateral calf, and again he had full range of motion and strength in the leg with pain over the proximal and distal fibula. We placed him on crutches with instructions to avoid putting any weight on the leg and to call if the pain increased. He called that evening, saying he was in the greatest pain that he had ever been in. We told him to go to the emergency room. His X rays were negative for a fracture, but he had increased pressure in the anterior and lateral compartments of his lower leg. He had surgery that night to relieve the pressure in each compartment. The anterior release was without complications, but when the lateral release was performed, the doctors found a major complication—a tear in a muscle, specifically the peroneus longus.

Phil Voorhis, MSEd, ATC

first, the deltoid ligament is much stronger than the lateral ligaments, and second, the fibula prevents severe eversion.

When the ankle inverts, the lateral ligaments are injured. The severity of the injury will depend upon the amount of force, the amount of taping, the type of shoe, and the strength of the muscles. During excessive eversion, the deltoid ligament will be injured.

Ankle injuries must be evaluated to determine their severity. Therefore, the shoe must be removed, and the sock must be cut off or removed. Upon examination of the ankle the AT may observe swelling and discoloration. He will determine the severity of injury based on the athlete's ability to move the ankle. If there is no decreased range of motion or strength, the athlete may be allowed to play with the ankle protected by a special brace or tape. Any decrease in range of motion will be treated with PRICES. A referral to the team physician is necessary when there is crepitus, rapid swelling, or bony deformity, because a fracture is likely in any of those instances.

Another type of ankle sprain is the syndesmosis sprain. This injury is also called a *high ankle sprain*.

What Would You Do If...

A hockey player with an ankle sprain tells you that she does not need the help of an AT. She intends to use kerosene applications twice a day.

The **syndesmosis** is the structure that binds the distal end of the tibia and fibula together, and when the ankle is either severely everted, or rotated, the talus can force the tibia and fibula to spread apart and sprain the ankle. Syndesmotic ankle sprains often take longer to heal.

Ankle Dislocation

An ankle dislocation can occur either anteriorly or posteriorly. An anterior dislocation occurs when the heel of the foot strikes the ground forcefully. A posterior dislocation occurs with a blow to the anterior aspect of the leg while the ankle is in plantar flexion. The athlete will be in obvious pain and will refuse to move or allow the foot to be touched. There will be deformity and an inability to use the foot. Swelling will rapidly appear. It is important to act quickly in the case of an ankle dislocation. The AT should call 911, splint the lower leg and ankle, apply ice, and remove the athlete from the field. In addition to damaging the ligaments, nerves and blood vessels can be injured; this means a physician must put the bones back in place.

Tissue Injuries

The weight-bearing lower extremities are prone to various tissue injuries. These include contusions, toe injuries, and anterior compartment syndrome.

Contusions

Soccer and field hockey players are prone to contusions of the lower leg—thus the invention of the shin guard. The impact of a ball, stick, or foot on the shin will cause swelling, pain, and discoloration. The athlete may limp and have limited range of motion. The AT will recommend ice and rest until full range of motion is restored. The athlete will need additional padding, such as a donut, to protect the area from further impacts.

Toe Abnormalities

Toe deformities, such as **hammertoes** (see figure 15.6), can become a problem for athletes. A hammertoe means that the middle joint of the toe is flexed and the metatarsal phalangeal and distal phalangeal joints are hyperextended. This deformity can become a problem, especially if a callus forms at the top of the flexed joint. **Hallux valgus**, also known as a **bunion**, is caused by excessive valgus stress (pressure toward the midline of the body) at the great toe (see figure 15.7). This deformity is often caused by poorly fitting footwear, usually shoes that are too tight. A common toe injury is an **ingrown toenail** (see figure 15.8) whereby the nail grows

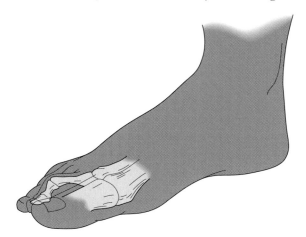

Figure 15.6   Hammertoe.

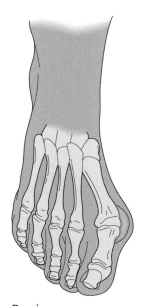

Figure 15.7   Bunion.

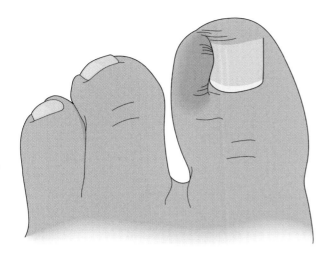

Figure 15.8 Ingrown toenail.

into the surrounding soft tissue. Ingrown toenails are often the result of poor trimming of the nail, such as trimming in a rounded fashion rather than straight across or trimming the nail too short. In severe instances, a physician may need to extract a portion of the nail to reduce pain and inflammation.

Heel Bruises

Beneath the calcaneus exists a thick fat pad that helps to absorb shock as we walk. If there is too much impact on the heel, a contusion can result. This heel bruise is debilitating because we strike with our heel first as we walk and the fat pad is tender when it is bruised. The area must be treated with ice and padded to help absorb shock to give it time to heal.

Anterior Compartment Syndrome

Anterior compartment syndrome is sometimes mistaken for shin splints, but as the name implies, it is an anterior compartment injury. The muscles to the anterior aspect of the tibia are enclosed in connective tissue. When the tissue in the compartment swells due to overuse or a severe impact, the swelling increases the pressure on the connective tissue, which causes severe pain that increases with activity and does not subside when there is no activity. The AT will note heat, red skin, loss of foot motion, and hardness of the area. An inability to move the foot and severe pain are critical indicators of this problem. The athlete must be seen by a physician immediately to prevent nerve damage from the pressure. The physician will make an incision in the leg to relieve the pressure, and the athlete can return to activity while wearing a supportive brace or bandage.

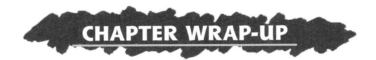

CHAPTER WRAP-UP

Summary

In addition to fractures, sprains, and strains, injuries caused by stress and overuse are common in the lower leg, foot, and ankle. The bones, ligaments, and tendons must be aligned to prevent injury and to allow the joints to function. PRICES is used to care for injuries of the lower extremity. Proper footwear and good hygiene are necessary for preventing toe abnormalities.

Key Terms

Define the following terms found in this chapter:

Achilles tendon	ingrown toenail	plantar surface
bunion	Jones fracture	shin splints
calcaneus	lateral malleolus	soleus
gastrocnemius	medial malleolus	syndesmosis
hallux valgus	metatarsals	talus
hammertoe	phalanges	tendinitis
heel spur	plantar fasciitis	

Questions for Review

1. On an anatomical picture of the foot, label the anatomical structures discussed in this chapter.
2. What area of the ankle is vulnerable to sprain and strain injuries?
3. List all of the injuries that can happen as a result of an inversion of the ankle.
4. Make a list of ways to care for the feet that are critical in the prevention of injury.
5. Why are there more lateral than medial ankle sprains?
6. Crepitus over the Achilles tendon is a sign of what injury?
7. What causes medial tibial stress syndrome?

Activities for Reinforcement

1. Volunteer to work in a local podiatrist's office for an afternoon. What types of athletic injuries does the podiatrist regularly treat?
2. Spray the bottom of your foot with water and make an imprint on a paper towel. What type of plantar arch do you have? Is it the same as any of your classmates' plantar arches?
3. Visit one of the following Web sites and review the anatomy of the foot, ankle, and lower leg:

    www.sportsinjuryclinic.net/cybertherapist/front/ankle/ankleanatomy.php

    www.human-anatomy.net/anatomy-foot-pictures.html

    www.human-anatomy.net/anatomy-ankle-pictures.html

    www.scoi.com/anklanat.htm

Above and Beyond

1. Write a report on one of the following subjects, including the prevention, cause, treatment, and rehabilitation of the condition:
    - Plantar fasciitis
    - Anterior compartment syndrome
2. Using the resources listed in the following activity, write a report on one of these topics:
    - Orthotics and their uses
    - Walking and running gaits
3. Using one of the following Web sites or journal articles, write a report about a specific ankle or lower-leg injury:

    www.apma.org/

    http://podiatrychannel.com/ankleinjuries/

    Bauer, A., E. Bluman, M. Wilson, and C. Chiodo. 2009. Injuries of the distal lower extremity syndesmosis. *Current Orthopaedic Practice* 20(2): 111-116.

    Connor, C. 2003. Injury management update: use of an ultrasonic bone-growth stimulator to promote healing of a Jones fracture. *Athletic Therapy Today* 8(1): 37-39.

    Hadzic, V., T. Sattler, E. Topole, Z. Jarnovic, H. Burger, and E. Dervisevic. 2009. Risk factors for ankle sprain in volleyball players: a preliminary analysis. *Isokinetics and Exercise Science* 17(3): 155-160.

Mullen, J.E., and M.J. O'Malley. 2004. Sprains: residual instability of subtalar, Lisfranc joints, and turf toe. *Clinics in Sports Medicine* 23(1): 97-121.

Palmer, D. 2007. Assessment and management of patients with Achilles tendon rupture. *Advanced Emergency Nursing Journal* 29(3): 249-259.

Pease, J., M. Miller, and R. Gumoc. 2009. An easily overlooked injury: Lisfranc fracture. *Military Medicine* 174(6): 645-646.

Pohl, M., J. Hamill, and I. Davis, I. 2009. Biomechanical and anatomic factors associated with a history of plantar fasciitis in female runners. *Clinical Journal of Sport Medicine* 19(5): 372-376.

Refshauge, K., J. Raymond, S. Kilbreath, L. Pengel, and I. Heijnen. 2009. The effect of ankle taping on detection of inversion-eversion movements in participants with recurrent ankle sprain. *American Journal of Sports Medicine* 37(2): 371-375.

Thorogood, L. 2003. Proprioception exercises following ankle sprain. *Emergency Nurse* 11(8): 33-36.

Ubell, M.L., J.P. Boylan, J.A. Ashton-Miller, and E.M. Wojtys. 2003. The effect of ankle braces on the prevention of dynamic forced ankle inversion. *American Journal of Sports Medicine* 31(6): 935-940.

Vela, L., T.W. Tourville, and J. Hertel. 2003. Physical examination of acutely injured ankles: an evidence-based approach. *Athletic Therapy Today* 8(5): 13-19, 36-37.

Weaver, T.D., M.V. Ton, and T.V. Pham. 2004. Ingrowing toenails: management practices and research outcomes. *International Journal of Lower Extremity Wounds* 3(1): 22-34.

UNIT VI

Rehabilitation and Reconditioning of Athletics-Related Injuries

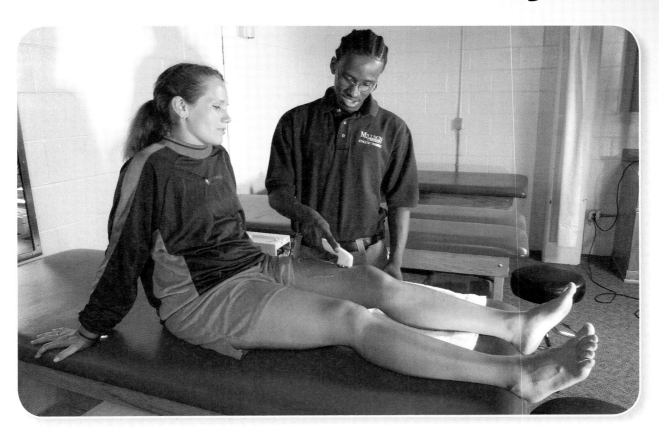

Patient Assessment and Treatment Methods

Objectives

Upon completing this chapter, the student will be able to do the following:

- Describe the components of a SOAP note for medical documentation and explain how it relates to the rehabilitation program.
- Identify the elements of physical function that should be included in a comprehensive therapeutic exercise program.
- Explain how to develop a therapeutic exercise program.
- Define passive, active–assistive, and active range of motion.
- Compare muscular strength and endurance and explain how to develop each.
- Compare and contrast therapeutic modalities and explain the benefits of each.

ATs understand that exercise is the most important aspect of a rehabilitation program. A logical and effective rehabilitation program, however, can only take shape after a logical and effective assessment of the problem. After assessment, the AT needs to formulate a problem list, establish rehabilitation goals, develop a treatment plan, and continually reassess the athlete's progress.

ASSESSING THE ATHLETE AND DOCUMENTING THE FINDINGS

Once an assessment is completed, a **SOAP note** will be written to document the findings. The SOAP note is a clean (no pun intended!), systematic way of documenting the assessment findings and recording an athlete's progress through a rehabilitation program. The acronym *SOAP* stands for **s**ubjective, **o**bjective, **a**ssessment, and **p**lan of action. We discuss each type of information next, and you can see a sample SOAP note in figure 16.1.

- *Subjective.* Detailed information about the history of the injury and the athlete should be recorded as well as chief complaints, signs, and symptoms. This information will be referred to in the future when following up on the injury. Subjective information is gathered by the AT, and it is only as good as the information given by the athlete.

- *Objective.* The objective data are a record of test measurements. Here the AT will state the information gained from inspection, palpation, and special tests.

- *Assessment.* In this portion of the SOAP note, the AT will state the type and severity of the injury and list problems associated with the injury. The statements should describe functional deficits resulting from the injury. The problems should be clearly and concisely identified. The AT should keep in mind that the goals of treatment are based on this list of problems.

Commonly identified problems include lack of range of motion, lack of strength, inability to perform certain functional movements, and pain with particular motions or activities. Developing a list of problems allows the AT to determine what needs to be corrected so that an athlete can return to participation as quickly and safely as possible. Once the AT understands what needs to be corrected, a plan of action can be developed.

- *Plan of action.* Here the AT will describe whether the athlete will be referred, treated, or monitored. Any rehabilitation procedures will be documented as well as the goals of the treatment.

Just as many of us have academic goals (e.g., getting an *A* in an athletic training and sports medicine class) and career goals (e.g., becoming an AT), an injured athlete must have rehabilitation goals. Therapeutic exercise goals must be both short and long term. In other words, one set of activities should be possible to achieve relatively soon, and another set should be achieved later in

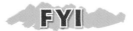

Therapeutic

The word *therapeutic* is used to describe something that has healing properties. In this case, a therapeutic exercise program means that the exercises help heal the body.

the program. The established goals should reflect the list of problems from the injury assessment, be objective, and have specific time frames. Moreover, the athlete should be involved with the goal setting, and her sport should be considered. Certainly a competitive bowler's goals will be different from a football player's goals.

PHASES OF TREATMENT

The extent of the injury and the phases of tissue healing should influence the selection of activities and goals to be included in the plan of action. Each program that is developed will follow a step-by-step **progression** that first attempts to control the initial response to the injury and then focuses on developing the elements of physical function. The elements of physical function that should be addressed in a therapeutic exercise program are

1. mobility,
2. flexibility,
3. proprioception,
4. muscular strength,
5. muscular endurance,
6. muscular power,
7. cardiorespiratory endurance, and
8. sport-specific function.

These elements allow athletes to be functional in their chosen sport.

Think of the phases of treatment as the IMPRESS program (see figure 16.2): **i**nitial injury phase, **m**obility restoration phase, **p**roprioception phase, **r**esistance training phase, **e**ndurance training phase, and **s**port-**s**pecific function phase. Athletes should always try to maintain their cardiorespiratory endurance as much as possible during the program.

Athletic Injury and Accident Report

Athlete's name: Jane Doe _____ Today's date: _6-1-11_ Injury date: _5-28-11_

Body part injured: ☒ L ☐ R _Ankle_____ Sport: _Cross country_____

Injury due to participation: ☒ Y ☐ N Other: _____

Subjective Information

Mechanism of injury: _The athlete reports having stepped in a hole while running. She believes she turned her ankle inward. She recalls hearing a popping sound._

Chief complaint: _Pain on lateral aspect of ankle, especially with walking. She reports an inability to walk with full weight on ankle._

Pain: _Pain rated as a 4 on a 0-10 scale. Pain is described as dull pain that becomes sharp when bearing weight._

Other: _The athlete reports having iced her ankle immediately for 30 minutes and applying an elastic wrap to the area. She saw her primary care physician on 5-29-11. An X ray was taken and no fracture was reported. Her physician recommended rehabilitation with the school's certified AT._

Objective Information

Inspection (observation): _Mild swelling is visible on the lateral malleolus; discoloration at lateral ankle, just below fibula._

Palpation: _Tenderness at distal fibular and sinus tarsi; no crepitus, warmth, or deformities noted._

Range of motion: _Plantar flexion—within normal limits; eversion—within normal limits; inversion—limited (9°); dorsiflexion—limited (11°)._

Strength: _Plantar flexion—normal; inversion—normal; eversion—fair; dorsiflexion—fair._
Neurological exam: Normal.

Special tests: _Anterior drawer—negative; bump test—negative; compression test—negative._

Girth: _Distal lower leg at malleoli 24.5 cm (left) and 21 cm (right)._

Functional testing: _Balance test limited to 10 seconds on involved limb compared with 45 seconds of uninvolved limb. The athlete walked without a limp in a straight line but began limping when attempting to walk in a lazy S fashion. Functional testing was stopped at that time._

Assessment

Disposition: _First-degree inversion ankle sprain with resulting weakness, swelling, and loss of function_

List of problems: _(1) Weakness of ankle musculature, (2) swelling, (3) abnormal gait, (4) lack of balance, (5) decreased range of motion_

(continued)

Figure 16.1 Sample SOAP note.

Plan of Action

Initial treatment: <u>Ice, compression, elevation 20 minutes. Athlete instructed to rest the area and maintain compression; also fitted for crutches and instructed in the use of crutch walking.</u>

The athlete will be: ❏ Referred to physician ❏ Referred to school nurse ☒ Treated by certified AT

Treatment will be: <u>__4__</u> days per week for <u>__3__</u> weeks

Treatment to consist of: <u>Ice application, strengthening exercises, and functional activity as tolerated. The area is to be iced postexercise.</u>

Short-term goals to be completed in <u>__1__</u> week(s): <u>(1) Eliminate swelling, (2) attain normal dorsiflexion and inversion ROM, (3) be able to walk in lazy S and Z pattern, (4) improve balance to 30 seconds, (5) reduce pain to 2 rating.</u>

Intermediate goals to be completed in <u>__1__</u> week(s): <u>Walk without aid of crutches.</u>

Long-term goals to be completed in <u>__2__</u> week(s): <u>(1) Obtain normal strength for all movements; (2) jog straight, lazy S, and Z patterns; (3) eliminate pain; (4) improve balance to normal.</u>

Long-term goals to be completed in <u>__3__</u> week(s): <u>(1) Run lazy S and Z pattern, (2) sprint lazy S and Z pattern, (3) return to practice.</u>

Parents contacted: ☒ Yes Date: <u>__6-1-11__</u>   ❏ No Explain: _____

Signature: <u>I. Train, ATC</u>

Figure 16.1   *(continued)*

Although we have presented these phases of therapeutic exercises as a step-by-step process, in practice the progression is not quite so clear. Each athlete is different and progresses at a different pace. For example, some people may be able to begin light strengthening exercises prior to the establishment of full flexibility. The sports medicine team will work with injured athletes to integrate them into practices before the establishment of full strength. Perhaps the most important thing to remember as a future AT is to be as progressive as you can when rehabilitating an athlete, but never do anything that would cause harm.

Initial Injury Phase

In the initial phase of treatment, the AT's primary goal is to control the amount of inflammation. Inflammation results from the body's response to

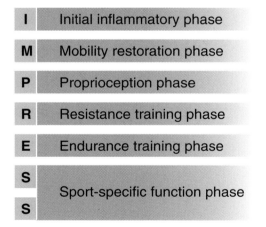

Figure 16.2   IMPRESS program for organizing a rehabilitation program.

an injury and is characterized by warmth, redness, swelling, and pain. It is the mechanism by which damaged tissue begins to return to normal. Although inflammation is necessary for tissue healing to occur, if it gets out of hand, chronic inflammation can result.

Pain can significantly interfere with a person's ability to function. It results from an initial injury or trauma, particularly when nerve tissue is damaged. Even if nerve tissue is not directly damaged, pain can indicate that tissue damage has occurred. During the inflammatory process the body releases chemicals that irritate nerve tissue; the swelling that results from the inflammatory process can put pressure on nerves, resulting in pain. Also, because the perception of pain warns the body of tissue damage, the body guards against further injury by causing muscle spasm. Muscle spasm itself can cause pain and thus a pain–spasm–pain cycle occurs.

Controlling inflammation in the initial phase is accomplished by preventing further damage, reducing swelling, reducing pain, and reducing edema. As we discuss in chapter 20, the critical treatment in this phase is PRICES. The injured area must be **p**rotected, **r**ested, **i**ced, **c**ompressed, **e**levated and **s**upported.

Mobility Restoration Phase

Once inflammation is controlled—as characterized by improved comfort and decreased swelling, **edema** (a thick swelling caused by excessive serous protein), and pain—joint mobility can be restored. This is done with therapeutic exercises that progress from passive range of motion to active–assistive range of motion to active range of motion. Once range of motion is back to normal, flexibility training can begin.

Restoring Range of Motion

There are three phases in restoring normal range of motion:

1. *Passive.* When the AT moves an athlete's body segment through the range of motion and

> ### The Real World
>
> When I worked at a physical therapy clinic, I helped rehabilitate a patient who had just had minor knee surgery. His physician gave us orders to accelerate him through the program because the patient was getting married in three weeks and planned to snow ski in Lake Tahoe, Nevada. The athlete worked hard and was very compliant. By the second week he had gained full range of motion and normal strength in his knee. His balance and proprioception continued to improve, and by the time he was ready to leave for his wedding, his knee was fully functional. It just goes to show you that when an athlete is motivated, he can accomplish anything.
>
> **Anonymous**

the athlete simply relaxes and produces no muscle contractions, **passive range of motion (PROM)** is being performed. Early pain-free PROM performed for an injury has been shown to be beneficial for tissue healing. However, PROM should not be done if it causes pain. In fact, most exercises should be done using pain as a guide—if the athlete complains of pain, the exercise should be stopped. PROM is most often used to keep the soft-tissue structures from becoming too tight following an injury.

2. *Active–assistive.* When the AT and the athlete move a body segment through the range of motion together, it is termed **active–assistive range of motion (AAROM)**. This is done when an injured athlete is strong enough (and pain is no longer a problem) to produce a muscle contraction but not strong enough to move the joint through a full range of motion by herself. AAROM should also use pain as a guide.

3. *Active.* When an athlete can move a body segment through a full range of motion without assistance, she is performing **active range of motion (AROM)**. AROM is necessary before strengthening of the joint can begin. Once AROM is established, flexibility training can begin.

Establishing Flexibility

For an injured athlete, restoring mobility means getting his flexibility back to normal. Note that range of motion and flexibility are not the same. **Flexibility** refers to the ability to move a joint through a full range of motion without restriction. Normal flexibility is needed for the body to function properly. In order to have normal range of motion, an athlete must have flexibility of the soft-tissue structures around a joint, including muscles, tendons, and skin. To develop flexibility, stretching exercises are often employed. These are covered in detail in chapter 17.

Proprioception Phase

Proprioception is the body's ability to get information to the brain in response to a stimulus arising within the body; it also refers to the body's ability to sense the position of its limbs at any moment. For example, an athlete who has gone airborne and then lands on an opponent's foot may injure her ankle if her brain does not sense that she is landing on someone's shoe and not the floor. Without proper proprioception, the body may not get the right muscles to fire at the right time to protect a joint. Because an athlete may have deficient proprioception due to an injury, many ATs believe that proprioception should be addressed in the early stages of a therapeutic exercise program, and thus many rehabilitation programs emphasize early proprioceptive training.

Proprioceptive training can be started early in a therapeutic exercise program by doing activities such as balance or coordination exercises.

Resistance Training Phase

Many programs can be used to improve an athlete's strength, or ability to exert force against a resistance, following an injury. When performing **resistance training**, not only will the muscles become stronger,

What Would You Do If...

You are assisting the AT in the athletic training room, and an athlete who has been doing extensive rehabilitation of her knee approaches you. She is disappointed that she is not allowed to return to practice even though she has normal range of motion and normal strength.

but surrounding tissues such as the ligaments and bone will become stronger as well. Resistance training thus is a significant phase in the rehabilitation process. It can be done in a variety of ways, including using free weights, resistive tubing, machines, and manual resistance. We cover resistance training in detail in chapter 17.

Endurance Phase

In addition to establishing or maintaining cardiorespiratory endurance, muscular endurance must be addressed. Not only do muscles need to be strong for athletic participation, they also need to have **endurance**, or the ability to perform movements over time. Cardiorespiratory exercises should be performed as early as possible as long as the injury is not aggravated. Developing muscle endurance with weight training often involves performing a high number of repetitions with a low amount of weight.

Sport-Specific Function Phase

A therapeutic exercise program is not complete unless the athlete is fully prepared to meet the demands of his sport. In this phase of the therapeutic exercise program, the athlete performs functional activities and is slowly integrated back into practices. Thus, it is necessary that the AT be fully aware of the requirements of the sport, the movement patterns involved, and the degree of strength, speed, power, and endurance needed for the athlete to be successful.

The **sport-specific function** phase is marked by activities that mimic those the athlete will perform on the playing field or court. Athletes are required to run, jump, cut, and throw. They should generally progress from light functional exercises to heavy functional exercises and then to limited practice. Practices are often restricted, and the athlete can participate only if she has full range of motion, normal strength, normal flexibility, normal coordination, normal cardiorespiratory endurance, and the consent of the team physician.

THERAPEUTIC MODALITIES

Although the essential element of any rehabilitation program is exercise, many athletes cannot perform even minimally because their injuries become too painful or swollen. If the injured part is not used, however, the muscles may weaken and further complications may arise. To decrease pain and help with normal recovery, the AT will use therapeutic modalities.

Therapeutic modalities include heat, cold, ultrasound, and electrical muscle stimulation. They can be categorized as thermal, mechanical, or electrical. All therapeutic modalities must be used with extreme caution and often only when prescribed by a physician.

Therapeutic modalities that require an electrical charge must be inspected annually to make sure they are operating properly. This entails having a bioelectrical technician inspect the modalities to make sure they meet the minimal safety standards.

Thermal Elements

Thermal elements transfer heat either into or out of body tissue. They are used to make the tissue either colder or warmer. The indications and contraindications for thermal modalities can be found in table 16.1.

Heating Modalities

Heating modalities warm the body tissue to create a specific physiological response that helps the healing process. Heating modalities should only be used after the initial inflammatory response to injury is finished. Chronic (long-lasting) sprains and strains are injuries commonly treated with heat. Increasing the tissue temperature causes an increase in blood flow and in tissue extensibility,

Table 16.1 Indications and Contraindications for Thermal Modalities

Type of modality	Indications	Contraindications	Precautions*
Heat	Chronic inflammatory conditions	Acute injuries	Heart disease
	Joint contracture	Areas with sensory deficits	
	Tightened tissue	Areas with circulation deficits	
	Chronic pain	Areas over tumors	
	Chronic muscle spasm	Peripheral vascular disease	
		Open wounds	
Cold	Acute injuries	Cold-related allergies	Areas with superficial nerves
	Pain	Open wounds	Areas with circulation deficits
	Swelling	Cardiovascular problems (heart disease)	
	Preparation for exercise	Areas with sensory deficits	
	Muscle spasms	Cold hypersensitivity	
	Inflammation	High blood pressure	
		Respiratory problems	
		Advanced diabetes or peripheral vascular disease	
		Infection	

*Precautions means you can use the modality with extreme caution.
Note: Disagreement exists among some experts as to whether modalities are contraindicated or can be used with caution.
Data obtained from Starkey (2004), Prentice (2009), Denegar, Saliba & Saliba (2010).

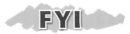

Indications

Indications are reasons why a modality can be used on the body.

Contraindications

Contraindications are reasons why a modality should not be used for treatment.

which helps to increase range of motion, increase healing potential, and reduce swelling. Heating modalities should not be used on acute injuries, areas of poor or impaired circulation, or areas of impaired sensation.

One of the most common heating modalities is a moist-heat pack such as the hydrocollator pack (see figure 16.3). These canvas packs are filled with a gel that retains heat after being activated in hot water. The packs are to be placed on an athlete only after they are wrapped in several layers of towels or placed in a special premade cover; otherwise they may cause burns.

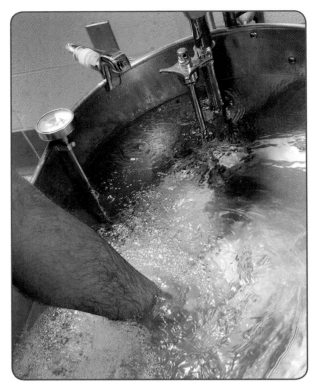

Figure 16.4   Whirlpool application to the leg.

A warm **whirlpool** is another common method of heating the tissue (see figure 16.4). Whirlpool application to an arm or leg can be performed for up to 20 minutes at a temperature ranging between 95° and 108° Fahrenheit (35-42 °C). The same contraindications apply for whirlpools as for hot packs. Further, the whirlpool should not be turned on or off while the athlete is in the water, and the athlete receiving treatment should be in view at all times (there is the possibility of electrocution or drowning if precautions are not taken). The athlete should not be placed in a whirlpool if the water turbulence irritates his injury, if he has skin conditions or infected areas, or if he has a fever.

A **paraffin bath** is commonly used when treating the hands or the feet. Because these body regions are uneven, the area is dipped in the liquefied paraffin and removed until the wax hardens on the skin (see figure 16.5). This is repeated 6 to 12 times and then the body part is wrapped with a plastic bag and surrounded by layers of towels. The parrafin is kept on the body for 20 minutes and then peeled off.

Modalities that heat the tissue are often used to prepare the area for stretching or range-of-motion exercises.

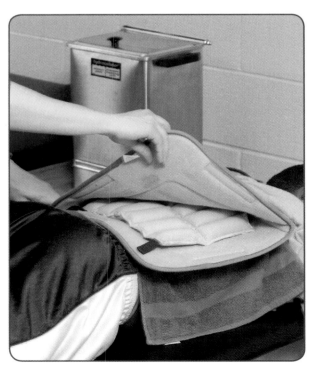

Figure 16.3   A hydrocollator pack being applied to an athlete. Note the extra layers of towels used to keep the back from getting too hot.

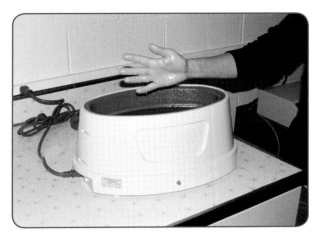

Figure 16.5 Paraffin bath showing a hand that was dipped into the wax and removed, allowing the wax to harden. This step is repeated 6 to 12 times.

Photo courtesy of Lorin Cartwright

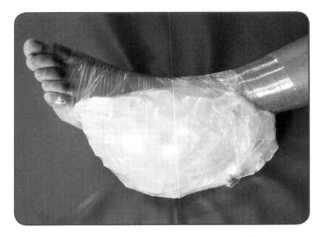

Figure 16.6 Ice packs are used for many injuries.

Cooling Modalities

Cooling modalities cool the injured tissue, which constricts (narrows) blood vessels, decreases inflammation, decreases cell metabolism, decreases pain, and decreases muscle spasm. Although cooling modalities are most commonly used to treat acute injures such as sprains and strains, they are also used during the rehabilitation process to decrease pain, thus allowing an injured athlete to perform exercises. **Cryotherapy** is the use of cold on the body to elicit specific physiological responses.

The most common cooling modality is the ice pack (see figure 16.6). Crushed or cubed ice in a plastic bag molds itself around injured body parts and can be easily secured in place. Ice packs should not be applied too tightly with an elastic wrap, and although the risk of frostbite is low, the athlete should be checked regularly. Cold should not be applied over open wounds, to areas of numbness, to someone who is overly sensitive to cold, or to an athlete who has cardiac or respiratory problems. The ice pack is applied for 20 to 30 minutes. When treating an acute injury, take the ice pack off after each 20- to 30-minute application and wait approximately 40 to 60 minutes before reapplying it. In other words, the ice is left off for twice the amount of time it was applied to the injured area. If the ice is left on too long, it can injure the skin or muscles.

What Would You Do If...

An athlete who injured his ankle yesterday has just entered the training room. He gets a hot pack and places it on his ankle.

Chemical cold packs are also popular because they can be stored in a freezer and reused. The AT must be careful, however, because chemical cold packs often get colder than 32° Fahrenheit (0 °C) and could freeze tissue. When using such packs, the AT will be sure to place a barrier such as a towel between the pack and the skin surface. It is also helpful to check the skin several times during the application to make sure the athlete is not breaking out in a rash or developing blisters. Finally, the AT should check to make sure the pack is not leaking—if it is, it should not be used.

Another common cooling method is an ice massage (see figure 16.7). Ice massage is performed by freezing water in a paper cup and then tearing the cup to expose the ice. The ice is then massaged over the injury site. Ice massage is not appropriate for acute injuries, but it is very helpful when treating chronic injuries after exercise.

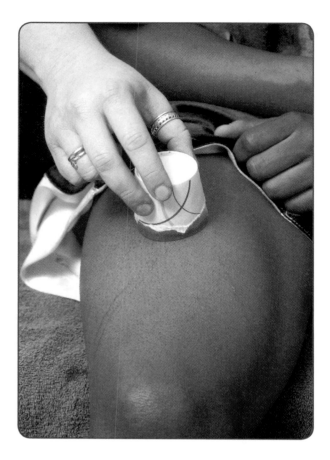

Figure 16.7   Ice massage.

Mechanical Elements

Mechanical elements produce a specific physiological effect with mechanical energy. They include ultrasound (acoustical energy), traction, massage, and intermittent compression devices. Indications and contraindications of mechanical elements can be found in table 16.2.

Ultrasound

Ultrasound may be categorized as a thermal modality because it can produce a deep-heating effect, but it can also cause nonthermal reactions in the tissue. As sound waves pass through the tissue, heat is produced through a process known as conversion. If the sound waves are sporadic or intermittent, heat may not be produced. Ultrasound waves are extremely high frequency and cannot be heard by the human ear. Figure 16.8 shows ultrasound application.

Common ultrasound frequencies used in treating athletic injuries include 1 megahertz (MHz), 2 MHz, and 3 MHz. These are much higher frequencies than the human voice can produce. The frequency, not the amount of intensity, determines the depth of penetration of sound waves into the tissue. The 1 MHz frequency penetrates deeper than the 3 MHz. Therefore, the 3 MHz frequency

Table 16.2   Indications and Contraindications for Mechanical Modalities

Type of modality	Indications	Contraindications
Ultrasound	Chronic inflammation	Areas with circulation deficits
	Acute injuries (nonthermal application)	Areas with sensory deficits
	Chronic injuries	Over tumors
	Muscle strains	Over growth plates in children
	Ligament sprains	Over heart, eyes, or nerve plexus
	Bruises, muscle spasm	Acute injuries, using the continuous heat setting
	Tightened soft tissue	Pregnancy
	Scar tissue	Vascular problems
		Over spinal cord

Type of modality	Indications	Contraindications
Traction	Spinal disk protrusion	Infection of the spine
	Degenerative disk disease	Osteoporosis
	Degenerative joint disease	Malignant tumors
	Soft-tissue stiffness	Acute injuries
	Nerve root compression	Pregnancy
	Muscle spasm	Rheumatoid arthritis
	Joint tightness	Fractured vertebra
	Intervertebral disk pain	Spinal hypermobility
		Cardiopulmonary problems
		Hiatal hernia (lumbar traction)
		Vascular problems
Massage	Promotion of relaxation	Nonunion fracture sites
	Muscle spasm	Over open wounds
	Pain	Over dermatological conditions
	Soft-tissue stiffness	Acute injuries
	When increased circulation is needed	Over tumors
	Edema	
Intermittent compression	Postacute edema	Acute injuries
	Lymphedema	Skin irritation
		When a fracture has not been ruled out
		Peripheral vascular disorders
		Compartment syndromes
		Infection
		Thrombophlebitis

Because machines vary, manufacturers' guidelines should always be followed.

Note: Disagreement exists among some experts as to whether modalities are contraindicated or can be used with caution.

Data obtained from Starkey (2004), Prentice (2009), Denegar, Saliba & Saliba (2010).

may be better suited for injuries that are closer to the surface of the skin.

The effects of heating the tissue with ultrasound are the same as for a hot pack. Ultrasound, however, can affect deeper tissue than a hot pack can. In fact, 1 MHz ultrasound can penetrate up to 5 centimeters of tissue. For the ultrasound to create heat, the machine must be set for a continuous emission—that is, sound waves need to be flowing 100% of the time. A pulsed setting interrupts the flow of sound waves and reduces the thermal effects.

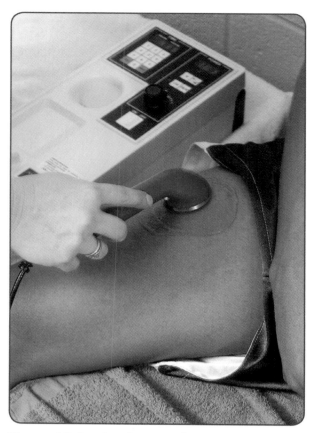

Figure 16.8 An ultrasound treatment provides benefits, but it must be used carefully or it can damage tissue.

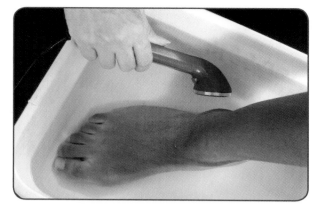

Figure 16.9 Indirect ultrasound application. Ultrasound can be applied underwater. This is especially helpful when the body area being treated is bumpy and the sound head will not stay flat against the tissue.

Traction

Traction is a pulling force. In this context it refers to deliberately attempting to separate the joints of the body if they have been compressed or if they have become stiff over a period of time. It is most commonly done to vertebrae. Traction can be performed to both the cervical and lumbar spine and can be done either mechanically (with a machine) or manually (by the AT). For example, if an AT were given permission by a physician to perform cervical spine traction on an athlete, he would have the athlete lie on her back and he would place one hand under the back of her head, the other under her chin. The AT would then gently pull on the neck to gradually separate the vertebrae. This technique would only be performed with extreme caution and only with a physician's permission.

Not only does traction separate bones that have been pushed too close together, it also causes minimal stretching of the ligaments and muscles in the area. It may also help the resolution of a disk protrusion, which we discussed in chapter 9. It is thought that separating the vertebrae creates a suction force that can cause the protruded disk matter to move toward the center of the disk where it belongs. Additionally, separating the vertebrae opens the space where the nerve roots exit the spinal cord (figure 16.10). By increasing this space, pressure can be removed from the nerve root, helping to decrease pain and facilitate healing.

When applying continuous ultrasound, the AT must move the sound head slowly and continuously. When pulsed ultrasound is applied, the sound head can be kept still. In either case, ultrasound must be applied using a coupling medium such as water, lotion, or gel. When the sound head is applied on the body part through the coupling medium, direct ultrasound is being applied. Direct application should be used only if the area is smooth. Irregularly shaped areas such as the hand, ankle, and elbow may need to have ultrasound applied indirectly (see figure 16.9). Indirect ultrasound is usually applied underwater in a plastic tub. When applying ultrasound underwater, the sound head must be fully immersed and about .5 to 1 inch (1.5-2.5 cm) away from the tissue, and the ultrasound intensity must be increased. There are many contraindications for the use of ultrasound; therefore, it should be used with caution and only when prescribed by a physician. Refer to table 16.2.

Intervertebral disk without traction

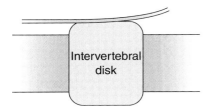

Intervertebral disk with traction. Note how the nerve root is no longer touched by the disk.

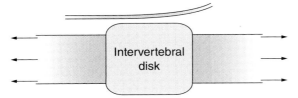

Figure 16.10   The effects of spinal traction. Traction pulls the joints apart and is helpful for relieving pressure on nerve roots at the spinal cord. Traction must be used cautiously and only if all contraindications have been ruled out.

As a precaution, patients should be monitored during their first treatment to ensure that no complications arise, such as increased pain, discomfort, muscle spasm, numbness, or tingling. Also, it is important to perform traction in a quiet area where the patient can relax. The indications and contraindications for cervical and lumbar traction are summarized in table 16.2. A physician should check the athlete before he receives traction and again before he returns to participation.

Massage

Massage is the methodical kneading and stroking of the soft tissues. It is used to increase circulation, decrease muscle spasm, and relieve swelling. If the goal is to decrease swelling, the massage strokes must move from below the injury site toward the heart. Massage strokes include effleurage, petrissage, vibration, percussion, and friction.

Effleurage consists of stroking the tissue with the palm of the hand in a smooth, rhythmical manner (see figure 16.11*a*). Effleurage is often done at the beginning and end of a massage session. **Petrissage** is often described as a kneading of the tissue in which the skin, muscle, and fasciae are squeezed between the hands (see figure 16.11*b*).

A **vibration massage** is designed to cause the tissue to tremble or shake vigorously. Many ATs use a mechanical vibrator to achieve these effects. The vibration technique is usually done at joints to help improve mobility. The **percussion massage**, or tapotement, uses a series of light chopping motions to the tissue. The AT's hands should be relaxed while this stroke is performed. Physiological effects created by the percussion stroke include increased circulation and relaxation (see figure 16.11*c*).

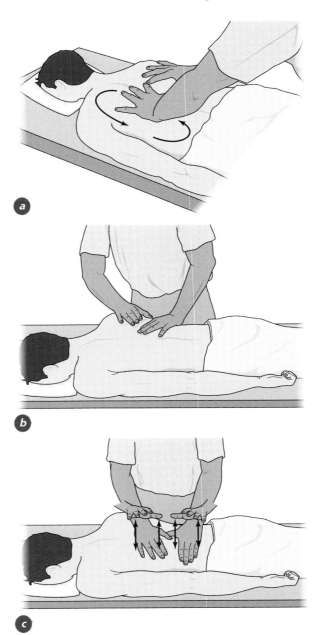

Figure 16.11   *(a)* Effleurage, *(b)* petrissage, and *(c)* percussion or tapotement massage strokes.

Friction massage requires enough pressure to affect the deep tissues. The deep penetration, pressure, and movement of the finger, thumb, or elbow into the tissue have many benefits. For example, friction massage helps to break up scar tissue and relieve muscle spasms. It is an excellent procedure for people who have a thick scar from a deep cut. Indications and contraindications are summarized in table 16.2.

Intermittent Compression

Similar to an elastic wrap, intermittent compression is useful for reducing swelling and edema following an injury (see figure 16.12). An **intermittent compression** device increases the pressure around the injury site and helps venous blood return from the injured extremity, which reduces the total swelling. Although this device is

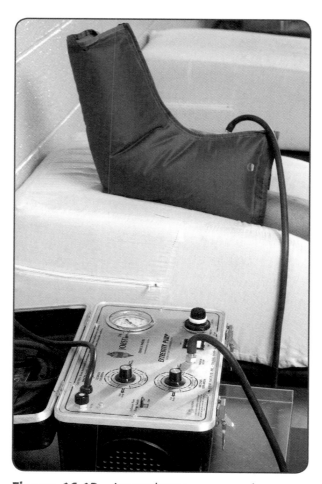

Figure 16.12 Intermittent compression combined with elevation is helpful for removing swelling from an injured joint.

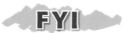

Nerve Root Impingement
A spinal nerve root impingement means that something, such as part of a disk or swelling, is putting pressure on the nerve where it exits the spinal cord.

Diastolic Blood Pressure
The diastolic blood pressure is the pressure in an artery while the heart is relaxed. It is the bottom number of a blood pressure reading.

extremely useful for acute injuries, it should not be used until a fracture has been ruled out, nor should it be used on compartment syndromes of the lower extremity.

Treatment time varies from 20 minutes to an hour. The pressure should not exceed the athlete's diastolic blood pressure, and it should be comfortable. Therefore, the athlete's blood pressure must be taken before the treatment, and his comfort and tolerance of the device should be checked regularly. Generally, the treatment consists of alternating compression for 45 seconds with 15 seconds off. A stocking is used to cover the skin before application to reduce the chance of skin irritation.

Electrical Elements

It may come as a shock to learn that electricity can be therapeutic. Many useful physiological changes occur when electricity is safely passed through tissue. Understanding these changes requires a basic understanding of electricity. Again, we must warn of the dangers that can exist with the use of electrical modalities (see table 16.3). Such modalities should be used only by people who have been trained and only after prescribed by a physician.

Electricity is the flow of electrons (negatively charged particles) through a circuit. A circuit is a path through which electricity flows, such as a wire in a house. Some circuits allow electrons to flow easily whereas other circuits offer more resistance. Given a choice, electricity will always choose the path of least resistance. In the body, the tissues create a circuit. Tissues with high water content, such as muscles, conduct electricity well, whereas bones do not.

Table 16.3   Indications and Contraindications for Electrical Modalities

Indications	Contraindications
Pain	During pregnancy
Edema	When there is an unknown cause of pain
Preventing muscle weakness	Over infected sites
Reducing muscle spasm	Over heart, eyes, carotid sinus, upper airway, wound care, open wounds, or tumors
Reeducating muscle function	Pacemakers
Increasing local circulation	Over some fracture sites

Because machines vary, manufacturers' guidelines should always be followed.

Note: Disagreement exists among some experts as to whether modalities are contraindicated or can be used with caution.

Data obtained from Starkey (2004), Prentice (2009), Denegar, Saliba & Saliba (2010).

The electron flow, or current, moves from a negative pole to a positive pole. Electrical currents can be either direct or alternating. With a **direct current (DC)**, electricity moves in one direction as it passes through the tissue circuit. Picture a simple DC electrical generator with two electrodes (positive and negative) placed on your forearm, one near your wrist and the other near your elbow. If the electrode pad nearest your wrist is the negative pole and the one nearest your elbow is the positive pole, then a direct current of electricity will flow from your wrist to your elbow.

With an **alternating current (AC)**, electricity moves back and forth between electrodes, changing the direction in which it moves through a circuit. The AC generator is sophisticated and is able to switch an electrode from positive to negative. Using the previous example, if an AC current were applied to the body, electricity would constantly change directions between electrodes, moving toward your elbow one moment and toward your wrist the next.

Direct and alternating currents are applied to the body in either an interrupted (i.e., pulsed) or uninterrupted (i.e., continuous) fashion. A pulsed current simply means that the flow of electricity is consistently stopped and restarted. A continuous current is not stopped until the treatment is terminated.

Many types of electrical currents are used during the rehabilitation process, and they all require electrical pads placed on the surface of the skin (see figure 16.13). The type of current used and how it is applied to the body depend on the goals of rehabilitation. For example, an AT may apply electricity to reduce

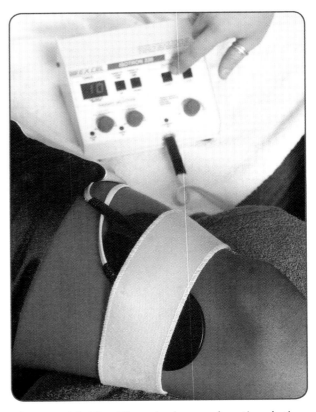

Figure 16.13 Electrical muscle stimulation helps reduce spasm and pain and can also help prevent weakness.

pain, muscle spasm, or swelling, or she may apply it to increase strength and healing potential. Types of electrical stimulation include high-voltage pulsed electrical muscle stimulation, low-intensity stimulation, interferential current, and transcutaneous electrical nerve stimulation.

Passing electrical current over the body can create several physiological effects depending on the type, intensity, and duration of the current. For example, high-voltage pulsed direct stimulation can cause a muscle contraction, which helps prevent a muscle from weakening when recovering from an injury. The muscle contractions can also create a pumping action to reduce swelling and edema. Applying electrical current to the body at an intensity that can be felt but is insufficient for causing a muscle contraction is often helpful for reducing pain. When the muscle is stimulated to contract, it does so without help from the athlete. Although this sounds terrific, it will not make a person physically fit or help him lose weight.

Low-intensity stimulation, also known as microcurrent, introduces a low level of electricity into the tissue; the athlete does not even feel the current passing through the body. Low-intensity stimulation is thought to mimic the body's natural electrical flow and promote tissue healing.

Interferential current is created when two electrical currents cross one another, thus interfering with the flow of electricity. Although this sounds counterproductive, the interference actually creates an appropriate current that stimulates the tissue to create a muscle contraction, thus reducing pain and edema. The majority of treatments to help reduce pain, however, use **transcutaneous electrical nerve stimulation (TENS)**. TENS creates an electrical current that moves across the skin, resulting in a pins-and-needles sensation. This stimulus of the sensory nerves can cause pain to be gated, or stopped in the spinal cord rather than transmitted to the brain where pain perception occurs.

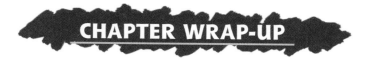

CHAPTER WRAP-UP

Summary

A SOAP note is used to document the findings of an injury assessment as well as to structure a plan of action for a rehabilitation program. In rehabilitation, ATs try to help an athlete regain normal function by regaining mobility, proprioception, strength, endurance, and sport-specific function. To aid the recovery process, ATs use therapeutic modalities such as heat, cold, ultrasound, electricity, and massage.

Key Terms

Define the following terms found in this chapter:

active–assistive range of motion (AAROM)

active range of motion (AROM)

alternating current (AC)

cryotherapy

direct current (DC)

edema

effleurage

endurance

flexibility

friction massage

intermittent compression

massage

paraffin bath

passive range of motion (PROM)

percussion massage

petrissage

progression

proprioception

resistance training

SOAP note

sport-specific function

traction

transcutaneous electrical nerve stimulation (TENS)

ultrasound

vibration massage

whirlpool

Questions for Review

1. What are the elements of physical function that should be redeveloped during rehabilitation of an injured athlete?
2. When should an AT use heat and when should she use cold? Is one more effective than the other?
3. What are some of the physiological effects of ultrasound? When should it not be used?
4. What are the components of a SOAP note, and how are they helpful for designing a rehabilitation program?
5. Explain why an AT would use traction on an athlete's spine.

Activities for Reinforcement

1. Your instructor will create injury scenarios for you and a partner. Take turns pretending to have an injury covered in one of the previous chapters while your partner fills out a SOAP note and develops a therapeutic exercise program to get you back to participating in a sport.
2. With a partner, review each modality discussed in this chapter and think of the types of injuries for which the modality could be used by an AT.
3. Invite an AT to class to discuss the rehabilitation process.
4. Take a class field trip to a rehabilitation center.
5. Work with an AT to create a functional throwing progression for a pitcher.
6. Work with an AT to create a functional progression for a running back.
7. Visit www.sportsinjuryclinic.net and select a link to learn more about treating specific injuries and using various therapeutic modalities.

Above and Beyond

1. Use the Internet to determine what the following conditions are and why some modalities are contraindicated in their treatment: thrombophlebitis, hiatal hernia, osteoporosis, and peripheral vascular disease.
2. Select a specific therapeutic modality from one of the following texts and write a report:

   Denegar, C.R., E. Saliba, and S. Saliba. 2006. *Therapeutic modalities for musculoskeletal injuries.* 2nd ed. Champaign, IL: Human Kinetics.

   Knight, K.L., and D.O. Draper. 2008. *Therapeutic modalities: the art and science.* Philadelphia: Lippincott Williams & Wilkins.

   Prentice, W.E. 2009. *Therapeutic modalities for sports medicine and athletic training.* 6th ed. Boston: McGraw-Hill.

   Starkey, C. 2004. *Therapeutic modalities.* 3rd ed. Philadelphia: FA Davis.

3. Select a rehabilitation topic from one of the following texts and write a one-page report:

   Barh, R., and S. Maehlum, eds. 2004. *Clinical guide to sports injuries: an illustrated guide to the management of injuries in physical activity.* Champaign, IL: Human Kinetics.

   Houglum, P.A. 2010. *Therapeutic exercise for athletic injuries.* 3rd ed. Champaign, IL: Human Kinetics.

   Prentice, W.E. 2011. *Rehabilitation techniques for sports medicine and athletic training.* 5th ed. Boston: McGraw-Hill.

chapter 17

Reconditioning Programs

Objectives

Upon completing this chapter, the student will be able to do the following:

- Explain the principles of strength training.
- Identify the various ways to develop strength.
- Compare muscular strength and endurance and explain how to develop each.
- Discuss the principles behind developing cardiorespiratory fitness.
- Identify appropriate exercises for rehabilitating specific conditions of the upper quarter, lower quarter, and trunk.
- Identify common safety procedures for weight training.

Reconditioning an athlete during rehabilitation is the same as conditioning in the sense that both programs use the same principles. The primary goal of reconditioning is to help the athlete get back to her preinjury level of fitness.

STRENGTH AND CONDITIONING PRINCIPLES

Injured athletes must get fit in order to successfully return to participation; therefore, their physical conditioning must be addressed. As discussed with the IMPRESS program in chapter 16, this includes strength, muscular endurance, cardiorespiratory endurance, and flexibility. Primary principles for strength and conditioning include progressive resistive exercise, overload, and specificity.

Progressive Resistive Exercise

When the goal is to develop an athlete's strength, **progressive resistive exercise (PRE)** is common. PRE involves progressively increasing the load (i.e., weight or number of repetitions) both during the training session and over a period of time. By advancing the resistance training appropriately, further injury can be avoided and the body can adapt to the demands of the activity.

Overload Principle

The **overload principle** means that for muscle to gain strength or endurance, it must be stressed beyond the demands of previous activity. For example, if an athlete bench-presses 50 pounds (23 kg) for 10 repetitions every other day for three weeks, she may not significantly improve her strength because she is not overloading the muscle. However, if she lifts 50 pounds (23 kg) for 10 repetitions one day and then lifts 55 pounds (25 kg) two days later, she probably will stress her muscles beyond the demands of the previous bench press.

Weight is not the only factor we can increase, however. Many variables can be adjusted to overload the muscle, including the frequency of the workouts, the intensity of the exercise, the length of the workout, and the type of exercise performed. The variable changed by the coach or AT will depend on the goal of the exercise. For example, if the athlete requires cardiorespiratory endurance for biking, the amount of time she spends biking during workouts should be increased. If the goal is to develop muscular endurance, she will need to lift less weight for a higher number of repetitions; if the goal is to develop strength, then she should use more weight and fewer repetitions.

Specificity of Training

Specificity means that the body systems will adapt to the specific demands placed on them. For example, if an athlete wants to become a better runner, his training should consist mostly of running. But if he wants to become a better hockey player, his training should consist mostly of hockey and ice-skating activities. When an athlete does nothing more than lift weights, it is doubtful that his body will improve its cardiorespiratory function; likewise, if he only rides a bike, his upper body probably will not become stronger.

In the context of strength training, a muscle gets used to the specific activities required of it. Take the athlete who bench-presses 50 pounds (23 kg) for 10 repetitions every other day for three weeks. Although lifting this amount of weight for the first few days is difficult, it will become easy by the third week. Her muscles will adapt to the specific exercise (bench press) and the demands placed on them (50 pounds for 10 repetitions).

TYPES OF MUSCLE ACTIONS

Muscles function in various ways. At times the muscles must contract simply to hold a joint still and not allow it to move. At other times the muscle must contract to move a limb through a whole motion, such as when a softball player throws a ball. There are three types of muscle actions: isotonic, isometric, and isokinetic. Regardless of which type an athlete performs, the goal is to overload the muscles to produce strength gains.

Isotonics

Isotonic contractions occur when moving a joint through a range of motion with a fixed amount of resistance. Performing an exercise with a free weight is a perfect example. Isotonic resistance training involves movement at the joint, and the muscles shorten and lengthen against resistance. When a muscle shortens against resistance, it is a concentric contraction; when a muscle lengthens against resistance, it is an eccentric contraction. Adolescent athletes should refrain from doing only eccentric weight training because it places a great deal of stress on the muscles and tendons.

Isometrics

When an **isometric contraction** is performed, there is no joint movement. Picture yourself pushing against a brick wall. Although the muscles in your arms and chest contract, no joint motion is produced. Because there is no motion at the joint, the joint is less likely to become irritated or painful. Therefore,

What Would You Do If...

You are asked by the AT to give a message to an athlete who is working out in the weight room. When you enter the weight room, you notice that the athlete is alone, performing a bench press with a weight bar that has about 200 pounds (91 kg) on it.

Resistance Training Progression for Healthy Adults

The ACSM (2009) has the following recommendations:

1. Concentric, eccentric, and isometric muscle actions should be included in a resistance training program.

2. People at the beginner and intermediate levels should use a load of about 65% of what they could lift only one time for an exercise, or **one-repetition maximum (1RM)**. More advanced athletes should use about 90% of 1RM.

3. Beginners should use one to three sets when starting a resistance training program.

4. Both one-sided (unilateral) and two-sided (bilateral) exercises should be performed during training. As an example, flexing one elbow while holding a dumbbell is a unilateral exercise, whereas flexing both elbows while holding a long bar with plates is a bilateral exercise. Also, exercises that use single-joint movements (e.g., only elbow flexion and extension) should be used as well as multijoint movements (e.g., a push-up that not only flexes and extends the elbow but also requires movement at the shoulder joint and scapula).

5. People at the beginner and intermediate levels should use both free-weight exercises and machines, whereas advanced athletes should focus on free weights.

6. Large muscle groups should be trained before small muscle groups. An example is working the deltoid and pectoralis major of the shoulder girdle before exercising the rotator cuff muscles.

7. Multijoint exercises should be performed before single-joint exercises.

8. A two- to three-minute rest between core exercises such as the bench press or squats using high loads is recommended. Only one to two minutes of rest is needed between sets of noncore exercises such as biceps curls.

9. Beginners should use slow to moderate speeds during resistance exercises. Intermediate lifters should use moderate speeds, and advanced athletes should use a variety of speeds, including fast speeds.

10. Novice lifters should exercise two to three days per week, and intermediate athletes should lift four days per week. In instances where an athlete may perform only lower-body exercises one day and upper-body exercises another day (split routine), each major muscle group should be trained twice per week.

The strength training guidelines should be modified for young athletes. The National Strength and Conditioning Association (NSCA) 2009 position statement suggests that for girls up to age 11 and boys up to age 13, the focus should be on proper technique for lifting movements. Also, the NSCA recommends one to three sets of three to six repetitions.

isometric exercises are extremely useful to prevent weakness in the early stages following an injury.

Isokinetics

When an **isokinetic contraction** is performed, speed of movement is controlled. Isokinetics are typically performed using sophisticated equipment that controls the speed at which an athlete will work—no matter how much force he exerts against the machine, he can only make it move at a predetermined speed. It is similar to trying to pull a canoe paddle through the water—you can pull easy or hard, but its speed does not change.

Kinetic Chain Movements

Besides isotonic and isometric contractions, there are other considerations when moving the body. There are times when a limb moves openly in space and other times when it is fixed firmly to the ground.

When you are moving your arm in the air, such as when throwing a baseball, your arm is functioning in an **open kinetic chain**. If you were to place yourself in a push-up position with your hands on the ground and bearing weight, you would be functioning in a **closed kinetic chain**.

As an AT chooses exercises for an injured athlete to perform, deciding whether to include open or closed kinetic chain exercises is important. Often open chain exercises are used early in a rehabilitation program because an athlete is not able to bear her body weight. Later in the program the athlete can bear more weight and closed kinetic chain exercises can be used.

MUSCULAR DEVELOPMENT PROGRAMS

Although many resistance training programs exist, the premise of each is the same. The purpose of such programs is to overload the muscles in a specific manner using isotonic, isokinetic, or isometric movements. However, most muscular development programs use isotonic movements and free weights.

Muscular Strength

Muscular strength is the ability to exert force against a resistance. Developing strength often also leads to developing muscular endurance and power. Generally, an athlete develops strength by using a heavy weight for a low number of repetitions. To accomplish this, the athlete may find it helpful to use a constant set method—that is, using the same amount of weight for the same number of sets and repetitions, such as 40 pounds (18 kg) performed in four sets of four repetitions. The ACSM released a 2009 position statement describing how to progress resistance training programs for healthy adults (see the highlight box on the previous page).

The **DeLorme method** of PRE is an example of an ascending pyramid method. It requires that the athlete perform three sets in a progressive manner. Let's say that the maximum an athlete can military press for 10 repetitions is 200 pounds (91 kg). In the DeLorme method, the 200 pounds is called the *10-repetition maximum* weight, or 10RM, and the athlete does three sets of 10 repetitions at 50%, 75%, and 100% of 10RM. Thus, the athlete would perform the first set of 10 repetitions at 50% of 10RM, or 100 pounds (45 kg). This would be considered a warm-up. He would perform the second set at 150 pounds (68 kg), or 75% of 10RM, for 10 repetitions. The third set would be performed at the maximum weight of 200 pounds (91 kg), which is 100% of 10RM. DeLorme's program of three sets of 10 repetitions continues to be a popular method of strength training.

Another common method of training is the Nautilus method of weight training. In this method, a person performs one set of an exercise to fatigue, or until she can no longer perform the exercise.

The **pyramid method** uses multiple sets (at least three and sometimes up to five or six sets) in which the weight is increased or decreased with each set (see figure 17.1). The athlete may use an ascending pyramid method when she wants to build up to lifting the higher amount of weight with less chance of hurting herself. It is thought that using a descending pyramid technique works the muscle against a higher amount of weight earlier, when it is not as fatigued. Performing multiple sets, for example by doing both sides of a pyramid, is thought to facilitate maximum strength gains. Provided that the muscle is overloaded, however, strength gains can be made regardless of the type of program the athlete follows.

Muscular Endurance

The ability of a muscle to perform repetitive movements for an extended time is referred to as **muscular endurance**. Activities that require a significant amount of muscular endurance include cross country running, cross-country skiing, and many swimming events. An athlete can develop muscular endurance using the programs for building strength. However, using a lower amount of weight and performing a higher number of repetitions develops muscular endurance more efficiently.

Circuit training is a popular and effective method of developing muscular endurance as well as over-

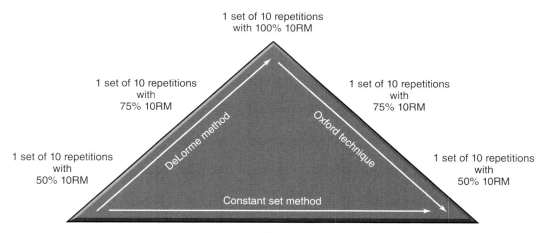

1 set of 10 repetitions
with 100% 10RM

1 set of 10 repetitions
with
75% 10RM

1 set of 10 repetitions
with
75% 10RM

DeLorme method

Oxford technique

1 set of 10 repetitions
with
50% 10RM

1 set of 10 repetitions
with
50% 10RM

Constant set method

3 sets of 10 repetitions with same weight for each set

Figure 17.1 Training programs. Pyramid training involves the use of about five sets of a given exercise. When an athlete ascends the pyramid (increases the weight per set), he is using the DeLorme method. When an athlete descends the pyramid (decreases the weight per set), he is using the Oxford technique. If he follows the bottom of the pyramid (maintains the same weight per set), he is using the constant set method.

all fitness. **Circuit training** involves exercising at multiple stations (usually 8-20) that often target a full-body workout (exercises to work all major muscle groups are selected). The athlete rotates from station to station either performing a given number of repetitions or exercising for a given length of time (e.g., 30 seconds) at each station. It is wise to select stations that target alternate body parts so that the same muscles are not used at consecutive stations.

Power

Muscular power refers to the ability to exert force quickly. Many programs that focus on developing power do so by using very heavy weights and a low number of repetitions; the movements, however, are performed quickly. For example, a football lineman must be able to react quickly once the ball is snapped by exploding off the line of scrimmage and pushing his opponent. The result is fast movement against resistance, but the play does not last long.

JOINT FLEXIBILITY

Stretching is performed to lengthen tissue that has been shortened from lack of use, such as when an athlete is immobilized in a cast. Stretching should

be performed if range of motion is limited because of soft-tissue tightness around a joint. A stretch should not produce pain; instead, it should be comfortable. Stretching should be done before and after heavy athletic activity, but it is necessary to perform a light warm-up (aerobic activity) before stretching—stretching a cold muscle might lead to injury.

There are three types of stretches. The first is **static stretching**—the muscle is isolated, stretched, and held in the stretch for approximately 30 seconds. The second is **ballistic stretching**. Ballistic stretching is when a specific muscle is isolated and quickly stretched and relaxed repetitively, as though the athlete is bouncing. This form of stretching is not recommended because it can aggravate an existing injury or cause a new injury. Static stretching is the way to develop flexibility; it should be done three times in each exercise session for 30 seconds at a time, addressing each muscle. Static stretching should be done after a light warm-up. **Dynamic stretching**, the third form, is done by simply moving a limb or part of the body through its range of motion. An example of dynamic stretching is swinging the leg forward and backward to stretch the hip.

EXERCISES FOR RECONDITIONING MUSCLES

Because there are many exercises for injuries, the AT and the athlete need to decide which exercises to perform. Although it is beyond the scope of this text to provide a comprehensive list of exercises, we provide information about basic exercises for reconditioning athletes following an injury and helping them develop general strength and mobility.

Reconditioning Techniques for the Lower Extremity

When rehabilitating the lower quarter, strengthening the region and establishing proprioception are major concerns. Balancing activities such as working on wobble boards and stork standing are excellent for regaining proprioception, even if the athlete can tolerate only partial weight bearing (see figure 17.2).

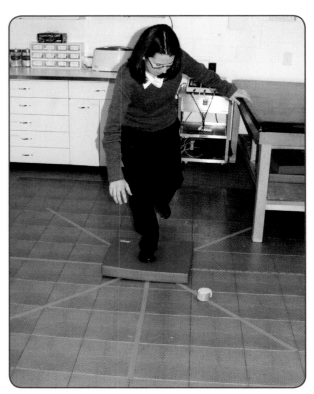

Figure 17.2 Balance exercise. The patient can initially stand still and then progress to reaching for objects placed on each line of the floor pattern.

Photo courtesy of Lorin Cartwright

Balance exercises should be progressed carefully. Typically an AT will have an injured athlete stand with a wide base of support (legs spread to shoulder width apart) on a firm, stable surface. If the athlete is successful, the AT will progress her to a narrow base of support (feet close together) and then to an unstable surface such as a foam pad. Once successful in this position, the athlete can progress to standing on one leg using a stable and then unstable surface. More dynamic balance exercises can be used afterward, meaning the athlete will begin moving her body while maintaining balance. Failure to properly progress an athlete's balance can result in a reinjury. See figure 17.2 for an example of a balance exercise progression.

The Foot, Ankle, and Lower Leg

Rehabilitation procedures of the foot, ankle, and lower leg involve reestablishing flexibility and strength with active range-of-motion activities such as calf stretches (see figure 17.3b) and writing the ABCs with the foot while it is hanging off the end of a table. Strength can be regained by using elastic bands while resistance is applied as the athlete inverts, everts, plantar flexes, and dorsiflexes his foot (see figure 17.3, c-f). If another person is not available, the bands can be made into loops and securely fastened around hooks mounted on the floor, wall, table leg, or table edge. Exercises such as these are excellent for many ankle sprains and strains.

The Knee, Hip, and Pelvis

To improve flexibility of the muscular structures around the knee, the athlete should perform static stretching of the involved muscle groups, specifically the quadriceps, groin, and hamstrings (see figure 17.4, a-c). These stretching exercises are especially helpful for improving range of motion. The knee and hip musculature can be strengthened initially by using the weight of the limb itself with straight leg raises and later progressing to resistive exercise tubing (see figure 17.4, d-f). Isotonic exercises with a knee and thigh machine can be done as well as forward lunges and wall squats. Beginning with straight leg raises helps to develop basic strength for athletes who are weak. As soon as possible, however, the athlete should perform strengthening exercises in a standing position (for example, with resistive tubing).

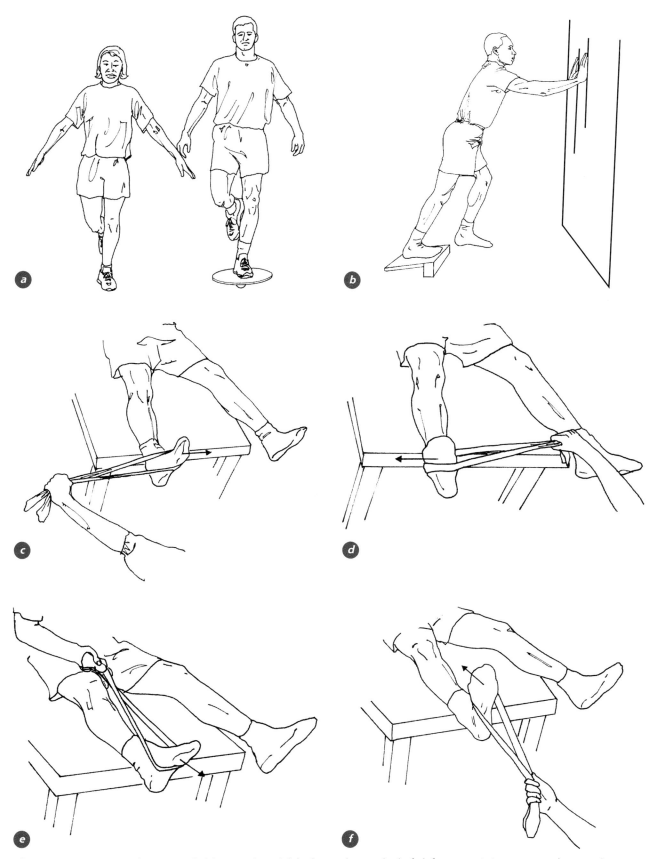

Figure 17.3 *(a)* Balance activities and wobble boards are helpful for regaining normal proprioception. *(b)* Calf stretches. Ankle strength can be improved using resistive tubing while the athlete moves the ankle into *(c)* inversion, *(d)* eversion, *(e)* plantar flexion, and *(f)* dorsiflexion.

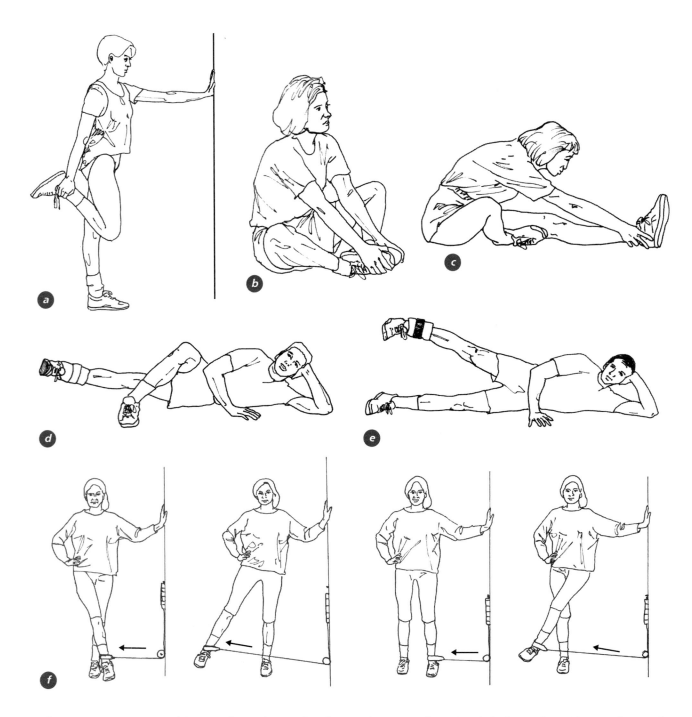

Figure 17.4 *(a)* Quadriceps, *(b)* groin, and *(c)* hamstring stretches. Straight leg raises *(d-e)* performed while lying down and *(f)* against resistive tubing while standing are helpful for regaining hip and knee strength. *(g-h)* In the later stages of rehabilitation, isotonic movement can be done with weight machines to develop quadriceps and hamstring strength. *(i-j)* Forward lunges and wall squats are a great functional way of strengthening the lower quarter.

a: Reprinted, by permission, from V.H. Heyward, 2002, *Advanced fitness assessment & exercise prescription*, 4th edition (Champaign, IL: Human Kinetics), 336.

c, d, e: Reprinted, by permission, from J. Griffin, 1998, *Client-centered exercise prescription* (Champaign, IL: Human Kinetics), 188, 241.

f, g, h: Reprinted, by permission, from V.H. Heyward, 1998, *Advanced fitness assessment & exercise prescription,* 3rd edition (Champaign, IL: Human Kinetics), 271, 272.

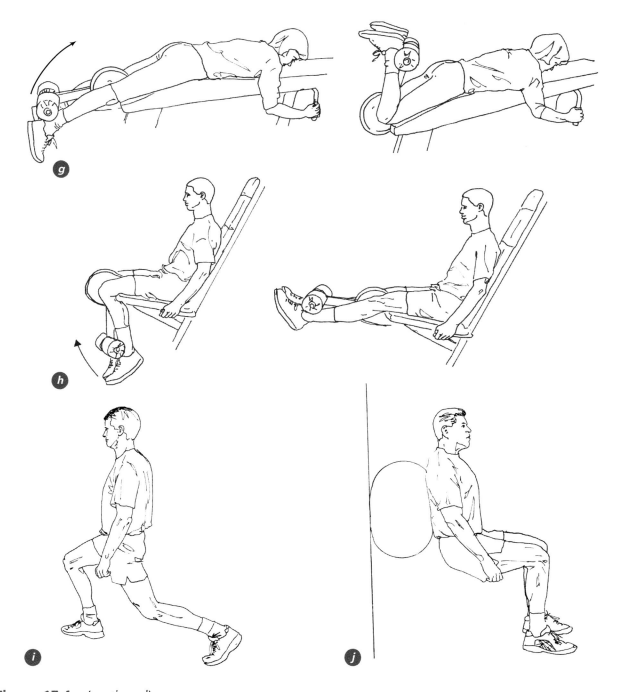

Figure 17.4 *(continued)*

To develop proprioception, a balancing program can be performed. This may begin with a timed stork stand and progress to wobble-board activity. An athlete can achieve knee and hip musculature endurance by swimming, biking, or running, provided these activities do not aggravate the injury. The AT should always observe the athlete to make sure she is not favoring the knee during activity. Getting the athlete back into sport activity involves performing sport-specific change-of-direction exercises at a slow running speed and gradually increasing the speed. For example, the athlete can run in a figure-eight pattern, between cones, or on the out-of-bounds lines on a basketball court. She will perform the exercises at slower speeds with less cutting and then progress to higher speeds and more cutting.

Reconditioning Techniques for the Axial Region

Rehabilitation procedures of the spine must be done with extreme caution. People who support a conservative approach to treating the spine argue that the athlete should progress only at a slow pace. The AT must perform a thorough assessment before rehabilitation begins and reassess during the rehabilitation process. The athlete must be taught normal posture and how to treat his back before he can achieve a proper recovery. If he is rehabilitating the lumbar spine, the AT will be concerned with reestablishing balance among mobility, flexibility, and lumbar strength. Muscular endurance, cardiorespiratory endurance, and sport-specific function are also concerns. Flexibility of the muscular structures around the spine involves either flexion or extension movements, depending on the problem at hand. A good general flexibility exercise for athletes seeking to improve trunk flexibility is shown in figure 17.5.

Flexion Movements

Flexion movements of the spine are useful for athletes who have lordosis or muscle strains of the back extensor musculature. Flexion movements for regaining flexibility include single and double knee-to-chest exercises (see figure 17.6). If an athlete has a disk bulge of the lumbar spine, this type of movement should not be performed.

Extension Movements

Extension movements of the spine are useful for athletes who have too little curvature in the lumbar spine or who have disk bulges. Extension movements for regaining flexibility and function include having the athlete lie facedown and push into trunk extension, first to the elbows and then progressing to using the hands for support (see figure 17.7).

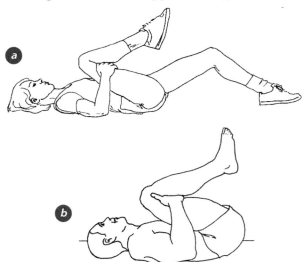

Figure 17.6 (a) Single and (b) double knee-to-chest flexion exercises are helpful for stretching the lumbar region.

a: Reprinted, by permission, from V.H. Heyward, 2002, *Advanced fitness assessment & exercise prescription*, 4th ed. (Champaign, IL: Human Kinetics), 337.

b: Adapted from M. Alter, 1998, *Sport stretch*, 2nd ed. (Champaign, IL: Human Kinetics), 165. By permission of Michael Richardson.

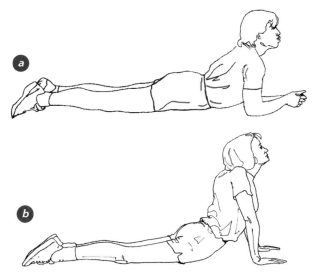

Figure 17.7 Extension movements of the spine are helpful for disk bulges.

b: Reprinted, by permission, from V.H. Heyward, 2002, *Advanced fitness assessment & exercise prescription*, 4th ed. (Champaign, IL: Human Kinetics), 340.

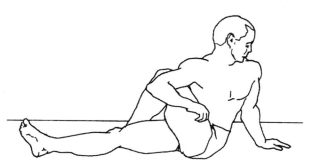

Figure 17.5 Trunk rotation stretch.

Adapted, by permission, from M. Alter, 1998, *Sports stretch*, 2nd ed. (Champaign, IL: Human Kinetics), 146.

Lumbar Strength

To regain strength of the lumbar spine, the athlete gets into a neutral spine position and then moves the extremities while maintaining this position. These lumbar-strengthening exercises can be performed while the athlete is lying on the floor on the back or facedown, on hands and knees, lying on an exercise ball on the back or facedown, and even in a standing position (figure 17.8, *a-b*). Great care must be taken to begin with simple movements and progress to harder ones. The AT must also help the athlete maintain a neutral spine by continually providing feedback during activity. Additionally, abdominal strength is vital for a strong back. A simple abdominal curl can be used (figure 17.8*c*). The lat pull-down is a must in any conditioning program and an excellent exercise to help develop back strength (figure 17.9).

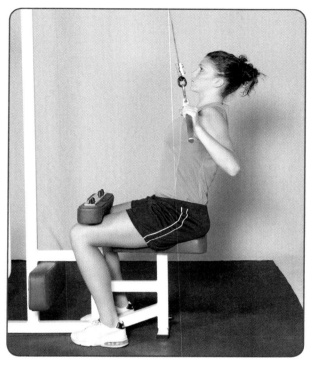

Figure 17.9 Lat pull-downs are helpful for general back strengthening.

Cervical Region

Neck stretches will restore the mobility of the cervical region. The athlete can do a neck stretch as pictured in figure 17.10*a*. In a seated position, the athlete grabs her left wrist and pulls it to the outside of her right thigh while bending her head to the right; then she grabs her right wrist and pulls it to the outside of the left thigh while bending her head to the left. Simple neck range-of-motion activities can also be performed. To strengthen the neck, resistive tubing can be attached to the head and cervical movements can be resisted (see figure 17.10, *b-c*). Any cervical stretching and exercise must be performed gently and gradually; otherwise further injury can result. Shoulder shrugs are also helpful for strengthening the trapezius muscle (see figure 17.11).

Reconditioning Techniques for the Upper Extremity

As with the lower quarter, when rehabilitating the upper quarter, strengthening the region and reestablishing proprioception are major concerns. Balancing activities, such as using a ball for wall push-ups, help to reestablish proprioception of this area (see figure 17.12*a*).

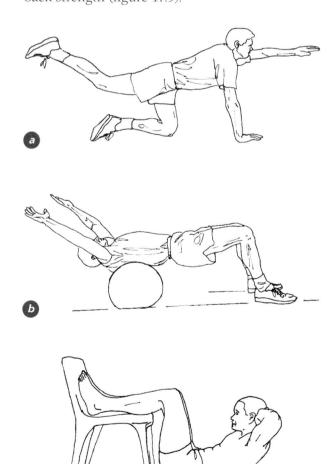

Figure 17.8 *(a-b)* Lumbar stabilization exercises; *(c)* abdominal curls.

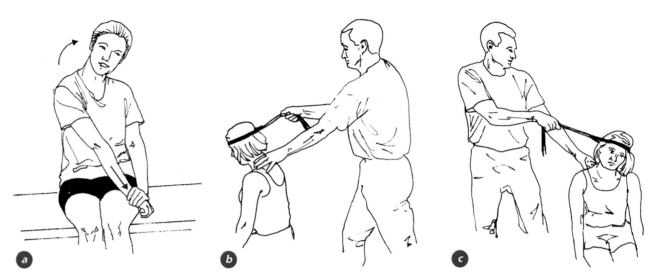

Figure 17.10 *(a)* Lateral neck stretches; *(b-c)* resisted cervical movements with rubber tubing.

a: Reprinted, by permission, from J. Griffin, 2006, *Client-centered exercise prescription* 2nd ed. (Champaign, IL: Human Kinetics), 200.

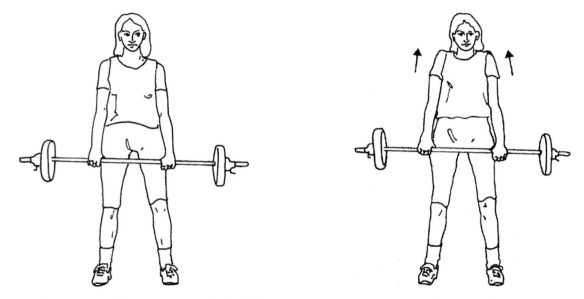

Figure 17.11   Shoulder shrugs are helpful for strengthening the trapezius muscle.

Reprinted, by permission, from V.H. Heyward, 1998, *Advanced fitness assessment & exercise prescription,* 3rd edition (Champaign, IL: Human Kinetics), 268.

The Shoulder

Basic rehabilitation procedures of the shoulder involve reestablishing flexibility and strength. To accomplish this, active range-of-motion exercises such as moving the arm into flexion, extension, abduction, and adduction can be performed as well as stretches that will improve flexibility of the anterior and posterior aspects of the region (see figure 17.12, *b-c*). The athlete can learn wand exercises and wall walking with the fingers, which she can perform on her own. By gripping the wand with both hands as she performs the wand exercises, the injured shoulder is helped by the good shoulder; as her fingers walk up the wall, they pull the arm up to work the injured shoulder. These exercises are helpful for athletes who need to work at home, but they will need some instructions about how

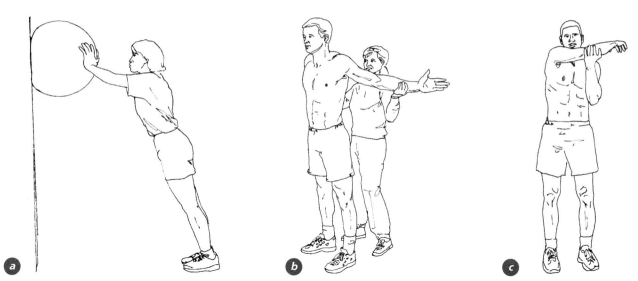

Figure 17.12 *(a)* Doing wall push-ups with a ball can help the athlete regain upper-extremity proprioception. *(b)* Anterior and *(c)* posterior shoulder stretches.

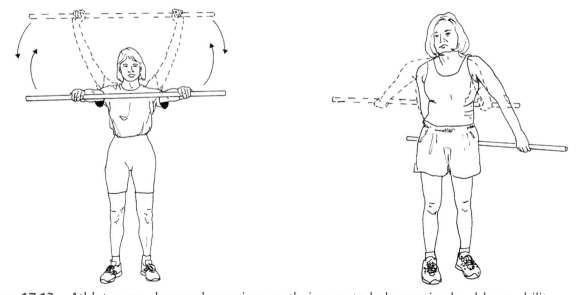

Figure 17.13 Athletes can do wand exercises on their own to help regain shoulder mobility.

a: Reprinted, by permission, from J.C. Griffin, 1998, *Client-centered exercise prescription* (Champaign, IL: Human Kinetics), 240.

to do so effectively (see figures 17.13 and 17.14). Pendulum exercises can also improve mobility (see figure 17.15).

The athlete can regain strength in the area by moving the joint through the major motions while resistance is applied using either free weights or elastic bands (see figure 17.16, *a-b*). Special attention should be given to the rotator cuff muscles. Internal and external rotation movements, as shown

in figure 17.16, *c* and *d*, are especially helpful when recovering from rotator cuff injuries or impingement syndromes.

In the later stages of strengthening, the bench press and military press may be performed either with dumbbells or with weights on a straight bar (see figure 17.16, *e-f*). These are excellent exercises for developing shoulder strength and should be included in general conditioning programs. A spot-

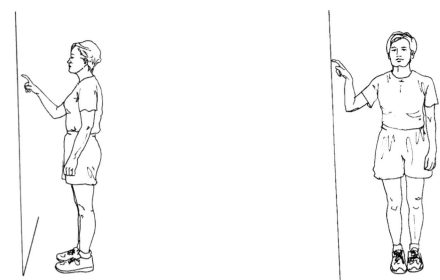

Figure 17.14 Wall walking is another good exercise for an athlete to perform when the goal is to gain range of motion.

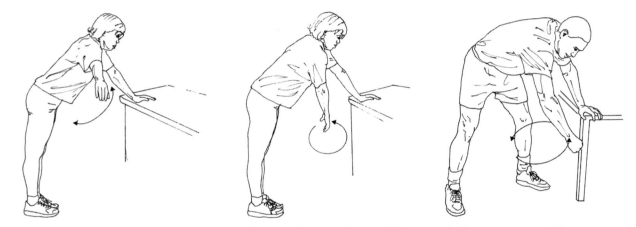

Figure 17.15 Pendulum exercises can be used soon after an injury to help restore mobility.

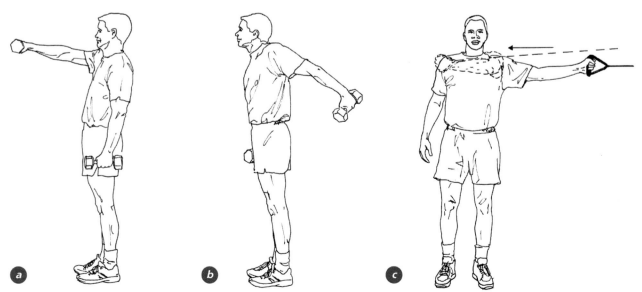

Figure 17.16 Shoulder (a) flexion and (b) extension against resistance. (c-d) It is important to strengthen the internal and external rotators of the shoulder. (e) Military press and (f) bench press with free weights.

c, d: Reprinted, by permission, from J. Griffin, 1998, *Client-centered exercise prescription* (Champaign, IL: Human Kinetics), 147.

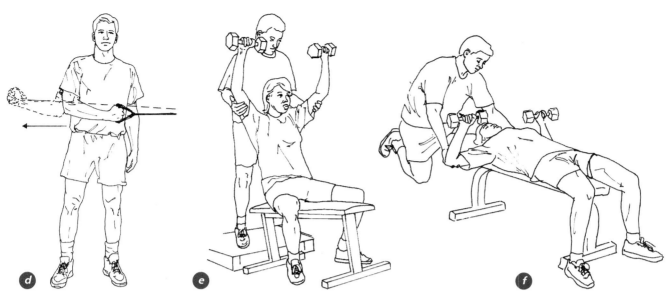

Figure 17.16 (continued)

ter is necessary for each exercise at all times regardless of the type of free-weight equipment used.

The Elbow, Wrist, and Hand

At the basic level, the AT is concerned with reestablishing elbow and wrist mobility, flexibility, and strength. Flexibility of the muscular structures around the elbow and wrist involves static stretching of the involved muscle groups (see figure 17.17a), specifically the extensor and flexor muscles. Strengthening of the elbow and wrist musculature can be done using handheld weights (see figure 17.17, b-d). To help the athlete bear weight on the limb, wall push-ups can be performed (see figure 17.17e). These are even helpful for some shoulder injuries.

The biceps and triceps must not be neglected; they can be strengthened by performing triceps pull-downs and biceps curls (see figure 17.18, a-b). Hand injuries may also require that an athlete attempt to improve her grip strength by squeezing a racquetball or tennis ball, or she can squeeze hand clay between her fingers (see figure 17.18c). As long as the injury is not aggravated, elbow and wrist muscular endurance can be achieved by performing a high number of repetitions while lifting weights or by swimming, biking, or running. The AT should always observe the athlete to make sure that she is not aggravating the elbow or wrist injury during activity. She can get back into sport activity by throwing, beginning with short distances at slow speeds and progressing to longer distances at higher speeds.

Focus on Function

Although we have presented the contents of this section according to body region, the reality is that many joints work together to achieve a functional outcome. When we perform an athletic movement of the upper extremity, for example, the legs and trunk are often required to move simultaneously. With this concept in mind, many ATs focus on function so an athlete is ready for the demands of the sport.

Functional exercises take many forms, but the premise is to use sport-specific movements. As an example, if an athlete is performing a lunge to strengthen the legs, he can easily include an arm movement, such as a military press, and perform it at the same time. Another example is to have an athlete balance on a foam pad while performing biceps curls—he is not only working on upper-body strength but also balance.

CARDIORESPIRATORY CONDITIONING

Just as proper resistance training taxes and overloads the musculoskeletal system and makes it stronger, properly administered aerobic training can enhance an athlete's **cardiorespiratory endurance** in preparation for returning to play.

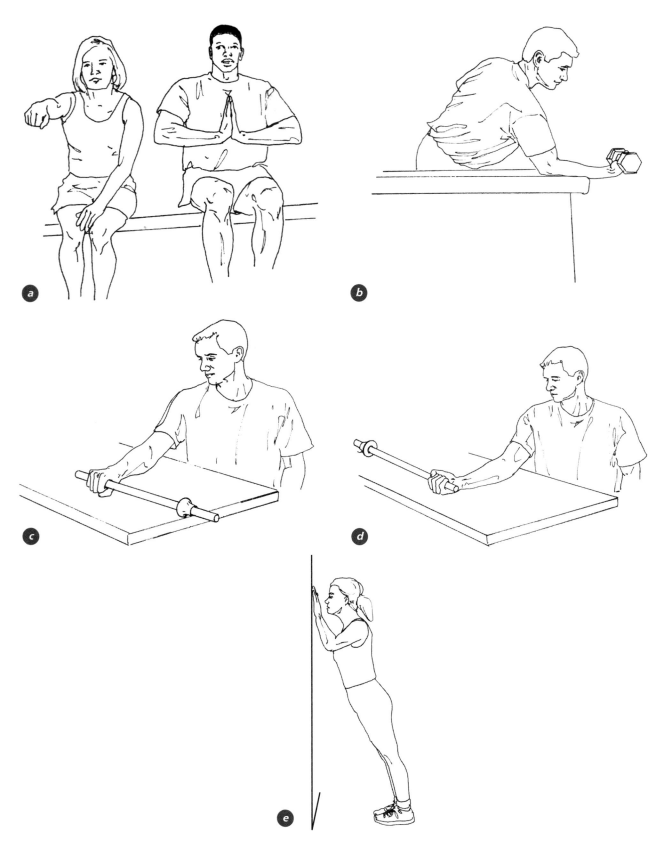

Figure 17.17 *(a)* Wrist extensor and flexor stretch. *(b-d)* Wrist and elbow strengthening exercises. *(e)* Wall push-ups help an athlete begin to bear weight on the upper extremity.

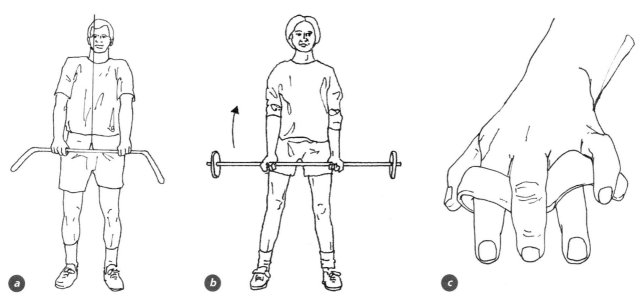

Figure 17.18 *(a)* Triceps pull-downs and *(b)* biceps curls are especially helpful for strengthening the upper arm. *(c)* Clay can be used to strengthen the fingers and hand.

b: Reprinted, by permission, from V.H. Heyward, 1998, *Advanced fitness assessment & exercise prescription,* 3rd edition (Champaign, IL: Human Kinetics),

The ACSM currently recommends training for three to five days a week in order to improve cardiorespiratory endurance. Training more than this can lead to overuse injuries because time must be taken to rest and recover throughout the week. The intensity of the exercise should elevate the heart rate to between 60% and 90% of the maximum heart rate. To determine maximum heart rate, subtract the athlete's age from 220. For example, let's determine the target heart rate for a 16-year-old cross country runner. The formula determines her maximum heart rate: 220 – 16 = 204. If she is new to running, we may choose to start easy and increase the intensity as she gets in better shape. Therefore, if she begins training at 60% of her maximal heart rate of 204 beats per minute, she must elevate her heart rate to about 122 beats per minute to get a training effect.

The duration, or amount of time, an athlete trains each session is another variable that can be controlled. To achieve maximum benefit, the exercise should be performed at the proper intensity for 20 to 60 minutes each session. As the intensity increases, the duration generally decreases.

The type of exercise selected to improve, maintain, or reestablish cardiorespiratory endurance for the athlete depends on several factors. Ideally, we would choose rhythmic activities that include large muscle groups and can be performed continuously. However, the available equipment and the type of injury affect that decision. If an athlete has an injured ankle and is not yet allowed to perform much weight-bearing activity, he may need to perform an upper-body aerobic exercise and work on the upper-body cycle machine, for example (see figure 17.19). Conversely, if he has an injured shoulder, he may need to limit upper-extremity exercises but can ride an exercise bike.

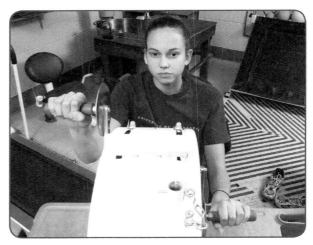

Figure 17.19 Exercises such as upper-body cycling can help maintain cardiorespiratory fitness if an athlete has a lower-extremity injury.

The Real World

A student of mine shared a video of a competitive power-lifter's weight training session. The athlete was performing a squat with about 550 pounds (250 kg) of weight on the bar. While he was squatting, his knee buckled and gave way. He collapsed to one side and lost control of the weight. Thankfully, his two spotters grabbed the bar, or he would have been badly hurt. Everyone watching the film got the message: Always train with a partner—or in some cases, two.

Bill Pitney, EdD, ATC

A WORD ON SAFETY

Safety during training should always be a chief concern. Don't let people using dumbbells act like dumbbells. Safety procedures must be established and faithfully followed.

Whether athletes are weight training or performing a cardiorespiratory workout, to prevent injury they need a proper warm-up to prepare the body for the demands of the sport and a cool-down to help the body recover from the exercise. The warm-up and cool-down should include light cardiorespiratory work followed by stretching of the major muscle groups. Just how long the warm-up or cool-down should last is hotly debated among professionals, and the length is likely to vary from coach to coach and athlete to athlete. Ten to 15 minutes for each, however, should be acceptable.

Athletes should follow several safety precautions when weight training. An athlete should always train with a partner, who should know the exercise to be performed as well as the number of repetitions and be ready to assist when needed. The athlete should not hold his breath while performing an exercise; instead, he should exhale during concentric contractions (while exerting force) and inhale during eccentric contractions. Any time a bar is used, the weights should be secured with a collar. Exercise form should never be compromised, especially when trying to lift a heavier weight. No horseplay in the training area should be tolerated—athletes must not be bumped while performing an exercise. Lastly, be conscious about moving weights and weight stacks; it is easy to injure a finger or hand if you inadvertently catch it between the weights.

Proper weightlifting form has several components. The athlete should be stable—that is, when she is standing, lying, or sitting on a bench, she should maintain balance. She should be able to control the weight at all times. This means she should raise and lower the weight at a slow, easy pace, usually raising the weight for two seconds and lowering it for four seconds. She should never cheat on her form just to be able to lift a weight.

When training for improved cardiorespiratory function, it is also a good idea to train with a partner. Training partners check on each other's water consumption and keep each other at an appropriate training level. Coaches and ATs should always monitor the heat index to be sure the environment is safe for training.

CHAPTER WRAP-UP

Summary

PRE, overload, and specificity principles should always be followed by the AT to ensure that a reconditioning program is both safe and effective. A complete conditioning program includes aerobic activity for cardiorespiratory endurance that allows the athlete to reach the target heart rate. Stretching should be static to avoid injury in the warm-up, which should gradually raise the heart rate before the exercise program. Stretching should also be done in the cool-down, which should gradually lower the heart rate back to normal. Safety rules and guidelines must be implemented and followed to avoid potential injury during weight training and conditioning.

Key Terms

Define the following terms found in this chapter:

ballistic stretching

cardiorespiratory endurance

circuit training

closed kinetic chain

DeLorme method

dynamic stretching

isokinetic contraction

isometric contraction

isotonic contraction

muscular endurance

muscular power

muscular strength

one-repetition maximum (1RM)

open kinetic chain

overload principle

progressive resistive exercise (PRE)

pyramid method

specificity

static stretching

Questions for Review

1. Explain the differences among strength, endurance, and power. How might an athlete develop each of these?

2. Define *isotonic*, *isometric*, and *isokinetic*. How are these movements different?

3. If an athlete needs to become more flexible, what is the best way to stretch?

4. Is it better to use multiple sets of an exercise to develop strength?

5. When would closed kinetic chain exercises be used rather than open kinetic chain exercises?

6. What intensity level would an athlete need to train at in order to improve cardiorespiratory conditioning?

7. Think of the functional demands of a baseball player compared with a basketball player. How might their conditioning programs differ in order to return to sport following time away?

Activities for Reinforcement

1. Find alternative exercises that can be done for the upper quarter, lower quarter, and axial region.

2. Work with an AT or strength and conditioning coach to design a strength and conditioning program for a soccer player.

3. Work with an AT or strength and conditioning coach to design a conditioning program for a football lineman.

4. Invite a strength and conditioning specialist to class to speak about training programs.

Above and Beyond

1. Visit one of the following Web sites to find information related to strength training and conditioning. Write a one-page summary of your findings.

   www.exrx.net/index.html

   www.nsca-lift.org/Publications/posstatements.shtml

   www.nsca-lift.org/youthpositionpaper/Youth_Pos_Paper_200902.pdf

   www.asmi.org/sportsmed/Performance/aerobic.html

2. Examine the following information related to weight-room facility rules offered by the College Strength and Conditioning Coaches Association:

   www.acsm.org

3. Visit the following Mayo Clinic Web page and learn more about exercises for core strength:

   www.mayoclinic.com/health/core-strength/SM00047.

4. Read one of the following articles and write a one-page summary:

   Hass, C., M. Feigenbaum, and B. Franklin. 2001. Prescription of resistance training for healthy populations. *Sports Medicine* 31: 953-964.

   Kraemer, W.J. 2003. Strength training basics: designing workouts to meet patients' goals. *Physician and Sportsmedicine* 31(8): 39-45.

   Wilmore, J.H. 2003. Aerobic exercise and endurance: improving fitness for health benefits. *Physician and Sportsmedicine* 31(5): 45-51.

chapter 18

Psychosocial Aspects of Athletic Training

Objectives

Upon completing this chapter, the student will be able to do the following:

- Have a broad understanding of and appreciation for sport psychology.
- Understand relaxation and imagery techniques that are often used with athletes.
- Explain the athlete's perspective of an injury and typical emotional reactions.
- Identify the types and symptoms of eating disorders.
- Describe practical strategies to help an athlete better cope with an injury.

Athletes and ATs are beginning to understand that physical considerations are not the only factors in sport injury and rehabilitation; psychological factors such as stress play a major role as well. Therefore, ATs and athletes should learn the basics of sport psychology.

Sport psychology is the study of how variables such as life stress, mood, and motivation affect sport performance and sport-related injury. Sport psychologists and sport psychology consultants try to improve the mental well-being of athletes. They have many roles, including the following:

- Researching to better understand how these variables affect athletes

- Teaching coaches, athletes, and ATs psychological techniques to improve performance
- Working directly with athletes in a clinical setting to help them deal with stress and improve sport performance

Many ATs are excellent at providing physical treatment and care to injured athletes. However, they also need to be aware that injuries can cause psychological problems that inhibit not only performance but also proper recovery. The most successful ATs have a clear understanding of an athlete's psychology, injured or not.

REFERRING AN ATHLETE FOR PROFESSIONAL HELP

Although ATs have basic skills in counseling athletes, sometimes an athlete will need to be referred to another professional that specializes in a certain form of help. Some issues that need referral include

- anxiety,
- depression,
- post-traumatic response,
- suicidal thoughts,
- eating disorders,
- overwhelming life stressors,
- life-altering significant injury,
- mental health disorders, and
- any situation the AT does not feel comfortable handling.

The AT can refer athletes to various experts:

- Psychiatrist—physician who specializes in mental health
- Psychologist—person who specializes in psychology and individual educational testing
- Social worker—person who specializes in group or individual therapy
- Sport psychologist—person who improves an athlete's performance using psychology

Anxiety

As you might imagine, high school athletes must deal with many pressures. Although few students could say they've never been stressed or anxious, athletes must cope with the expectations of their peers, coaches, and parents regarding their sport performance in addition to the everyday stress of school and social life. Because of these stresses, many athletes become anxious before sport participation. Although ATs are not sport psychologists, they spend a lot of time with the athletes and are in a good position to talk to them when necessary. The AT must be able to counsel an athlete who is too anxious.

Depression

Depression is a feeling of despair or hopelessness that causes behavior such as not wanting to be around other people, not being excited about things that might normally excite someone, not taking the initiative to do things, and not talking much to anyone. Many theories exist about what causes a person to become depressed. Professionals think that depression is caused by biological (e.g., genetics), environmental (e.g., a traumatic childhood), or sociological (e.g., losing a spot on a team) factors. Along with feelings of hopelessness, a depressed athlete may exhibit many other signs and symptoms, including lack of appetite, nausea and indigestion, headaches, dizziness, and susceptibility to colds and other illnesses.

Post-Traumatic Response

A **post-traumatic response** is a sustained emotional disorder that results from a traumatic experience. For instance, a football player who was involved in a serious car accident in which a friend died might experience depression, problems with personal relationships, and impaired concentration, or he might even attempt suicide. Post-traumatic stress does not just happen to athletes; for example, an AT may experience post-traumatic stress disorder (PTSD) after working with an athlete who suffered a serious spinal cord injury. She may become fearful and unable to work well. She might also sleep a lot, refrain from eating, and avoid situations that are similar to the one that caused the initial stress.

Suicidal Thoughts

Because of the many pressures that come with being a student, the AT working at a high school should be concerned about suicide. A person who attempts suicide has usually been through a stressful experience and is also suffering from depression. Warning signs of suicide include

- a change in an athlete's eating and sleeping patterns;
- statements indicating he wants to die;
- depression;
- anxiety;
- a recent loss, such as a death in the family, a broken relationship, or the loss of a job;
- a family history of suicide; and
- a lack of support from friends and family.

If a student suspects that someone may be suicidal, she should tell the school counselor that she is concerned about that person. If a student-athlete has made a suicide attempt, the AT should call 911. If the athlete has serious suicidal thoughts and is not thinking clearly, or if he exhibits suicidal warning signs but denies being suicidal, he should see a counselor as soon as possible.

People who are more likely to be at risk for suicide include

- those who have made previous suicide attempts,
- those who have a plan for their suicide,
- those who are gay or lesbian,
- those who have eating disorders, and
- those who are isolated.

An athletic injury need not be severe to create stress and discomfort for an athlete. In a recent study by Valovich and colleagues (2009), injured adolescent athletes who suffered an injury not only had loss of physical function and pain but also decreased social functioning. This means that injured adolescents are likely to have difficulty participating in social activities as a result of an athletic injury.

Eating Disorders

Unfortunately, some athletes may participate in sport to gain a thinner body. Excessive exercise may appear to be devotion to a sport when in reality it is the first sign of an eating disorder. Disordered eating leads to the conditions of amenorrhea, dysmenorrhea, and osteoporosis, which are discussed in more detail in chapter 25.

All athletes should understand that the body has two types of fat: essential and storage. Essential fat is necessary for the body to function. The minimum level of essential fat for males is 7% of body mass and for females it is 12%. Storage fat is excess fat—it's just hanging around with no purpose. If an athlete has love handles or a belly that he wants to get rid of, that's fine. But if male athletes dip under 7% body fat or if female athletes go below 12% body

The Real World

I once worked with a football player who became so anxious before games that he got physically sick. He would have to leave the training room while he was being taped because he had to vomit. Once the game started, he was fine and played extremely well. This player was definitely a candidate for relaxation training.

Anonymous

fat, they put their health and their performance in danger.

Anorexia nervosa is characterized by a pattern of starvation and a fear of being fat. **Bulimia nervosa** is characterized by bouts of bingeing followed by self-induced vomiting. Both of these eating disorders are signs of deeper psychological problems that must be addressed. An AT who recognizes an eating disorder must refer the athlete to a specialist on eating disorders for counseling. If the illness is severe, the athlete may need to be hospitalized.

According to Kratina (2005), anorexia has four chief symptoms:

1. Extreme fear of being overweight
2. Denial that one's body weight is seriously low
3. Resistance to maintaining a minimally acceptable weight based on height and weight
4. Loss of menstrual cycle

Bulimia affects 1% to 2% of young adult females and has three chief symptoms:

1. Regularly taking in large volumes of food and then feeling that control of eating has been lost
2. Serious anxiety about body size and shape
3. Regular engagement in inappropriate behaviors related to food, such as self-induced vomiting and fasting

According to the Academy for Eating Disorders (2010), the actual cause of eating disorders is not clear, but many factors contribute to their development. For example, low self-esteem and perfectionism appear to be risk factors for eating disorders. Treatment of eating disorders is complex and often requires a team consisting of a physician, mental health expert, dietitian, and counselor.

ATs and coaches can help prevent eating disorders among athletes by

- watching for the signs of eating disorders,

- not pushing weight loss or weighing athletes,

- ensuring that athletes with menstrual irregularities are referred for counseling (Kratina 2005),

- making sure that conversations about positive body image occur,

- examining their own body image perceptions so they don't affect the athletes (Kratina 2005),

- giving accurate information about weight and body composition (Kratina 2005), and

- sharing that eating disorders are more commonly found among women but that some men also have eating disorders (Kratina 2005).

Death of an Athlete

Despite all of the injury prevention strategies and all of the measures taken by ATs to ensure the safety of athletes, sometimes things go terribly wrong. Although it may not happen on the court or on the field, the death of an athlete is a tragic event that leaves coaches, athletes, and parents with a devastating loss. An athlete who needs to talk about the loss of a teammate may confide in the AT, who holds a position of help and trust.

The AT should understand that the athlete may express a great deal of anger during this time. The emotions that an athlete goes through when a peer dies are similar to those she will experience when she is injured.

The Real World

Many ATs deal with eating disorders as part of the job. One of my softball players was severely anorexic. I teamed with our psychologist and physician and encouraged the athlete to receive inpatient treatment. After three weeks and a gradual return to the sport, it appeared that the treatment was successful. The athlete graduated with honors, finished her softball career, and went on to get a master's degree. Sadly, this athlete stopped by my office six years later with a feeding tube in her nose. Eating disorders are a crippling disease.

Gretchen Schlabach, PhD, ATC

Significant Injury

To understand the psychology of an injured athlete, we examine the classic five-stage theory presented by Kubler-Ross in the late 1960s. These stages represent the emotional response of an athlete and how he may act after an injury or loss. The stages are denial, anger, bargaining, depression, and acceptance. This theory has been widely referred to in much of the literature on psychological response to athletic injury. Although many athletes will progress through these stages in sequence, keep in mind that everyone is different, and some may exhibit these stages out of order.

- *Denial.* When an athlete is first injured, it is not uncommon for her to deny that there is a serious problem. Many athletes will tell themselves that things will soon be better. Unfortunately, when the athlete does not soon improve following a significant injury, she will feel anxious. She may also be emotionally disorganized, and the AT may hear her make unrealistic statements such as "I will be fine, I'll be walking by tomorrow" when that may not be the case.

- *Anger.* Another response is anger, especially when the athlete realizes that the injury is real and potentially serious. He will often direct this anger at the nearest person, who may be a student assistant or AT. The athletic training staff and other members of the sports medicine team must not take the anger personally. They must remember that this is not a personal attack but rather an emotional release. Listen to the athlete, and continue to respect him as an individual.

- *Bargaining.* Once an athlete's anger has diminished, she will begin to bargain with the AT, coach, team physician, God, and even herself. She will attempt to make a deal with the AT, such as "If I can play at least one quarter of the basketball game, I will do all of my exercises until my ankle is healed." When limits are set with the injured athlete, she may become depressed.

- *Depression.* The student assistant is in a good position to see if the athlete is depressed. The depression phase brings a lack of motivation and a feeling of hopelessness. This becomes a big challenge for the athletic training staff because athletes can become noncompliant with their treatment, which is a concern of both sport psychologists and ATs. The AT needs to be supportive, motivational, and understanding to get the athlete to comply with the treatment plan. In addition, if the AT takes the time to educate the athlete about the injury and why certain signs and symptoms exist, he can help her become more compliant with the rehabilitation program.

● *Acceptance.* When an injured athlete finally takes responsibility for her injury, she has come to the stage of acceptance. Accepting an injury means that the athlete has finally realized what it will take to get back to normal—or that she may never get back to normal, depending on the seriousness of the injury.

Many athletes become anxious when it comes time to return to participation. The AT must see to it that the athlete in a rehabilitation program progresses gradually from simple to more complex exercises to build his confidence. Moreover, an AT is wise to allow the athlete opportunities to be with his teammates so that he can maintain contact and not feel isolated. In addition, a decisive therapeutic exercise program helps the athlete eliminate many fears of returning to play.

RELATIONSHIP BUILDING

ATs are likely to deal with athletes from various racial and sociocultural backgrounds. Though the details of these backgrounds may not be fully understood, ATs should work to build positive relationships with all athletes, parents, and coaches. The most effective ATs are good listeners. Being a good listener means that the AT is fully invested in that athlete at that time. Thinking about other things or being distracted will take away from the positive relationship-building process.

An athlete needs to feel that the AT respects her and knows what to do and when to do it. Having mutual respect for one another will develop trust, which is important to the athlete. The AT must convey that doing everything possible in the best interest of the athlete is critical in creating trust. Doing what is in the best interest of the athlete does not mean the athlete will agree. The AT must also be consistent when working with athletes so that

What Would You Do If...

The AT has asked you to come up with some ideas to make the athletic training room bright and cheerful.

there is no perceived preferential treatment toward one athlete or another.

One thing an AT can do is try to see things from the athlete's perspective. For some athletes, an injury can be traumatizing. Before retuning the athlete to competition, the AT will want to do some desensitizing work or refer the athlete to a social worker and make sure the athlete is mentally ready to return and has no fear of getting injured.

Some athletes will be relieved at getting hurt and not being able to play. These athletes may not have been totally invested, and the AT may have to work to get the athlete to determine if participation is what he wants. If an athlete is not invested, then they are more prone to injury, and they also find ways to malinger and use time of the AT that is not needed.

Other athletes may view their injury as a reason to avoid working hard. These athletes will find ways to fake an injury or be less than enthusiastic about doing rehabilitation. The AT needs to have a keen awareness of this type of athlete. Being able to push this athlete to fight through the supposed injury and get the athlete back into competition is a delicate balance. Being an AT does not mean making athletes happy; it's about doing the right thing. The AT also must be careful to avoid assuming that the athlete is faking it each time he complains of being injured.

For other athletes, the injury may make them feel that they are no longer part of the team. These athletes need to be assured that there is a need for them to attend practices and encourage their teammates.

There will be times when athletes try to convince the AT to allow them to return to competition. If the AT has a good relationship with the athlete, it will be easier to explain why the athlete should not return. If there is no respect or trust, the athlete will look for another resource.

Another aspect ATs need to consider when working with athletes is gender. A study by Drummond and colleagues (2007) found that in many instances an athlete will be more comfortable speaking with an AT of the same gender, particularly if the injury or illness relates to a sensitive issue. For example, if a female athlete is experiencing cramps and bleeding during her menstrual cycle, she will likely be more comfortable speaking with a woman. ATs should plan ahead and have personnel of both genders available for athletes to speak with.

PRACTICAL SUGGESTIONS

There are some practical things the AT can do in the athletic training room to help injured athletes cope with the injuries they have sustained. These include modeling, maintaining a good physical environment, and encouraging relaxation.

Modeling

Modeling means that an injured athlete is able to observe a successfully rehabilitated athlete with a similar injury. The idea is that once he sees someone who is doing well with a similar injury, he may become less discouraged and more motivated to work at his rehabilitation program. The AT and the student assistant should become positive, upbeat influences—another aspect of modeling. They should be cheerful and helpful to the athletes, and they should treat the athletes as they would want to be treated.

Physical Environment

Imagine going into a doctor's office that is dark, noisy, and smelly when you walk through the door. Would you want to be there? Would you ever go back? Would you be comfortable performing exercises there? The same is true of the athletic training room. It is important to have a bright, clean, cheerful, and physically inviting atmosphere in which to treat athletes. In such an environment, the athletes may not feel that what they're doing is work; rather, it may be pleasant for them.

Relaxation

If you go to a high school track meet, take a look at the athletes preparing for an event. You will see some of them listening to their headphones, others standing quietly with their eyes shut while gently moving their bodies through various patterns, and others lying down taking deep breaths or stretching. Helping athletes relax helps them alleviate stress and cope with the demands of sport and sport injury. Several relaxation techniques that can be found in the literature include breathing techniques, meditation, imagery, music therapy, massage, and muscle relaxation. Among these techniques, we discuss imagery and muscle relaxation.

Imagery

In the world of sport psychology, imagery is also known as visualization, mental training, and mental rehearsal. Imagery is used in athletics to help reduce stress. Several specific imagery techniques can be employed, but generally an athlete pictures herself successfully completing a game, match, play, or event. Many sport psychologists describe the mental imagery process as creating a motion picture. The person doing the imaging is the writer, the actor, the producer, and the director all at once. She creates the scene, the athletic movement, and the outcome that can help her visualize success. Imagery can also be done in the athletic training room to aid in rehabilitation.

Muscle Relaxation

Progressive muscle relaxation is one of the most common methods used to help athletes relax. This relaxation method originated in the early 1900s with a physician named Edmund Jacobson. The routine consists of a series of muscle contractions and relaxations. The athlete assumes a comfortable position, probably lying down, and begins by contracting a muscle group (e.g., calves) at 100% effort for about 5 seconds and then relaxes them for a longer period of time, sometimes up to 45 seconds. Next, the athlete contracts the same muscles at 50% effort, followed by a rest period. Finally, he gently contracts the muscle group for 5 seconds and then rests. The athlete should select each main muscle group and work his way through his body, concentrating on smooth, rhythmic breathing.

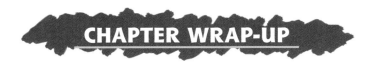
CHAPTER WRAP-UP

Summary

Athletes experience not only physical injuries but also psychological stresses that can be hard to manage. Sport psychologists can help athletes overcome many of the stresses they encounter with imagery and muscle relaxation techniques. Because ATs get to know athletes well and work with them every day, they can also help the athletes overcome anxiety. However, the AT must understand what an athlete will experience emotionally following an injury as well as the warning signs of mental health concerns.

Key Terms

Define the following terms found in this chapter:

anorexia nervosa

bulimia nervosa

depression

post-traumatic response

sport psychology

Questions for Review

1. State what is meant by sport psychology, and describe how sport psychologists might help an athlete who is experiencing anxiety.
2. What is depression, and what are the warning signs you should look for if you think someone is depressed?
3. Explain an athlete's perspective of an injury and the typical emotional reactions that he will display.
4. What are some of the warning signs that a student may be suicidal?
5. What are some warning signs of eating disorders, and how should an AT deal with this issue?

Activities for Reinforcement

1. Discuss with your head AT the various community agencies that an athlete could be referred to if she needed counseling.
2. Visit a suicide prevention hotline center.
3. Invite a sport psychologist to speak with the class.
4. Visit Active Insight, the online journal of sport psychology, at www.athleticinsight.com, and find resources related to sport psychology.
5. Visit the Web site for the Association for Applied Sport Psychology at www.aaasponline. org/index.php. Then discuss the association with your classmates.
6. Check out sport injury brochures, newsletters, and Web searches to find psychological tips for helping an athlete return to full activity following an injury.

Above and Beyond

1. Read one of the following articles and write a one-page summary:

   McLeod, T., R. Bay, J. Parsons, E. Sauers, and A. Snyder. 2009. Recent injury and health-related quality of life in adolescent athletes. *Journal of Athletic Training* 44(6): 603-610.

Stiller-Ostrowski, J., D. Gould, and T. Covassin. 2009. An evaluation of an educational intervention in psychology of injury for athletic training students. *Journal of Athletic Training* 44(5): 482-489.

Walker, N., J. Thatcher, and D. Lavallee. 2007. Psychological responses to injury in competitive sport: a critical review. *Journal of the Royal Society for the Promotion of Health* 127(4): 174-180.

2. Investigate goal setting and how to set attainable goals.
3. Investigate and review articles about athletes who are injury prone.
4. Investigate visual imagery and how an athlete might use it to improve performance.
5. Read about attention-seeking athletes and report about the subject to your class.

UNIT VII

Providing Emergency Care

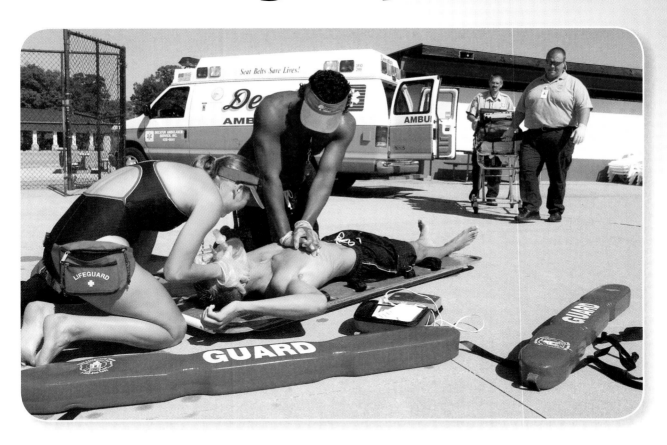

chapter 19

Planning for Emergencies

Objectives

Upon completing this chapter, the student will be able to do the following:

- Describe the principles of developing a crisis plan.
- Explain why crisis plans are necessary.
- Design a basic crisis plan.
- Understand the role of the student assistant during a crisis.

In this chapter we focus on how to plan for emergencies and explain the role of the AT during a crisis. There may be times when student assistants will have to help a coach or AT care for a seriously injured athlete or deal with a potentially hazardous situation. To be sure that the sports medicine team and coaches perform to the best of their abilities, it is necessary to have a crisis plan in place before an emergency happens.

Recognizing the importance of crisis plans, NATA has created a position statement for emergency planning in athletics. This position statement suggests that every athletic organization should develop and document a written crisis plan that is practiced regularly. The plan should identify the roles and responsibilities of various personnel as well as the type and location of necessary emergency equipment. The crisis plan should be specific for various locations (athletic fields or buildings), and mechanisms for clear communication should be established. Facilities that might be used to provide care to injured individuals should be included in the plan, and local EMS personnel should consult in the design of the plan. The crisis plan should identify who will document the actions taken during the emergency as well as how the plan will be evaluated. Many people within the community and athletic organization have a responsibility to participate in creating and implementing a crisis plan, and the finished plan should be reviewed by the school's administrators and legal counsel.

MEDICAL EMERGENCY CARDS

In most instances an emergency situation will not be a mass casualty but will only involve one person at a time. To assist with the quality of care provided to the person, good planning involves using medical emergency cards. These cards are required by many school districts. They contain important medical information as well as contact information in case of an emergency. See figure 19.1 for a sample card.

THE CRISIS PLAN

The **crisis plan** will enable the central **sports medicine team** to cope with emergency situations. It should be shared with all school personnel (i.e., ATs, team physician, coaches, school nurse) and emergency medical responders. The crisis plan should be practiced regularly in all facilities. Also, the sports medicine team should anticipate problems that could arise in various circumstances and with various personnel.

Most often the AT deals with a controlled situation and the crisis plan is simple. The plan becomes intricate when there are serious injuries. Before an emergency occurs, the sports medicine team should answer the following questions:

1. *Who is in charge of assessing an injury and beginning first aid until the proper help arrives?* In order, the person in charge is (1) the team physician, (2) the AT, (3) the coach, and (4) the person with the most training in first aid and CPR. Do not delay rendering care while waiting for the AT to arrive. A student assistant who is certified in first aid and CPR can begin giving care until someone who is better trained takes over. Once the team physician or AT arrives, the first person at the scene should give a full account of what has been done and then be ready to perform other duties as assigned.

2. *Is a phone available and is the emergency number known?* Emergency phone numbers change when the team travels to away games. It is important to confirm the numbers before the start of a game—do not wait until something happens. If the trainer uses a cellular phone, the battery must be charged and the bill must be paid on time. If the telephone service is cut off, how can you call for help? It is also important to have home and work phone contacts for all parents. For sporting events it is helpful to have a land line available (in case cell phone service is disabled for some reason). Also, if a bomb threat is made at a facility, it is important to use a land line to contact EMS since a cell phone may trigger an explosion if the bomb is real.

Doe, Jane **Emergency medical card** **Date of issue: 03/04/11**		
Address: 456 7th St. Anywhere, IL 01234	**Date of birth:** 01/02/96 **Sex:** Female **Blood type:** B +	**Emergency contacts:** John Doe **Relationship:** Father 555-123-4567 Cell: 555-345-5437
Preexisting conditions Asthma	**Medications** Advair twice a day Epinephrine as needed	**Emergency contacts:** Janet Doe **Relationship:** Mother 555-789-1234 Cell: 555-345-5432
Allergies Peanuts Sulfa drugs Bee stings	**Physician** Dr. John Eod Phone: 555-543-2109	**Other** Insurance carrier: NatCoverage PPO

Figure 19.1 An emergency card should be available so an AT can quickly determine whether an athlete has any preexisting conditions or needs medications in a crisis.

What Would You Do If...

A football player has suffered a head injury. At the scene, you are asked to locate the player's parent. Upon arriving at the sideline the parent becomes argumentative, saying, "There's nothing wrong. I came all this way to watch the game—put the boy back in!" Then the parent says to the son, "Why did you let that player do that to you? Are you dumb?"

3. Who will call for an ambulance? Ideally, the person who calls the ambulance is not directly responsible for giving care or getting supplies. To ensure that the caller does not panic and gives the right information, copy the emergency telephone procedures form (see appendix G) and keep the list readily available for the caller to use. The ideal order of people who should call for an ambulance is as follows: coach, student assistant, and athletic director.

4. Who will control the crowd? Crowd control is best done by someone who is not directly responsible for giving care or getting supplies. It is difficult for those giving care when people are hovering over them, so anyone who is not a caregiver needs to be moved away. On the field, team captains must take charge and move the team away. If possible, the team should practice or play on another field while care is being given so they will not get in the way of the caregivers. A coach, student, game supervisor, or athletic director usually is available to control the crowd. Parents should be allowed to talk with their injured son or daughter, and someone should be prepared to give them support, drive them to the hospital, or remove them from the scene if necessary.

5. Is spectator safety accounted for? An emergency plan must always consider the safety of the spectators. To that end, several facility-related items must be in place. First, the plan must prepare to move large masses of people from one location to the next. Consider, for example, a lightning storm occurring during a football game. An announce-

ment must be prepared to communicate the situation to the spectators and tell them where to go and how to get there.

Second, signs must be in place to show people how to exit a facility. Any ushers or facility staff must provide directions that are consistent with the announcement and the signs.

Third, appropriate lighting will be necessary to ensure the movement of people from one area to the next. Emergency lighting systems are used in public facilities for this reason. If the power goes out, the emergency lighting is activated, allowing people to see the exits and signs.

6. Is a safe facility available for inclement weather? If spectators must be evacuated because of environmental conditions, a safe location must be identified in advance so their safety is secured. An ideal area to occupy in the event of lightning, for example, is a substantial, enclosed building with indoor plumbing, electricity, and telephone communication. In the event of a tornado, an area that is free of windows is ideal, as is an area belowground within the structure.

7. Who will bring supplies and equipment, and what supplies are needed? Be sure that the supplies in the training kits, golf carts, splint bags, and so forth are always stocked and the equipment is in working order. If the AT or coach receives a report of an injury, conducts an on-field evaluation, and determines that the athlete will need to have an injury splinted and crutches, having a student assistant who can read the universal signals that tell what equipment to bring out to the injured athlete can save valuable time (figure 19.2). If the AT discovers that she needs more equipment than she has brought to the accident scene, she can simply signal the assistant, who is stationed within sight but as close to the athletic training room as possible, to bring whatever is necessary.

8. Is an automated external defibrillator (AED) available? An AED is necessary to restart the heart in instances of sudden cardiac arrest. A consensus statement from the Inter-Association Task Force on emergency preparedness and management of sudden cardiac arrest in high school and college athletic programs recommends that an AED be available at practices and games.

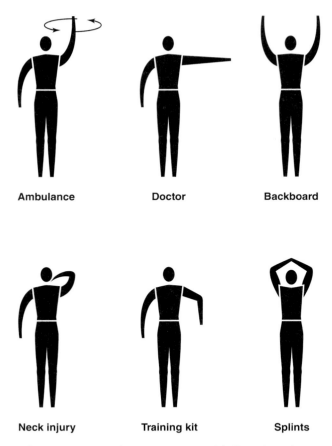

Ambulance   Doctor   Backboard

Neck injury   Training kit   Splints

Figure 19.2 The AT can use sideline signals so that prompt care of the athlete can occur. The student assistant will read the signals of the AT and jump into action, getting equipment, getting the team physician, or calling for help.

9. *Who will transport or assist the athlete from the field of play?* Sometimes an athlete is too severely injured to move. We discuss these situations in chapter 22. But most often the injured athlete can be moved, and the AT can assist him from the field, perhaps with a golf cart, a stretcher, or crutches. If the athlete is too tall or too heavy for the AT to assist alone, the trainer can recruit a couple of athletes and direct them in getting their injured teammate to the sideline. If the injured athlete is taken to the hospital, someone from the school must travel with him. This person can be the athletic director, a coach, or an AT. If the injured athlete in need of the ambulance is from an opposing team, the visiting coach is responsible for contacting the athlete's parents. Be sure that both the athletic director and school principal know which

hospital the athlete has been sent to, because they will get phone calls from people who are concerned about the athlete.

10. *Where is the safest and easiest access for emergency services to the area where the injured athlete is?* The area around the injured athlete should be clear of materials, cars, and so forth, and any locks barring access to the area should be unlocked.

11. *Who will direct the emergency services to the injured athlete?* A coach, student, or athletic director usually is available to direct an ambulance to the area. A person should be stationed at every possible point where the ambulance might approach the scene, and each of these people should be instructed in the proper technique for signaling and guiding the emergency vehicle.

12. *Who will notify the parents that their child has been injured?* It is always best to let the athlete call and tell her parents that she has been injured. If she is in no condition to call, the AT, coach, or team physician should do so. Ask the athlete which family member is best to talk with (i.e., the person who will remain calm and be able to make medical decisions). The caller will tell that person what happened, what is being done, and who is caring for the athlete. He will find out which hospital is preferred by the family and will tell the parents where to meet emergency personnel. The AT should see to it that an emergency card, which gives emergency personnel permission to treat each athlete, is with every athletic team at all times.

13. *If more than one athlete is injured, what area will be used for triage, and how will athletes get to this facility?* Most often the **triage** area, which is where decisions are made about which injuries must be treated first, is the training room or nurse's office. There may be times when the normal triage facilities are not available (e.g., fire, locked doors), so an alternative must be set up and its location communicated. In many instances where a large catastrophe has occurred at the school, the gymnasium may be used as a triage facility.

The AT plays a huge role in triage. The AT's medical background and preparation in injury assessment allow him to help determine which people are suffering the severest injuries and need to be treated first.

What Would You Do If...

At a gymnastics meet an athlete loses control, flies off the high bar, and lands on her back. The AT does an assessment and determines that she could have a spinal cord injury. You are instructed to call 911. A person comes out of the crowd and stops you, saying, "There is nothing wrong with the athlete."

Communication is essential. Make sure everyone on the emergency team has a walkie-talkie with charged batteries. Getting people who are hurt to the triage site may not be an easy task, especially if the injuries have occurred in an area that is difficult to reach because of locked doors and no keys, multiple stairways, or remoteness. Plan ahead of time for the best way to move the injured, such as by wheelchair, crutches, backboard, stretcher, executive chair with wheels, or whatever is available.

14. What personnel are available in the event of a mass casualty? How many faculty members, coaches, or students have been trained in first aid and CPR? Who can assist? If they are not on campus, can they be reached to help? At the beginning of the school year, a seminar should be held to train all faculty in first aid and CPR. Get a list of those faculty members who want to be a part of the emergency medical responder team. Decide who will be responsible for first aid kits, flashlights (in the event electricity goes out), the crisis plan, and first aid care for each area of the building (see the highlight box on this page for a list of items needed in an emergency). It is important to have people in

charge of the section of the building where they normally work. There may be times when there is no outside access to parts of the building, such as in the case of an explosion; therefore, there must be people inside who know what to do.

15. Who will fill out an accident report form and get statements from other witnesses? It is best to have someone document what is being done as it is going on.

16. How will the emergency medical response team work around known obstacles? Try to anticipate obstacles that will be fairly common in an emergency situation, such as cars obstructing a driveway, stairways, pools, poisonous gas, locked doors, smoke, no lights, no phone, foul weather, equipment failure, communication problems, lots of injuries and no help, and so on. The plan should include each of these obstacles and any others you can think of. If the plan is to remove an athlete from the field by a golf cart but it is snowing and the golf cart will not go, be prepared with an alternative plan. Make sure that all the people in the response team have keys to the areas they will be responsible for. Everyone should have access to a walkie-talkie and a lantern.

17. How will the crisis plan change for each facility (e.g., pool, gym, outdoors, game, practice, ski hill, ice arena)? Make sure people who are capable of carrying out the crisis plan are located in each facility for which the response team is responsible.

18. How will the facilities be evacuated? Evacuation is difficult because there are generally spectators who know nothing about the facility. Within the building, evacuation instructions should

Items Needed in an Emergency

- Walkie-talkie or cellular phone
- First aid kit
- Wound care supplies
- Splints
- Scissors
- Eye care supplies
- Dental injury supplies
- Gloves
- Pen light
- Tweezers
- Pocket mask
- Hand antiseptic
- Elastic wraps
- Tape
- Stethoscope
- Blood pressure cuff
- Ice
- Crutches
- Backboard
- Towels
- Notepad

be posted in every room. The outdoors must be evacuated when lightning storms, tornadoes, or hurricanes are headed into the area. The evacuation plan should include the site where each team should go for protection and accounting purposes. Hold practice evacuations so that everyone becomes familiar with the procedures.

19. *What should be done if someone forgets what to do?* The crisis plan should be available to all members of the emergency medical response team and coaching staff. Because all team members have walkie-talkies, if someone forgets what to do, another member can read the plan page by page to help get through it.

20. *Who should talk to the press?* The school system normally designates who will give information to the press and to the faculty and student body. Let the information person give the facts to the press. An in-school fact sheet can be given to all staff members to keep rumors to a minimum.

21. *Who will give counseling to those who need it?* School counselors are usually designated to help with counseling. Most situations do not require counseling, but often it is helpful to talk over a situation and review what happened.

PRACTICING THE CRISIS PLAN

As previously mentioned, you must practice a crisis plan so that people can learn their roles and so that potential problems can be recognized early and then corrected. The following is an example of a practice session. Appendix F contains a reproducible sheet to assist you in practicing your crisis plan.

First, athletic training staff should consider meeting with EMS personnel to discuss everyone's role. Second, once the roles have been clarified, identify a date in which a mock injury scenario can be

practiced. In this situation, a student assistant can pretend she is an injured athlete who needs emergency medical care. The AT can initiate the crisis plan, and a coach can contact EMS, alerting them that this is the practice drill for the crisis plan. The AT can assess and monitor the athlete and direct another student assistant or coach to bring specific medical supplies (e.g., splints). At this time, another member of the crisis team should place people at appropriate locations to direct EMS personnel into the school. Once EMS arrives, the crisis team can determine the following:

- Did an appropriate person assess the victim and direct someone to call EMS?
- Was the assigned person able to find the nearest phone and give appropriate information to EMS?
- Were assigned people able to find and deliver appropriate medical supplies to the emergency site?
- Were people able to locate themselves appropriately so that EMS could enter the site and get to the victim?

These questions allow the crisis team to identify problems. However, the practice is not quite finished. The crisis team should perform the following mock actions:

1. Call the athlete's parents.
2. Complete an injury report.
3. Identify who will speak with the press.
4. Identify how counseling services will be activated.

At the very least, the practice session should facilitate communication among the people involved in managing a crisis and help uncover obstacles. Any problems should be discussed and decisions should be made about how best to solve them.

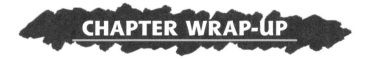

The Real World

One of the rules in cross country is to never touch a runner unless it is absolutely clear that she will not be able to finish the race; otherwise you will disqualify her. We had spent a long day working a cross country meet, and the last race of the day was a combined boys' and girls' middle school race. I was responsible for an area on an uphill slope. As a young girl approached the hill, she began to cry. I encouraged her to keep going. Instead, she lay down on the grass and kept crying. I again encouraged her to get up and finish the race, but she just lay there.

Suddenly she stopped crying and appeared to have fallen asleep. I stood next to her and tried to elicit a response by talking to her, but she did not respond. At this point I had to touch her. I checked her breathing and heartbeat, and everything was normal. I radioed to our central location to try to get more information. Her coach didn't know if the girl had any illness that would put her in this condition. The coach was on her way to us when the girl's grandmother arrived. The grandmother stated that she was a nurse, and the girl would be fine with more air. Suddenly the anxious woman slapped her grandchild across the face so hard her head rocked. Then she began giving the girl mouth-to-mouth breathing. I radioed for help, but before anyone else arrived, the girl became conscious and walked away with her grandmother. I never saw her again. To this day I wish I had had the authority to intervene, and I still wonder if the girl was ill or if she just hated running.

Anonymous

CHAPTER WRAP-UP

Summary

To be the best AT, coach, or student assistant, it is important to have a crisis plan, good evaluation skills, and good treatment skills. The crisis plan has 18 parts that will make caregivers more effective. Once the plan is designed, it is critical to practice it. Practice will prepare the caregivers and help them foresee many problems. The student assistant can help by being trained to fill a role in the crisis team and by obtaining first aid and CPR training.

Key Terms

Define the following terms found in this chapter:

crisis plan
sports medicine team
triage

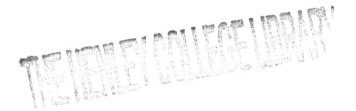

Questions for Review

1. Why is a crisis plan important?
2. Who should be included in a crisis plan?
3. What types of things can a student do in the event of a crisis?
4. What do you think is the most important part of a crisis plan and why?
5. Why is it important to practice a crisis plan?

Activities for Reinforcement

1. With another student, design a crisis plan for an athletic facility on the day of an event.
2. Design a crisis plan and go through a practice drill.
3. Make a list of the people on the athletic training team. Determine who will do each of the following: Give first aid, call the ambulance, get first aid supplies, keep the crowd back, direct the ambulance, and call the parent or guardian.

Above and Beyond

1. Find an existing crisis or emergency action plan and use the NATA position statement on emergency planning in athletics to evaluate how well constructed the emergency action plan is. Examine the NATA position statement and use it as a guide to create a venue-specific emergency action plan. Here is the source for the position statement: Andersen, J.C., R.W. Courson, D.M. Kleiner, and T.A. McLoda. 2002. National Athletic Trainers' Association position statement: Emergency planning in athletics. *Journal of Athletic Training* 37(1): 99-104.
2. Examine the following Web site, which contains an article on emergency action planning, and prepare a brief presentation for your class: www.thesportjournal.org/article/introducing-risk-assessment-model-sport-venues.

chapter 20

Emergency Assessment and Procedures

Objectives

Upon completing this chapter, the student will be able to do the following:

- Explain the difference between primary and secondary assessment.
- Explain the difference between signs and symptoms.
- Explain the CABs of a life-threatening emergency.
- Define the procedure used to restart breathing once it has stopped.
- Explain the types of illnesses or injuries that cause breathing and the heart to stop.
- Explain when CPR is used.
- Explain how external bleeding is controlled.
- Explain what precautions can be taken to prevent communicable diseases.
- Ask the basic questions for obtaining the history of an injury or illness.
- List the common vital signs, and explain how they help identify an injury or illness.
- Determine whether an injury can cause shock.
- Describe the procedures that the AT uses when testing an athlete's injury.

Athletes who become injured or ill trust the AT, coach, team physician, and student assistant to render appropriate care, which is called *first aid*. In this chapter, we discuss how to conduct a primary and secondary assessment and provide first aid for life-threatening and non-life-threatening injuries. Various life-threatening injuries and conditions are listed in the following highlight box. In subsequent chapters we cover many routine athletic injuries and their care.

An AT can begin emergency procedures only after determining the problem. Taking care of an athlete who is injured or ill is like putting together the pieces of a puzzle. The AT takes the pieces of information gathered during an assessment—the mechanism of injury, history, primary assessment, secondary assessment, and vital signs—and completes the puzzle to determine what is going on with the athlete.

In the unusual case that the AT is working with unfamiliar athletes, he should begin with an introduction. Next, it is important to ask permission to treat the athlete, although in most cases the athletes are teenagers and cannot refuse treatment because of the policies that many school districts and states have about who can refuse treatment. In addition, it is customary for parents to sign waivers to allow treatment in their absence. However, if a parent of an injured teenager has refused permission to treat, then no treatment should be given. In that case it is important for the AT to document the refusal of permission to treat by having the athlete sign the refusal in front of a witness. Refusal of treatment is rare but must be followed.

When investigating an athlete's injuries, the AT will ask her questions and observe her for signs and symptoms. A **sign** is objective evidence that a rescuer can measure or sense, such as sweating, breath odor, temperature, blood pressure, breathing rate, and heart rate. A **symptom** cannot be seen, smelled, or heard; it is subjective evidence of what the athlete feels. Examples of symptoms are pain, nausea, and anxiety. Many signs and symptoms prompt an AT to activate EMS (i.e., call 911). The list provided in the highlight box on the next page identifies the most common signs and symptoms related to emergency situations. The AT must talk to the athlete throughout the assessment process as a way of reassuring the athlete. The last sense to be impaired by unconsciousness is hearing, so the AT should continue talking to the athlete at all times. Even if the athlete is unconscious, talking to her is helpful.

PRIMARY ASSESSMENT

The assessment of each injury is divided into two categories: primary and secondary. The **primary assessment** deals with injuries that are life threatening, or injuries involving the **ABCs**—**a**irway, **b**reathing, and **c**irculation. The secondary assessment involves all non-life-threatening injuries. Luckily, most athletic injuries are not life threatening.

The order in which the assessment is done is crucial to ensuring that life-threatening injuries will be cared for first. Current American Heart Association guidelines stress that **C**ompressions come first, and then you focus on the **A**irway and **B**reathing (CAB). The primary assessment is done in the following order: (1) Check the scene to determine that it is all right to approach the athlete safely, (2) assess responsiveness by lightly tapping or shaking (not so hard that the neck gets twisted or jostled) and talking to the athlete, (3) recognize that

---

Life-Threatening Injuries

1. Cardiac arrest (heart has stopped)
2. Respiratory arrest (breathing has stopped)
3. Internal bleeding
4. Shock
5. Burns
6. Heat-related illness
7. Cold-related illness
8. Asthma attack
9. Diabetic emergency
10. Drowning
11. Electrocution
12. Falls from height
13. Poisoning
14. Severe bleeding
15. Anything else that causes breathing or cardiac impairment

Sources: American Academy of Orthopedic Surgeons (1999), American Red Cross (1993), Anderson, Hall, and Martin (2000) American Heart Association (2010).

Signs and Symptoms That Require EMS

1. Athlete is unconscious at any time.
2. Athlete is having trouble breathing or has stopped breathing.
3. Athlete is dizzy or light-headed.
4. Athlete has bleeding that will not stop.
5. Athlete has pain or pressure in the abdomen.
6. Athlete vomits, passes out, or coughs blood.
7. Athlete has fallen from height.
8. Athlete has possible head, neck, or back injuries.
9. Athlete has lost sensation or cannot move extremities.
10. Athlete has seizures, regardless of history.
11. Athlete has been poisoned.
12. Athlete has chest pain or heartbeat has stopped.
13. The amount of care required is beyond the AT's ability.
14. Athlete has broken bones, false movement, or crepitus.
15. Athlete has slurred speech.
16. Athlete has difficulty remembering things.
17. Athlete has no pulse in an extremity.

Sources: American Academy of Orthopedic Surgeons (1999), American Red Cross (1993), Anderson, Hall, and Martin (2000).

lack of responsiveness, no breathing, or abnormal breathing indicates a cardiac emergency, (4) call 911 and obtain an AED if available, (5) start CPR by initiating chest compressions, (6) open the airway and provide two breaths, and (7) check for severe bleeding. Conducting 30 compressions should take 18 seconds. The student assistant should become certified in first aid and **cardiopulmonary resuscitation (CPR)** so that when an emergency happens, she will be better prepared to help.

Checking the Scene

The first step is to prevent any more injuries than already exist, which includes making sure you do not get hurt. Approach an athlete only when the scene appears safe. If, for example, an athlete goes down during a football play, you will need to make sure the play has stopped so you do not step onto the field and accidentally get hit by a player.

Determining Responsiveness

The first step is to determine whether an athlete is conscious and able to respond. To check responsiveness, the AT will gently talk to and tap the athlete.

An unconscious athlete may be able to hear the AT and may be able to respond to a voice if she does not have a severe head injury. The response may be no more than a squeeze of a hand, but even such a feeble sign is an indication that the athlete is hearing and reacting. No one near the athlete should speak negatively about the athlete when she is unconscious because she may be able to hear. Reasons for unconsciousness include poisoning, respiratory arrest, cardiac arrest, hemorrhaging, diabetic illness, heat-related illness, cold-related illness, and head injury.

If an athlete is able to respond clearly and logically to the responsiveness check, the AT will know that the airway, breathing, and circulation are OK. At that point in the primary assessment the AT can skip the CABs (steps 3-7 in the primary assessment) and proceed to check for severe bleeding. It is important to recognize that if the athlete does not respond, however, the AT must check the CABs. If other rescuers are present they should be directed to call 911 and obtain an AED if one is available.

Initializing the CAB Sequence

If the respiratory or circulation system is impaired, the athlete's life is in danger, and the AT must respond quickly to give the athlete the best chance for survival. Quick action and early chest compressions without interruptions are recommended.

• *Circulation.* Based on the response and recognition of cardiac arrest, rescuers should start CPR immediately. It is no longer recommended that pulse or breathing detection be performed first, as early chest compressions are critical for survival. There may be spurting blood; a steady, heavy flow of blood; or blood pooling. This type of bleeding is severe and is an emergency that requires immediate attention from the AT.

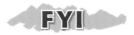

Conscious

A conscious athlete is one who quickly responds to outside stimuli such as talking, tapping, or shouting and is aware of his environment.

Respiratory Arrest

An athlete in respiratory arrest has stopped breathing.

Diabetic Illness

Diabetic illness is a disease in which sugar is not metabolized properly. The chemical insulin, which helps break down sugar, may be lacking, or the tissues may have a resistance to the insulin that is present.

• *Airway.* An untrained or solo rescuer should provide hands-only CPR, and not interrupt compressions to check the airway or breathing. A trained rescuer, or second rescuer who is able, should make sure the airway is open. To do so, the AT will place one hand on the athlete's forehead and two fingers of the other hand under the athlete's chin. Simultaneously lifting the chin while controlling the head will open the airway by pulling the tongue away from the back of the throat. This is called the *head-tilt chin-lift procedure.*

• *Breathing.* To check breathing, the AT will use a technique called *look, listen, and feel.* The AT will *look* at the chest and watch for the chest to rise and fall, *listen* for breathing by placing an ear close to the mouth, and *feel* for hot breath on his cheek. Checking for breathing should take about 10 seconds, and should be done by a trained rescuer. The look, listen, and feel step has been removed for lay rescuers.

BREATHING EMERGENCIES

Any situation in which breathing has stopped or is compromised is considered life threatening. Breathing emergencies can involve any part of the respiratory system, and the compromise of any part of the respiratory system can cause death. Direct traumas, such as rupture of the diaphragm, punctured lungs, anaphylaxis, or an illness like asthma can cause a breathing emergency. Drowning, suf-

focation, or an airway obstruction can also cause an athlete to stop breathing. If the brain does not receive oxygen, cells begin to die. The longer the brain goes without oxygen, the greater the number of cells that die; eventually whole portions of the brain die until the death of the athlete results. As little as 4 minutes without oxygen can cause permanent brain damage. The sooner lifesaving efforts begin, the better the chances are that the athlete will survive without brain injury. Most often EMS will have a response team to the location within 4 to 10 minutes. If proper care begins immediately, the chances of survival are 98%. If care is delayed by 4 minutes after breathing has stopped, the chances of survival are significantly reduced.

Illnesses such as asthma that cause a breathing emergency can most often be dealt with by elevating the athlete's head and, when appropriate, helping the athlete take her medication. A punctured lung must be cared for in a different manner (see page 90).

Cardiopulmonary Resuscitation

If an AT determines that an athlete is not breathing when the primary survey is performed, mouth-to-mouth rescue breaths may be initiated. In mouth-to-mouth breathing, which is also known as rescue breathing and CPR, the AT places a protective barrier over the athlete's mouth and exhales into the athlete's lungs, causing the chest to rise. Initially, two rescue breaths are given. The American Heart Association recognizes that for healthcare providers the sequence of emergency care can be tailored to match the problem the patient is having.

What Would You Do If...

You are a spectator at a soccer game. The temperature is cool. A parent who is videotaping the game is pale and sweating. The man's wife, who knows that you are a student assistant, asks you to take a look at her husband. You check his pulse, and it's so rapid that you cannot count that fast. The man insists there is nothing wrong with him. The AT is on the sideline, watching the game.

Pediatric Cardiopulmonary Resuscitation

Pediatric cardiac arrest occurs primarily from asphyxia, or respiratory inefficiency, so the American Heart Association continues to support the use of rescue breathing and chest compressions if the victim is a child. With pediatric victims, the AT will still utilize the CAB sequence and provide rescue breaths along with the chest compressions. If there is a pulse and no breathing, then mouth-to-mouth breathing is performed. Rescue breaths last one to one-and-a-half seconds, and one breath is given every three seconds (one breath every five seconds for an adult). After giving a breath, the AT will always turn her head and look at the athlete's chest. This not only helps the AT see if the athlete has begun to breathe but also slows things down so that AT does not hyperventilate. Placing one's mouth on another's mouth or nose can transmit some diseases, and several devices are available that act as a barrier between the AT and the injured person. At least one of these devices should be a part of every emergency kit.

AT will initiate chest compressions after the initial rescue breaths and after checking for a pulse. A total of 30 chest compressions are given, followed by two rescue breaths. This procedure is continued until the athlete begins breathing or the AED arrives and is ready to be applied to the victim. The compressions are given at a rate of about 100 per minute at a depth of at least 2 inches. The AT may need to use only one hand to get the necessary depth for a child.

Adult Cardiopulmonary Resuscitation

If the victim is an adult, the AT will initiate chest compressions if CPR is warranted. A total of 30 chest compressions are given, followed by two rescue breaths. This procedure is continued until the athlete begins breathing or the AED arrives and is ready to be applied to the victim.

Chest compressions are conducted by overlapping hands, placing the heel of one hand on the victim's sternum, and quickly compressing the chest down to at least 2 inches (5 cm) for an adult. Compressions and breaths should be given at a 30:2 ratio. The rate of compressions should allow for 100 chest compressions in a minute.

The number of compressions and breaths has been updated from a previous ratio of 15:2. If there

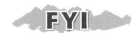

Diaphragm

The diaphragm is the muscle that separates the chest and abdominal cavities and assists in breathing.

Asthma

Asthma is a condition in which the air passages narrow in response to an allergen such as pollen, dust, or mold. Exercise may also trigger an attack. The air passage may close entirely.

Anaphylaxis

Anaphylaxis is an allergic reaction in which the air passages narrow in response to a foreign protein, such as bee venom, or to a drug, such as medication to which the person has been sensitized.

Blood Pressure

Blood pressure is the pressure that the blood exerts against the walls of the vessels as it moves through them. The blood pressure of an average teenager is 110 to 120 systolic (when the heart beats) and 65 to 80 diastolic (between beats).

Hyperventilation

Hyperventilation is rapid and deep breathing consisting of 24 breaths or more per minute.

are two rescuers, the ratio of 15:2 can be done, but this is a more advanced skill. We recommend obtaining CPR certification for the professional rescuer, or basic life support, so you are capable of performing both single- and two-person CPR.

Please note that the CPR guidelines change frequently. We urge readers to visit the Web sites of the American Red Cross, American Heart Association, and National Safety Council to learn when the parameters are updated.

Obstructed Airway

An athlete's airway can become obstructed in a number of ways, but the tongue is the number one airway obstructer. In an unconscious athlete, especially one lying on her back, the tongue likely will relax and obstruct the air passage. Other possible obstructions are food, gum, mouth guards, broken teeth, blood, vomit, and chewing tobacco. (To prevent airway obstruction, we recommend barring food, gum, and chewing tobacco from practices

What Would You Do If...

In the cafeteria a student tells a joke and another begins to cough forcefully just after laughing. The student continues to cough, and her face is turning red and tears are rolling down her cheeks. The athletes next to you say, "She's choking. Do something!"

and games.) A conscious athlete with an obstructed airway will grab at his throat. If the athlete is unconscious, the AT will have to open his airway, check his breathing, and begin giving breaths before discovering that there is an airway obstruction. An airway obstruction may be partial or total.

A **partial airway obstruction** occurs when an object covers the air passage but still allows some air to flow in and out of the lungs. The athlete will grab for his throat—the **universal choking sign**—as an indication that he has a problem with the air passage (see figure 20.1). To determine if this obstruction is partial or total, the AT will ask him if he can speak, cough, or breathe. If he can, he has a partial airway obstruction. An athlete who has a high-pitched whistling noise coming from his throat has a total airway obstruction.

A **total airway obstruction** occurs when an object blocks the entire air passage and does not allow enough air to flow into the lungs for the athlete to take a breath. Under such conditions, the athlete may have a high-pitched whistling noise coming from her throat, which comes from a small amount of air pushing past the object in the throat. A conscious athlete will demonstrate the universal choking sign. She will show redness of the face and tearing. In the event that an athlete is conscious but has a total airway obstruction, the AT will lean the athlete forward and perform five back blows by slapping the person between her scapulas. After five back blows, abdominal thrusts are performed. Abdominal thrusts are performed by standing behind the athlete and placing one fist against her abdomen, just above the navel. The AT reaches around with the other hand, placing it over his fist. Once the AT's hands are in place, inward and upward thrusts are performed to dislodge the object. In the event that an athlete is unconscious and an AT determines that the airway is blocked, the athlete is evaluated as an unconscious victim and CPR may need to be performed, as described previously.

CARDIOPULMONARY EMERGENCIES

There are two cardiopulmonary emergencies that concern the AT: heart attack and cardiac arrest. Both are life-threatening emergencies that must be dealt with immediately.

Heart Attack

A **heart attack** is also called an *acute myocardial infarction* and occurs when the heart muscle is damaged by a blockage of a vessel to the heart, a clot, stress, or an injury to the heart muscle that does not allow the heart to receive the blood it needs to function. A student assistant may think, "I'm going to work with healthy young athletes, so I probably won't have to know much about heart attacks." However, consider the people in the stands and athletes who have an undiagnosed heart problem. The student assistant may be the one called upon to help a heart attack victim.

Signs of a heart attack are breathing difficulty, shortness of breath, breathing faster than normal, a pulse rate that is faster or slower than normal

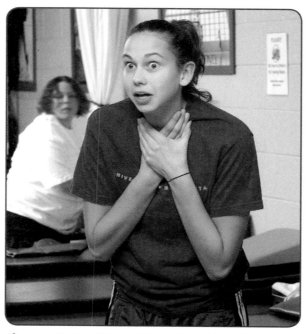

Figure 20.1   The universal choking sign.

What Would You Do If...

Your high school's track star is doing some preseason sprints to get into shape. She suddenly drops to the ground and stops moving. When you arrive, you see she is not breathing, and you cannot find a heartbeat. Your friends say you must be mistaken—the athlete is only 15 years old. You check again, and there is no breathing and no heartbeat.

or irregular, skin that is pale or bluish, profuse sweating, vomiting, sudden unexplained fainting (**syncope**), and elevated blood pressure. Symptoms of a heart attack include nausea, persistent chest pain or discomfort that is not relieved by rest or by changing positions, anxiety, a general feeling of weakness, and light-headedness.

The victim often describes a feeling of someone standing on or tightening a belt around his chest. This crushing chest pain is termed **angina pectoris**. It is common for people to be embarrassed by chest pain if it turns out there is nothing wrong. Many people having heart attacks die because they do not go to the hospital, thinking they have nothing more than an upset stomach. It is better to go to the hospital and let the experts rule out a heart attack than it is to die or have irreparable heart damage.

Treatment of a heart attack begins with recognizing that a heart attack is occurring. The AT must assess the athlete quickly, get the victim to stop her activity, and call EMS. The AT should also monitor the victim until help arrives and make her as comfortable as possible.

Sudden Cardiac Arrest

Cardiac arrest occurs when the damage to the heart muscle is so severe that it interferes with the heart's electrical system, causing the heart to stop beating. A heart attack and sudden cardiac arrest (SCA) are not the same. According to the National Center for Early Defibrillation, SCA is one of the leading causes of death among adults and accounts for 225,000 deaths each year in the United States. If the damage is too severe, lifesaving measures will not start the heart again. This, however, is a deter-

mination that an AT cannot make—he must treat the cardiac arrest whether he thinks the damage is severe or not. The symptoms of SCA occur so quickly that there may not be enough time to seek help. Symptoms include irregular heartbeat, and the athlete will often have a history of fainting and dizziness.

If an athlete is in cardiac arrest, the AT must begin treatment immediately to save the athlete's life. He will place the athlete on a hard, flat surface and begin giving CPR (see figure 20.2). An ambulance must be called because professional medical care is critical for the athlete's survival.

Unfortunately, an AT can rarely restart the heart by performing CPR; it will probably be necessary to stimulate the heart with an electrical shock or injected medication. Thankfully, AEDs are becoming standard equipment at public locations, and many ATs have an AED on-site during practices and games or at least have them in a known location for easy access. AED use is also often included in CPR courses. An AED will deliver an electrical

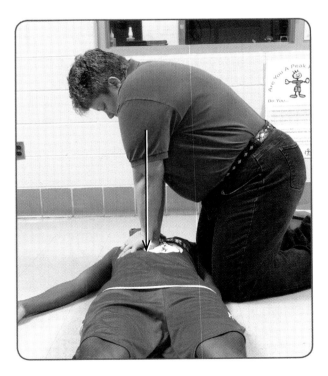

Figure 20.2   CPR is given to a person who is not breathing and who has no heartbeat. The AT will administer 30 compressions and two breaths. For effective compression, the AT's shoulders must be over the victim's sternum.

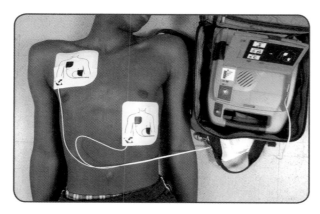

Figure 20.3 AED pad placement.

shock to the victim to restart the heart. The AED requires that an AT attach electrodes to the victim in specific locations on the chest, usually at the victim's right upper chest and left lower side (see figure 20.3). The AED will first monitor the victim's heart and determine if a shock is necessary. The AED then indicates that a shock is advised, and the AT administers the shock once everyone is clear of the victim. The AED is used in conjunction with CPR procedures to circulate the athlete's blood and provide oxygen to the brain.

HEMORRHAGE

A hemorrhage is a discharge of blood, externally or internally, that may be severe enough to cause death. The average adult has 6 quarts (5.7 L) of blood, and the loss of 10% can result in death.

External Bleeding

External bleeding occurs when a person suffers a laceration, incision, amputation, avulsion, puncture, or abrasion (see page 42). If the blood is spurting from a wound, an artery has been cut. Blood that is flowing rapidly but not spurting is most likely from a vein.

Control of Bleeding

The body's blood-clotting mechanism easily controls most bleeding. However, some areas of the body, such as the head, abdomen, thighs, and chest, have a greater blood supply than other areas and therefore may bleed profusely. A large pool of blood indicates that the athlete has suffered a severe blood loss. The AT must act immediately or the athlete could die.

To control bleeding, the AT will follow these procedures in order:

1. Apply **direct pressure** to the wound, using a hand to squeeze the area tightly.
2. Elevate the body part, but only if no fractures are present and direct pressure has not slowed the bleeding.
3. Apply a pressure bandage when bleeding is controlled or if another injured athlete needs care.
4. Apply pressure to a **pressure point**. This will slow blood flow to the extremity but will not stop it entirely. Use this measure only if all the other measures fail. (See figure 20.4.)

Internal bleeding must be dealt with by a physician. The AT will call for the ambulance. We discuss the signs and symptoms of internal bleeding in chapter 8.

Wound Care

After bleeding is controlled, the AT must care for the wound. First, the wound is inspected to determine if sutures (stitches) are needed. Sutures will be needed if the wound is deep and the edges are gaping apart. When an athlete needs sutured, she must be referred immediately to a physician because sutures should be applied within 12 hours of the incident. In this instance, the wound should be covered with a nonstick sterile dressing and covered with a bandage to keep the dressing in place.

If sutures are not needed, proper steps of wound care should be followed. The AT will first take precautions to prevent disease transmission (see the next section) by applying gloves. Once preventive measures are in place, the wound should be cleaned.

The athlete should be instructed to first wash the wound with antimicrobial soap and water. Once washed, the wound should be cleaned again with

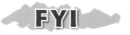

Elevate

Elevate means to lift above the level of the heart.

Bandage

A bandage is a strip of cloth used to hold a dressing in place.

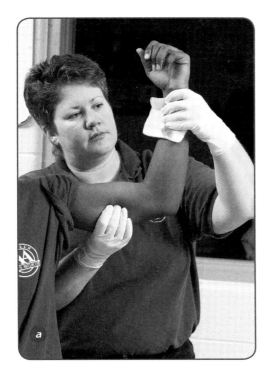

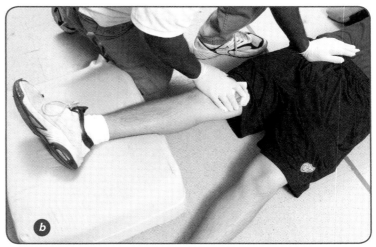

Figure 20.4 The pressure points at the *(a)* brachial and *(b)* femoral arteries.

a 10% Betadine solution. If debris is present in the wound, irrigation with sterile saline may be needed to dislodge the particles. The saline should be squirted at a slight angle onto the wound and should drain away from the wound.

An antibiotic cream should be applied to prevent infection. The antibiotic cream should be applied to a sterile dressing and then the dressing applied to the wound.

Methicillin-Resistant *Staphylococcus Aureus*

Athletes should change their wound dressing daily and observe for any signs of infection. An infection can be life threatening, particularly if the infection is resistant to standard antibiotics. A serious infection that is becoming more common is methicillin-resistant *Staphylococcus aureus*, also known as **MRSA**.

The Real World

I was sitting in the training room doing some paperwork with a senior student assistant when I looked up to see a football player being helped through the doorway. He was staggering, and he was a bloody mess—he had fallen into a glass door. I immediately dialed 911, and I told him to lie down and elevate his legs because I could see that he was showing signs of shock and hysteria. He was holding his wrists, each of which had a deep cut down to the tendons. He had a third severe laceration, a 2.5-inch (6 cm) gash across his forehead. I put on gloves and grabbed a pole of gauze. I applied direct pressure to the forehead and the worst of the two wrist lacerations.

Then things got complicated. I literally had my hands full, so my student assistant (a first responder) gloved up to help me. I thought, "This will be a great experience for her." As she was standing next to me putting on her gloves, she said, "I'm going to faint." Before I could tell her to sit down, she did faint, striking her head on the floor, and she had a petit mal seizure caused by the bump. I could see she was breathing, so I kept my pressure on the wounds, kept an eye on her, and waited for the police and paramedics to arrive. It was quite the scene. The other athletes in the area were freaked out. Everything turned out OK, though. We got the bloody football player bandaged and off to the emergency room where they stitched him up. My embarrassed assistant just ended up icing the large lump on the back of her head.

Steve Marti, ATC

According to the Centers for Disease Control and Prevention (CDC), signs and symptoms of MRSA include swelling, pain, redness, warmth, pus drainage, and a yellow or white core or center to the wound. The athlete is also likely to have a fever. In many instances the wound will first appear as a small spider-bite lesion. Athletes suspected of having MRSA or other infections should be examined by a physician right away. Treating MRSA involves strong antibiotics along with having the wound drained by a physician.

PREVENTING COMMUNICABLE DISEASE TRANSMISSION

When dealing with bleeding wounds, the AT must protect herself and the athlete from infection. We tend to assume that athletes are free from communicable diseases because they look and act healthy, but this is not necessarily true.

An athlete may hide certain medical conditions to avoid discrimination. If an athlete chooses to reveal such a condition, it should be noted on the records from the physical.

Communicable diseases are transmitted, either directly or indirectly, by contact with an infected person. Although most viruses and bacteria cannot live long in the absence of a host, the AT and the athletes should take sensible precautions against possible infections. They should make it a habit not to share drinking glasses or towels, and they should try to avoid people who are contagious, such as someone who is sneezing a great deal from a cold. Some viruses, namely HIV and HBV (the viruses that cause AIDS and hepatitis B, respectively), may be present in bodily fluids from oozing wounds or needles. Thus, the athletic training team should take precautions when handling body fluids or when handling cloth, paper, or surfaces that have been soaked with body fluids (e.g., blood, urine).

Special precautions must be taken against the spread of HIV and HBV, which may be present in blood or other bodily fluids. Not only the athletic staff but every staff member of the school should be trained in **universal precautions** and follow procedures set forth by the Occupational Safety and Health Administration (OSHA) to prevent the spread of bloodborne diseases. A person with HIV or hepatitis B may show no signs or symptoms of the disease and may not even know she has the disease, yet the disease may be transmitted through contact with her blood. Therefore, universal precautions must be used every time bodily fluid is present. To take universal precautions, five simple rules must be observed:

1. Carefully wash your hands after any contact with an injured athlete.

2. Use rubber gloves to create a barrier between you and the athlete. Figure 20.5 illustrates how to properly remove gloves.

3. Thoroughly clean any tables, counters, or playing surfaces in an athletic training room or court with a disinfectant such as a 1:10 solution of bleach and water.

4. Deposit in a red biohazard bag any material, including clothes, gloves, or gauze pads, that is contaminated.

5. Dispose of any used needles or syringes in a specially made sharps container. If an AT is contaminated by body fluids, she must document the incident and report it to her supervisor as soon as possible.

Athletes should observe other standard precautions, which, for example, will help to prevent the spread of common cold and flu viruses. The AT should not allow players to dip their cups into a team cooler to get water; this practice allows saliva to be mixed into the cooler. Every athlete should drink from his own glass or squeeze bottle. Athletes should avoid tasting each other's food, borrowing utensils, and sharing drinking glasses. They should also avoid sharing personal items such as combs, towels, and clothes, and they should shower after each practice. Teams must also be prepared to replace uniforms that are potentially soiled with a pathogen.

In addition to taking universal precautions, ATs can be vaccinated against certain diseases. They can be vaccinated against HBV, for example, by receiving a series of three vaccine injections over a

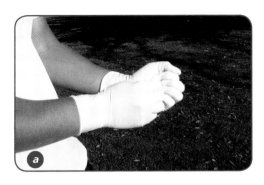
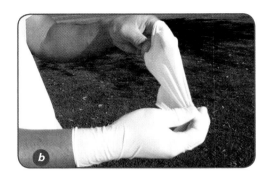
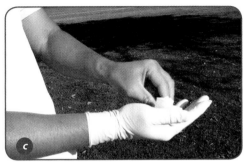
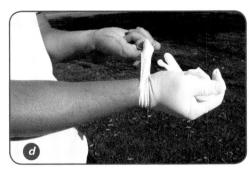

Figure 20.5 When removing latex gloves, *(a)* place all waste in one hand, and with the opposite, pinch the latex near the wrist; *(b)* pull the first glove off with the waste inside the glove; *(c)* place the first glove into the second hand; *(d)* slide a finger under the inside edge of the second glove; and pull the glove off. Discard the gloves in a biohazard container.

seven-month period. According to OSHA, the HBV vaccine is 90% effective in preventing infection.

SECONDARY ASSESSMENT

The secondary assessment is an evaluation of injuries that are not life threatening. The AT performs a secondary assessment after she has completed the primary survey and taken care of any life-threatening injuries. In the secondary assessment, she will check the following in order: history, head, vital signs, arms, chest, abdomen, hips, and legs. If at any time during the secondary assessment the airway, breathing, or circulation changes, the AT will immediately give care and abandon the secondary assessment.

HIT

Most of the time an AT is dealing with a specific complaint, such as "My thumb hurts." When doing an assessment on a specific body area, he uses the

H	**History**—Take a history by asking questions and checking vital signs.
I	**Inspection**—Observe the surroundings and injured body part.
T	**Testing**—Do specific testing to determine the severity of the injury.

Figure 20.6 Athletic injury assessment follows a predictable sequence: taking a history, inspecting the area, and testing.

HIT technique (see figure 20.6). The acronym *HIT* stands for **h**istory, **i**nspection, and **t**esting. The trainer takes a history to gather information about the situation and the injury, inspection is a visual examination of the body part, and testing includes touching, specific evaluations, checking the range of motion, and neurological testing. We will refer to the HIT technique throughout this text.

What Would You Do If...

The AT is doing an evaluation. Every time the AT touches a body part, the athlete responds by saying, "That hurts!" The AT tells you to get a backboard and call 911.

History

Taking a history includes both asking questions and checking vital signs. In taking a **history**, the AT will obtain information about what is happening and about the athlete's previous injuries and illnesses because they may play a role in the present problem (see the following highlight box). If the athlete is unconscious, reviewing records of her physical and talking to other athletes who saw the injury may be helpful.

The AT will check the athlete for a medical alert tag and the records from the physical for information that may help determine the cause of the current condition. The same questions can be used to take a history for any injury and illness. We refer to the questions for history of injury in the following chapters, so copy the list and keep it handy. Questions that apply to a specific body area will be listed in the appropriate chapter.

The **vital signs** checked in the secondary assessment are body temperature, skin color, breathing rate, heart rate, response to pain, pupillary reaction, ability to move, and capillary refill. The AT can also assess breath sounds and blood pressure if a stethoscope and blood pressure cuff are available. Table 20.1 outlines abnormal vital signs.

Heart Rate

Heart rate is measured at **pulse points**, where an artery lies close to the skin (see figure 20.7). The

Table 20.1   Abnormal Vital Signs

Vital signs	Abnormality	Indication
Pupils	Constricted	Drug or medication overdose or bright light
	Unequal	Head injury or illness
	Dilated	Drug or medication overdose, death, shock, heatstroke, or darkness
Pulse	Rapid and weak	Shock, internal bleeding, diabetic coma, or heat exhaustion
	Rapid and strong	Heatstroke, anxiousness, or physical exercise
	No pulse	Blocked artery or cardiac arrest
	Slow pulse	Heart problem, drugs, or medications
Skin color	Red	Heatstroke, inflammation, or diabetic coma
	White	Shock, heat exhaustion, insulin shock, or low blood pressure
	Blue	Cardiac arrest or breathing difficulty
Body temperature	Hot and dry	Heatstroke
	Cool and moist	Heat exhaustion
	Chills	Cold exposure or illness
	Hot and moist	Fever
Breathing	No breathing	Cardiac arrest, respiratory arrest, or head injury
	Decreased breathing rate	Chest trauma or head injury
	Increased breathing rate	Drugs or medication, shock, heart injury, or anxiety

pulse points of the carotid artery and the radial artery are used most often. The carotid artery can be found by placing two fingers on the Adam's apple and then sliding them toward the shoulder until the fingers go into a depression in the neck. The radial artery is located on the volar aspect (palm side) on the thumb side of the wrist. Once the pulse is found, the AT will count the number of times the heart beats in a minute—this is the **pulse rate**. The normal pulse rate for an average teenager or adult is between 60 and 80 beats per minute. A highly trained athlete, however, may have a pulse rate as low as 40 beats per minute and still be perfectly

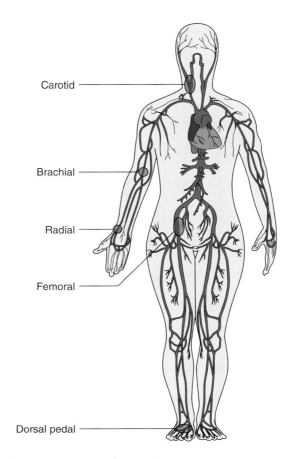

Figure 20.7 Pulse points.

healthy. A person may also have a pulse rate below the norm because of medication (legal or illegal), heart abnormalities, or internal injuries. Rapid pulse rates may be due to shock, hyperventilation, medication (legal or illegal), anxiety, or recent physical activity.

Breathing Rate

Breathing rate is determined by counting the number of times the chest rises and falls in a minute. The normal breathing rate for a teenager or adult is between 12 and 20 breaths per minute. Breathing rates can be slower than normal due to a head injury, lung injury, medication (legal or illegal), shock, diabetes, and hyperventilation. Breathing rates that are rapid may be the result of shock, medication (legal or illegal), anxiety, heat-related illnesses, or recent physical activity. Athletes may also have **dyspnea**, or difficulty breathing. This is common among athletes with asthma, cystic fibrosis, shock, pneumonia, lung

Questions for History of Injury

The following questions should be asked as part of the history:

1. What happened?
2. When did it happen?
3. Has this happened before?
4. Where was the pain initially?
5. Did you hear or feel a pop, snap, crack, slip, or give?
6. Were you able to continue participating?
7. How soon did it swell?
8. Does it feel unstable?
9. What relieves the pain?
10. How severe is the pain?
11. What does the pain feel like?
12. What treatment was applied immediately? Later?
13. Have you had a previous injury to this body part?

If the problem relates to an illness rather than an injury, ask the following questions:

1. Are you allergic to any medications?
2. What have you eaten today?
3. Are you allergic to anything else?
4. Have you had anything to drink today?
5. What events led to this situation?

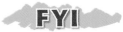

Breath Sounds

Breath sounds are heard through the chest wall with a stethoscope. No breath sounds means that the athlete is not breathing or the lungs are seriously injured.

Cystic Fibrosis

Cystic fibrosis, a disease that affects the pancreas and lungs, is inherited.

Shock

Shock is a condition in which inadequate oxygen is reaching the tissues of the body because of insufficient blood flow.

Pneumonia

Pneumonia is an inflammation of the lungs caused by an infection or irritant.

---

injuries, allergic reactions, airway obstructions, or upper-respiratory illnesses (colds or flu). The AT will not tell the athlete when she is checking his breathing rate because it is often hard for a person to breathe naturally if he knows he is being watched. He may hold his breath or breathe faster, invalidating the count. The AT will check the pulse and, while pretending to be taking the athlete's pulse, count the breathing rate. **Apnea** is the temporary cessation of breathing, and it is a serious symptom in an athlete because it may indicate a head injury. An athlete who has an unusual breath odor should be checked for possible poisoning, intoxication, or diabetes.

When the AT uses a stethoscope to listen to the lungs, she will listen to each side of the chest for one cycle of breathing and compare them. Then she will listen to the lower lung portions for one cycle to ensure that there are no immediate problems with the lungs.

Blood Pressure

The heart pumps the blood to move blood cells, nutrients, and oxygen throughout the body. Blood pressure is the pressure that the blood exerts on the walls of the blood vessels, especially the arteries. **Systolic pressure** is the pressure when the heart is contracting, and **diastolic pressure** is the pressure when the heart is relaxed between beats. **Pulse pressure** is the difference between the diastolic and systolic pressures. The blood pressure of a normal teenager is 110 mmHg (milliliters of mercury) systolic and 65 to 80 mmHg diastolic. Blood pressure can increase because of a head injury, recent activity, medication (legal or illegal), and illnesses. Blood pressure will drop because of heart failure, hemorrhage, shock, certain medications (legal or illegal), and illnesses.

Blood pressure is measured with a stethoscope and a blood pressure cuff, which is sized in proportion to the athlete's arm (see figure 20.8). The cuff is placed on the upper arm and pressurized until no blood can flow through the superficial arteries. As the pressure in the cuff is slowly released, the person listens through the stethoscope, which has been placed on the inside of the elbow, and watches the dial on the cuff. The first time a sound is heard, the person reads the dial; that is the systolic pressure. When the sounds stop, the dial is read again; that is the diastolic pressure. If a stethoscope is not available, systolic blood pressure can be taken by feeling (palpating) for a radial pulse, although this method is less accurate. As the blood pressure cuff is released, the person reads the dial when he feels the radial pulse, and

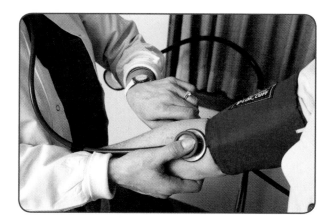

Figure 20.8 Place the stethoscope over the artery and listen as the pressure is released from the blood pressure cuff. The systolic pressure is read from the dial when the first pumping sound is heard. The diastolic pressure is read when the last pumping sound is heard.

that will be the systolic pressure. When taking a blood pressure reading, bear in mind that an athlete who has just finished exercising will have a higher-than-normal blood pressure, as will an athlete who is upset. If the AT is having trouble getting a blood pressure reading, he will check the athlete for the following:

- A heartbeat
- Shock
- Placement of the stethoscope
- Blockage of the artery

Body Temperature

Normal **body temperature** is 98.6° Fahrenheit (36.6 °C). An athlete's body temperature can rise if she has an infection or heatstroke, and it may drop if she is in shock or exposed to cold. Electronic temperature-measuring devices, which are quick and accurate, are now available. The temperature can be taken with an oral thermometer, which is left in place for three minutes. It is also possible, although unreliable, to take a temperature by placing a thermometer in the armpit for 10 minutes. It is not possible to measure a person's temperature or even tell if she has a fever by feeling her forehead, but the AT may feel an athlete's forehead to determine if she is hot, cold, sweaty, or dry.

Skin Color

Skin color can give information about what illness or injury may have occurred. Four color changes are significant: cherry red is an indication of heatstroke or carbon monoxide poisoning, a bluish tinge is an indication of poor oxygen supply,

yellow is an indication of liver illness, and a lack of color or a paleness of the nail beds and lips is an indication of shock or lack of circulation. The AT will also check for color changes in the whites of the eyes (sclera), the inside of the lip, and the fingernail and toenail beds, especially if the athlete has a dark complexion.

Understanding Diversity

It may be difficult to evaluate pallor or jaundice in people with darker skin. The AT may use nail beds, the sclera of the eye, or the inside of the lip to determine skin color changes (Purnell and Paulanka 2003).

Capillary Refill

Capillary refill is an indication that blood is flowing to the fingertips and toes (see figure 20.9). It is determined by pressing on the nail and measuring how long it takes the color to return to normal (approximately one second). When the AT is checking capillary refill, he will check both arms or both legs at the same time. That way he can tell if there is a difference between them, which may indicate a fracture or a blood clot in one of the body parts.

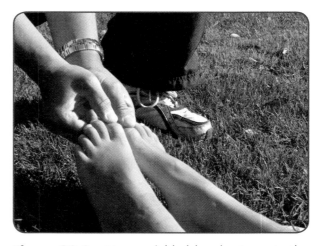

Figure 20.9 How quickly blood returns to the tip of a finger or toe after pressing on the nail bed and then releasing pressure is a measure of the blood supply to the finger. Poor capillary refill can mean restricted blood vessels or poor blood supply.

Pupil Response

The pupils of the eyes change size in response to light. When light shines into the eye, the pupils **constrict**, or get smaller, to decrease the amount of light entering the eye. In the dark, the pupils enlarge, or **dilate**, to allow more light into the eye. When the eyes do not respond normally to changes in light, a serious problem is indicated. If the pupils dilate when light shines into them, the athlete may have been poisoned or medicated, or she may even be dead. Pupils that constrict when there is darkness are an indication of heatstroke or poisoning. If the pupils are unequal in size (one is large and one is small), the AT will suspect a head injury, although a small percentage of people normally have unequal pupils. People who are blind may or may not have pupillary response, depending on the origin of the blindness. Figure 20.10 illustrates pupil responses.

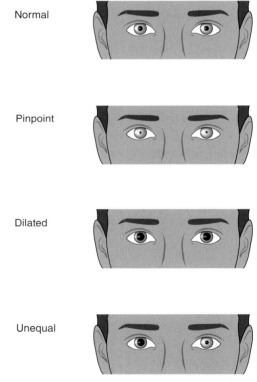

Figure 20.10 In response to light, the pupils normally get smaller. Pupils that dilate in response to light indicate a serious head injury, use of medication, or death. Pinpoint pupils are an indication of medication. Unequal pupils indicate a head injury on the same side as the enlarged pupil.

What Would You Do If...

An athlete has been kept out of basketball practice because of ankle pain. She has not been able to walk but has no swelling or discoloration. During the week she has been going to rehabilitation and has received other forms of therapy. While driving past her house, you see her playing basketball with several other people, and she has no problem running or jumping. Upon noticing you, she says, "Don't tell anyone. I just don't like to run."

Ability to Move

It is important to find out if the athlete can still move. This will help to determine what injury may have occurred and how to treat the athlete. **Paralysis**, the inability to move, is caused by an injury to the brain or spinal cord. The inability of an athlete to move one side of the body is known as **hemiplegia**, which is an indication of a head injury on the side opposite to the paralyzed side of the body. The extent of the paralysis depends on the location of the injury—the higher in the spine the injury occurs, the greater the extent of limb impairment. The inability to move the legs is called **paraplegia**, and the inability to move the arms and legs is called **quadriplegia**. Paralysis may be temporary; regardless, a physician must care for the athlete.

Response to Pain

People respond differently to being injured. Pain cannot be used to determine the severity of an injury, because people have different tolerances for pain and will respond to the pain of an injury in different ways. Paralysis, medication, and shock can also disguise pain reactions. In addition, it is important to understand that injuries to internal organs tend to refer pain to specific areas of the body. For example, an injury to the spleen may result in pain around the athlete's left shoulder. See figure 20.11, *a* and *b*, for referred pain sites from internal organs.

Inspection

The AT will observe the athlete's body and surroundings for clues as to what may have happened, which

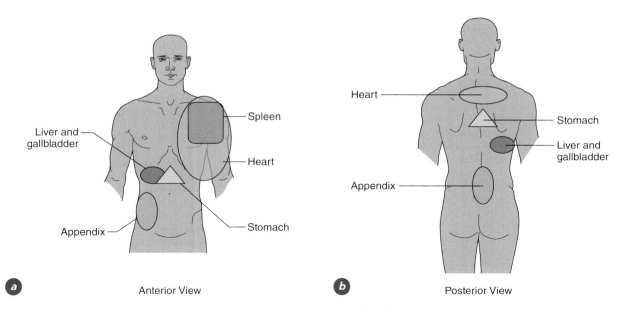

Figure 20.11 *(a)* Anterior view and *(b)* posterior view of referred pain sites from internal organs.

will suggest treatment options. If a chair has been tipped over, it is possible that the athlete fell out of it. Think about the injuries that could occur from a fall while sitting on a chair. Now think about the injuries that could occur if the athlete fell while standing on the chair. Are they the same? An empty bottle should raise red flags. Is this a poisoning, or was the athlete taking medication for an illness? An arm that bends where it never did before means what? The questions that are the hardest to answer are the ones on which the AT will concentrate. An even greater problem will be trying to get other athletes to talk about how the injury occurred. Some athletes may not want to help because they do not want to be involved, they fear lawsuits, or they just do not care.

Testing

Most often an AT will do the primary survey quickly, and during the history portion of the assessment the athlete will indicate what happened. At that point the AT can assess the body

The Real World

One day I arrived at work just as a fellow employee pulled into the parking lot, so we walked together across the street to the hospital. We saw a casually dressed man lying in the grass between the curb and the sidewalk, apparently unconscious. As we approached him to check his breathing, he opened his eyes and said loudly, "Please don't call an ambulance, just let me lie here." I wondered why we shouldn't call for help, but we couldn't just leave him there, so I stayed with the man while my colleague went to the emergency room, just inside the nearest building, to report the problem. The man's skin felt cool and clammy to the touch, and when I checked his pulse, I noticed an alert tag on his wrist, which said he had epilepsy. He must have had a seizure and fallen on the grass. He said he was very tired, and his speech was slurred. EMS arrived in only a few minutes and took him to the emergency room. When I went to check on him later that morning, he had been released to his family's care. What a way to start the morning! It just goes to show that you must be prepared for anything at all times.

Bill Pitney, EdD, ATC

part involved. She can do specific tests to determine the severity of injury before swelling and muscular contractions occur, which will cause the body part to become immobile and make it difficult to determine the extent of the injury. The tests will also help determine how the athlete should be moved, if he should be splinted, or if medical help is immediately necessary. Testing should be stopped if the swelling is exceedingly rapid, if crepitus is felt, or if there is deformity or excessive pain.

Palpation

During **palpation** the AT will examine the athlete by touch, feeling for depressions, fluid leakage, bumps, crepitus, and things that are not symmetrical. He will look for signs of pain on the athlete's face, decreased strength, decreased sensation, and false movement. Crepitus and excessive pain are reasons to stop palpation and splint the body part before moving the athlete. Palpation is done in the following order:

1. Head
2. Chest and thorax
3. Abdomen
4. Upper extremities
5. Lower extremities
6. Special tests

Listening to the Heart

Listening to the heart and obtaining useful information requires a lot of practice. For most ATs, listening to the heart will be limited to establishing that there is a heartbeat and determining a heart rate.

Range-of-Motion Testing

Range of motion must be tested at the injured segment as well as at the joints above and below the injury. The testing should be performed both actively and passively (see figure 20.12). That is, the injured

athlete moves the injured segment if he is able (active) and the AT also attempts to move it (passive).

An athlete with a suspected broken bone, a bone with deformity, or a spinal cord injury should not be put through range-of-motion testing. Suspected broken bones should be splinted before an injured athlete is moved.

Range of motion should be measured from the anatomical position with a **goniometer** (see figure 20.13). When documenting test results, the AT should be sure to note the position the athlete was in when she took the measurements. For example, the report should state that the athlete was supine (lying on her back) or prone (facedown). This allows the AT to take follow-up measurements with the athlete in the same position, thus making them more consistent. It is vital that the range of motion of an injured limb be compared with that of the healthy limb.

Strength Testing

Performing resistive range-of-motion testing helps to measure the strength of an area of the body. Muscular strength testing is often done with a technique called *manual muscle testing (MMT)*, which is

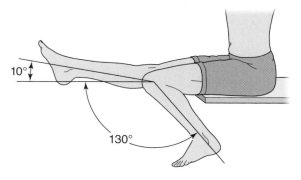

Figure 20.12 Anterior–posterior range of motion.

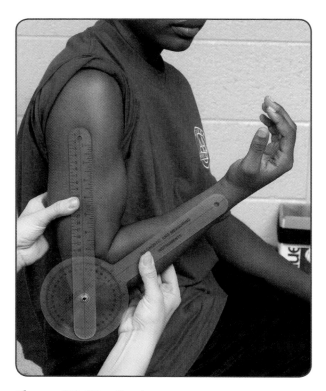

Figure 20.13 Goniometer use.

an objective way to determine the level of a person's strength. It is based on a grading system of zero to normal. A grade of *zero* indicates an inability to even twitch a muscle. *Trace* means an ability to perform a muscle twitch. A grade of *poor* indicates that an athlete can move a segment through full range of motion only if gravity is eliminated. *Fair* means the athlete can move a segment through full range of motion against gravity but with no other resistance. *Good* means that the athlete can move the segment through full range of motion, against gravity, and with some resistance applied by the AT. A grade of *normal* indicates that the athlete can move the segment through full range of motion, against gravity, and with full resistance from the AT. Some ATs use MMT without grading by simply comparing the resistive range of motion of an extremity with that of the extremity on the opposite side. The MMT strength-grading system allows ATs and other health care providers to document strength consistently and thus communicate the athlete's condition efficiently and effectively. The MMT strength-grading system can be found in table 20.2.

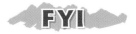

Crepitus

Crepitus is a crackling feeling under the skin.

False Movement

False movement is movement where there normally is none, such as in the middle of the forearm.

Testing to Rule Out Neurological Problems

Once strength and range of motion have been assessed, the injured athlete can be evaluated for neurological problems, which might include an inability to feel or move a body part. Each nerve that exits the spinal column is responsible for sensation and movement at a particular area of the body. By exposing these specific areas to a light touch or pricking stimulus and by asking the athlete to try to move the area, an AT can determine if a specific nerve may be involved in the injury. If a spinal cord injury is suspected, the athlete must be backboarded before moving him.

Table 20.2   Manual Muscle Testing to Determine Strength Level

Strength classifications (number or grade)		Description
5	Normal	The athlete can move the joint through a full range of motion against gravity and against full resistance from the AT.
4+	Good+	The athlete can move the joint through a full range of motion against gravity and against a significant amount of resistance from the AT.
4	Good	The athlete can move the joint though a full range of motion against gravity and against some amount of resistance from the AT.
3+	Fair+	The athlete can move the joint through a full range of motion against gravity and against minimal resistance from the AT.
3	Fair	The athlete can move the joint through a full range of motion against gravity with no applied resistance from the AT. If any resistance is applied, full range of motion is not achieved.
2	Poor	The athlete can only move the joint through a full range of motion if gravity is eliminated or against gravity with assistance from the AT.
1	Trace	When asked to move the joint, the athlete will not be able to do so. However, a muscle contraction should be observable.
0	Zero	When asked to move the joint, the athlete will not be able to do so. Moreover, a muscle contraction will not be visible.

Data obtained from Kendall, McCreary, and Provance (1993), Konin (1997), Starkey and Ryan (1996), and Magee (1997).

SPECIFIC CONDITIONS

Specific conditions that must be considered during a secondary assessment include shock and fractures. Here we discuss the common signs and symptoms and the necessary care of each.

Recognizing Shock

Shock is a condition in which inadequate blood and oxygen are supplied to vital organs. The body has five organs that must always receive an adequate blood supply to maintain life: the brain, heart, lungs, liver, and kidneys. When an athlete becomes seriously injured, the body tries to protect the vital organs by increasing blood flow to the organs while decreasing blood flow to the arms and legs. There are three reasons why a body goes into shock:

1. The blood vessels in the head, chest, and abdomen enlarge, getting ready to carry more blood. If the blood vessels in the arms and legs constrict and do not move blood into the vessels of the head, chest, and abdomen, blood pressure in these vessels decreases because the vessels have enlarged while the volume of blood has not increased. This means that the supply of oxygen to the vital organs is reduced.

2. The body will go into shock if the heart stops. Obviously, if the heart stops, no blood is flowing to

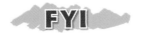

Cyanosis

Cyanosis is a blue coloration of the skin caused by lack of oxygen.

Backboards

Backboards are platforms that extend from the head to the toes. An athlete is secured to a backboard (backboarded) when a spinal cord injury is suspected.

---

the vital organs. When this happens, restarting the heart, not shock, is the first concern.

3. The body goes into shock if there is significant blood loss. If blood is leaking from the vessels, there is a smaller amount of blood to pump. If too much blood is lost, the organs will not get enough oxygen and nutrients to sustain life, they will shut down, and the athlete will die.

If shock is not recognized early and treated rapidly, it can cause death. Signs of shock include agitation (usually the first sign); rapid, weak pulse; decreased blood pressure (100 mmHg or lower); cold, clammy skin; sweating; cyanosis; increasing unconsciousness; and pale skin. Symptoms are nausea, thirst, anxiety, and dizziness. Table 20.3 describes the kinds of shock and what causes each.

Table 20.3 Types of Shock

Type of shock	Characteristics
Psychogenic (fainting)	Temporary loss of nervous function, causing blood vessels to dilate
Septic	General infection, causing circulatory failure
Neurological	Loss of control over the nervous system, causing blood vessels to dilate (spinal cord injury)
Cardiogenic	Cessation of heartbeat (cardiac arrest)
Hemorrhagic or hypovolemic	Loss of blood (internal bleeding)
Metabolic	Loss of fluids through vomiting, diarrhea, or urination (diabetics)
Respiratory	Cessation of breathing, causing a change in oxygen supply in the blood, which causes organs to shut down because of oxygen loss (asthma)
Anaphylactic	Cessation of breathing caused by a toxin (bee venom) in the system, causing changes to the oxygen supply within the body, which causes the organs to shut down

Treating Shock

Treatment of shock includes all of the following procedures: Treat the original injury; keep the athlete warm; if the arms and legs are not broken, elevate them 10 to 12 inches (25-30 cm) above the heart; measure breathing and pulse rate every five minutes; do not give anything to eat or drink; if vomiting occurs, turn the victim on her side and clear the airway; and get the victim to the hospital as soon as possible.

If the athlete has head or neck injuries and is in shock, she must be placed on a backboard and sent to the hospital for care. She can be covered with a blanket to maintain her body heat, but keep her lying flat. An athlete with respiratory injury can have her head elevated if there are no head or neck injuries; this will make it easier for her to breathe. Table 20.4 shows appropriate measures for treating each kind of shock.

Assessing and Managing a Fracture

When assessing an athlete with a possible fracture, the AT must check capillary refill, pulse rate in the extremity, and sensation of the body part. The athlete should never be asked to use the body part because this could cause further injury. If the trainer finds poor circulation, lack of sensation, or decreased capillary refill, the athlete may have seriously injured the nerve or vessels to that body part, and he requires immediate attention by the team physician. If the trainer cannot tell for sure whether the part is fractured, she should splint the area to be safe.

Types of Splints

Several types of splints can be used to manage fractures. A traction splint is used when the femur has been fractured, because the muscles in the thigh are so strong that they can cause the limb to shorten if proper splinting is not used. The traction splint pulls the bone ends apart and into alignment, which causes muscle tissue to relax, thus decreasing the pain. A rigid splint, which is made of a stiff material, is applied to the side, front, or back of an extremity. The splint must be padded and bandaged securely to the limb to hold the fracture in position. Examples of rigid splints are box splints, boards, and aluminum splints.

A semirigid splint is a moldable splint that hardens in place to hold a fracture; an example is a vacuum splint. Soft splints remain soft after the splint is applied to a fracture; examples include pillows, slings and swathes, and air splints. The trainer must check his supply of air splints regularly—they get holes and may not be usable in an emergency. Figure 20.14 illustrates various splints.

Table 20.4 Shock Care

Type of shock	Elevate feet?	Elevate head?	Do secondary assessment?	Position of patient for transportation
Psychogenic	Yes	No	Yes	Supine
Septic	Yes	No	No	Supine
Neurological	No	No	Yes	Supine
Cardiogenic	No	Yes	Yes	Head up
Hemorrhagic or hypovolemic	Yes	No	Yes	Supine
Metabolic	Yes	No	No	Supine
Respiratory	No	Yes	Yes	Head up
Anaphylactic	No	No	No	Supine

Data obtained from Prentice (2011), Bergeron and Greene (1989), Karren, Hafen, Limmer & Mistovich (2004) and American Red Cross (2006b).

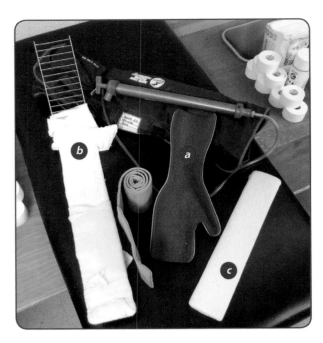

Figure 20.14 *(a)* A vacuum splint is applied and then air is withdrawn from it to mold it to a suspected fracture. *(b)* Aluminum splints are padded and molded to a specific body part. *(c)* Economical board splints are also padded. *(d)* Finger splints are made of various materials and are small enough to splint a finger.

Moving After Splinting

Once a body part is splinted, the athlete can be moved (assuming she has no other major problems), and body parts can be elevated for shock. On the way to the hospital, the AT must make sure the athlete is as comfortable as possible and prevent the splinted fracture from bouncing around in the transport vehicle. A fractured arm can be placed in a sling with a pillow between the arm and the athlete's lap. A fractured leg can be wrapped in blankets, which act as a comfort barrier, and strapped to the other leg.

PRICES METHOD

Most sprains, strains, and splinted fractures can be cared for with the **PRICES** method—**p**rotection, **r**est, **i**ce, **c**ompression, and **e**levation, and **s**upport.

The body part must be protected from further injury, and rest allows the body to heal. Ice, compression, elevation reduce the swelling, and external support restricts movement at the site.

Protection and rest are necessary to prevent further injury. Protection involves splinting or padding an area. Rest is self-explanatory. The athlete should avoid being active on the injured area.

Ice is applied for no longer than 20 to 30 minutes at a time because longer applications can cause frostbite. There should be at least 40 to 60 minutes between ice applications. Essentially, time without ice should be twice the time of ice application between icings. An acute injury should be iced no more than three times a day. For an acute injury, the ice should be crushed and placed in a plastic bag or should be a solid chunk in an ice cup. When applying ice to a body part, the athlete may experience pain and the sensation of extra pressure before the body part becomes numb.

Compression is pressure applied to the injured body part to prevent swelling. It is achieved with pads and snug application of elastic wraps or tape. Before elevating the body part, the student assistant or AT should arrange sufficient blankets, towels, or padding to lift the body part 10 to 12 inches (25-30 cm) above the heart. The body part can then be gently lifted while the support is slid underneath.

Support relates to providing necessary ambulatory aids such as crutches, canes, or walkers. With less severe injuries, support may take the form of a brace to allow ambulation with some stability to the area, such as a foot or ankle.

Another way to view appropriate steps of care is doing **No HARM** to an injured athlete. No HARM means that during the first 48 to 72 hours after an injury, the athlete should have **no h**eat applied to the injured area because this can cause more bleeding and swelling, no **a**lcohol ingested because this can cause more swelling, no **r**unning or activity because this may cause further injury, and no **m**assage to the area because this also can increase swelling.

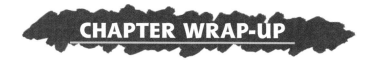

CHAPTER WRAP-UP

Summary

An injured athlete must be assessed immediately so that prudent care can begin. The AT will assess the athlete for life-threatening injuries first: He will check the ABCs, or the athlete's airway, breathing, and circulation. An athlete who has no ABCs needs immediate care and emergency medical assistance. Everyone, including the AT, coach, and student assistant, needs to observe universal precautions when working with bodily fluids. When determining the nature and severity of an injury, the AT will conduct a complete assessment of the athlete. The secondary assessment begins with HIT. Some injuries may cause the athlete to go into shock, which can be fatal. Treatment for shock depends on its cause. Sprains, strains, and splinted fractures are usually treated with PRICES.

Key Terms

Define the following terms found in this chapter:

ABCs	goniometer	PRICES
angina pectoris	heart attack	primary assessment
apnea	heart rate	pulse points
body temperature	hemiplegia	pulse pressure
breathing rate	history	pulse rate
capillary refill	HIT	quadriplegia
cardiac arrest	MRSA	sign
cardiopulmonary	No HARM	symptom
resuscitation (CPR)	palpation	syncope
constrict	paralysis	systolic pressure
diastolic pressure	paraplegia	total airway obstruction
dilate	partial airway	universal choking sign
direct pressure	obstruction	universal precautions
dyspnea	pressure point	vital signs

Questions for Review

1. What are the ABCs?
2. What is the most common airway obstruction?
3. How can an AT prevent the exchange of bodily fluids between the athlete and herself?
4. What medical conditions or illnesses would cause the heart to stop beating?
5. What methods are used to provide oxygen to an athlete who is not breathing?
6. Explain how a secondary assessment is performed.
7. Make a list of all the questions you can think of to ask during the history portion of an injury assessment. Compare your list with your partner's list. Did you forget any questions?
8. List three reasons why an athlete may go into shock.
9. What injuries can be determined from assessing an athlete's vital signs?
10. Explain the HIT technique.
11. Under what circumstances should you avoid testing (touching, specific evaluations, checking range of motion, and neurological testing) a body part?
12. What injuries are treated with PRICES?
13. What does the acronym *No HARM* stand for?

Activities for Reinforcement

1. Take a class in first aid and CPR and become certified.
2. Invite the local EMS to demonstrate CPR and electrical monitoring of the heart.
3. Find a Web site related to sport injuries and review the common steps of care for an injury.
4. Examine the following Web site and identify the types of splints that can be used by medical professionals: http://medicalsplints.com.
5. List the vital signs, and explain what each one can tell you about an injured athlete.
6. Make a list of items you could use to splint a fracture if regular splints were not available.

7. Practice taking someone else's blood pressure reading.

8. Make a list of various joints and their anterior–posterior range of motion.

9. Compare the range of motion of your classmates' knee or elbow joints. Why do you think some people have more or less range of motion?

10. Invite local EMS personnel to show how an AED works.

11. Visit the Web site of the National Center for Early Defibrillation and learn more about sudden cardiac arrest: www.early-defib.org/03_01_01.html.

Above and Beyond

1. Examine a current first aid and CPR text and give a presentation about people who are most likely to suffer a heart attack and how to prevent one.

2. Determine which cardiac and pulmonary conditions cannot be helped by using CPR. What are the reasons for the failure of CPR in each instance?

3. Access the OSHA Web site's bloodborne pathogen link at www.osha.gov/SLTC/ bloodbornepathogens/index.html and summarize the most up-to-date disease prevention strategies.

4. Find a Web site to learn about sudden cardiac arrest and present your findings.

5. Examine the following Web sites from the CDC and learn more about MRSA:

    www.cdc.gov/mrsa/index.html

    www.cdc.gov/mrsa/symptoms/index.html

6. Access the following OSHA Web site and examine the guidelines for dealing with blood-borne pathogens: http://osha.gov/pls/oshaweb/owadisp.show_document?p_table=STANDARDS&p_id=10051.

chapter 21

Environmental Situations and Injuries

Objectives

Upon completing this chapter, the student will be able to do the following:

- Explain how to care for heat-related illnesses.
- Describe how the body gets rid of excessive heat.
- Explain how heat-related illnesses can be prevented.
- Describe the person who is more prone to cold- and heat-related injuries.
- Explain the treatment of cold- and heat-related injuries.
- Explain how to prevent insect bites.

We live in a changing environment. Some days are rainy, and others are clear and sunny. Athletes like to practice in the same environment in which they will perform on game day. Some days, however, surprise the body with weather it is not accustomed to, such as a day in October with uncommonly high temperatures, which may cause problems for heat-sensitive athletes. In addition, for some athletes, an insect bite can lead to a life-threatening illness. In this chapter, we discuss the first aid necessary to care for an athlete who becomes ill due to environmental factors.

HEAT-RELATED PROBLEMS

Hyperthermia is an exceptional rise in body temperature. Body temperature rises when the athlete is exercising, the environmental temperature is excessive, the athlete has an infection, or the body's temperature-regulation system has failed. The body regulates temperature via the hypothalamus gland, which is located in the brain. As blood flows through the hypothalamus, heat receptors indicate a need to increase or decrease body temperature to maintain the body's core temperature at a constant

98.6° Fahrenheit (36.6 °C), which is the temperature at which the body's systems normally function. Through the hypothalamus, the body maintains a delicate balance in temperature, attempting to cool the body if heat production causes the body temperature to rise or trying to conserve body heat if the body temperature is decreasing. If body cooling exceeds heat production, the blood vessels in the arms and legs constrict, reducing the flow of blood passing close to the surface, where it would lose heat more rapidly. If body temperature begins to rise, the blood vessels in the extremities dilate so that more blood flows close to the surface in an attempt to rid the body of excess heat.

Heat-related illnesses range from mild heat cramps to severe heatstroke, which is considered a medical emergency. Heat exhaustion is considered a moderate illness.

The Real World

I was working on paperwork in the training room during the football season when our placekicker entered the room writhing in pain and screaming that something had bitten him on his hand. When I asked him if he knew what had bitten him, he didn't know, but it was obvious from the swelling and red marks on his middle finger that something had. I asked him what he had been doing when the bite occurred, and he said that he was retrieving his practice balls and had gone into a shrubbery bed to get one of them. Because the ball was in an odd location, he had put his hand on the trunk of a large tree to balance himself. He said he felt an immediate sting and then excruciating pain in his finger and hand. Then he came straight to the training room.

I radioed my college intern on the field and asked him to go to the tree and see if he could identify what had bitten the kicker. A few minutes later the intern radioed back that the tree was covered with furry caterpillars. Because the kicker was starting to exhibit the signs and symptoms of anaphylaxis, I decided to contact his parents and send him to the emergency room. I also radioed out to the field and asked my intern to capture one of the bugs in a cup and bring it inside so that it could be transported to the hospital.

An hour or so later the athlete returned from the hospital after being treated for the bite. The physicians in the emergency room had identified the culprit as a pus caterpillar and confirmed that its sting is indeed nasty and painful. Our kicker was careful to watch where he placed his hands the rest of the season, and our staff learned something new about the little creatures our athletes sometimes run into.

Jim Berry, ATC

Heat Cramps

Heat cramps are involuntary muscle contractions caused by dehydration and a loss of sodium as a result of profuse sweating. A poor daily diet may also contribute to the problem. The calf and abdominal muscles are the muscles most likely to be involved. Heat cramps should be treated by having the athlete drink water, stretch the involved muscle, and apply ice to the muscle to alleviate pain.

Heat Syncope

Heat syncope is a brief period of fainting and dizziness that occurs during exposure to high temperatures, especially when athletes must stand for a long time or immediately following activity in the heat. Heat syncope is more likely to occur during the first few days of practicing in hot environments. If heat syncope occurs, the athlete should move to a cool environment, elevate her feet, and rehydrate by drinking cool fluids.

Heat Exhaustion

Heat exhaustion is caused by prolonged exercise in a hot, humid environment to the point of severe dehydration. Symptoms of heat exhaustion include fatigue, dizziness, nausea, headache, muscle cramps, shortness of breath, and distorted vision. Signs of heat exhaustion are excessive sweating; rapid, weak pulse; decreased blood pressure; skin that is cold and pale; and normal body temperature. To treat heat exhaustion, cool the athlete by removing him from the hot environment (get him into the shade), face a fan toward him, and apply cold, wet towels. Encourage him to sip water if he can. If he loses consciousness or his case is severe, refer him to a physician—if prompt medical attention is not given, the athlete's condition may progress to heatstroke.

What Would You Do If...

The wrestling team practices in a facility where there is no direct fresh air. The temperature increases by the end of practice.

Heatstroke

Heatstroke is a dangerously high body temperature that is caused by the hypothalamus shutting down. Hypothalamus dysfunction can result from exercising in a hot, humid environment, severe dehydration, excessive weight loss, obesity, or untreated heat exhaustion. Symptoms of impending heatstroke are feeling extremely hot, feeling confused, having a headache, and experiencing dizziness. Signs of heatstroke are little or no sweating; hot, dry skin; core body temperature higher than 104° Fahrenheit (40 °C); low blood pressure; rapid, weak pulse; rapid breathing rate; dilated pupils; and unconsciousness. A comparison between heatstroke and heat exhaustion symptoms is found in the highlight box on this page.

If the AT suspects heatstroke, she will call 911 for emergency assistance and will begin cooling the body as quickly as possible. According to the NATA position statement on exertional heat illnesses, the best intervention to reduce the athlete's core body temperature is to take any equipment and clothes off the athlete and immerse him in a cold bath. He should be immersed up to his neck in a tub with the water temperature between 35° and 59° Fahrenheit (1-15 °C), with cold, wet towels applied to the neck, armpits, feet, and groin. Elevating the legs will help prevent shock. If the athlete is not treated immediately, death or irreversible brain damage will occur.

The most effective way to measure an athlete's core body temperature is with a rectal thermometer. When an athlete is immersed in cold water while treated for heatstroke, the rectal temperature should continue to be monitored. Once the athlete's temperature is reduced to 102° Fahrenheit (39 °C), the athlete can then be removed and her vital signs monitored. If the athlete is not treated immediately, death or irreversible brain damage will occur.

Exertional Hyponatremia

Exertional **hyponatremia** refers to a dangerously low blood sodium level that causes intracellular swelling and many signs and symptoms. According to the NATA position statement on exertional heat illnesses, these signs and symptoms include vomiting, disorientation, headache, lethargy, seizures, and swelling of hands and feet. The decreased blood sodium level is the result of ingesting large amounts of water while the body loses sodium via sweat. This condition is more common when events last longer than four hours, such as marathons and other ultraendurance events. This is a medical emergency and death can result if it is not treated.

An AT who suspects an athlete has hyponatremia should activate EMS immediately. Fluids should not be given unless a physician is consulted.

Sunburn

Athletes should also be concerned with sun exposure and burning the skin. Sunburn occurs when the body is exposed to ultraviolet (UV) light, which is not seen by the human eye. When the skin is exposed to UV light, extra melanin is produced. Melanin is the dark pigment in the skin that produces a tan. The body produces melanin to prevent sunburn, but it has a limited ability to protect the skin. If exposure to UV light continues, the skin can burn, resulting in redness, swelling, blistering, headaches, and fatigue. Sunburn can cause dehydration and make an athlete more prone to heat illnesses. Another problem with sun exposure is the increased risk of skin cancer.

Signs of Heatstroke and Heat Exhaustion

Heatstroke	Heat Exhaustion
Unconsciousness	Conscious
Shallow breathing	Rapid, shallow breathing
No sweating	
Red, dry skin	Profuse sweating
Rapid bounding pulse	Pale, clammy skin
	Rapid weak pulse
High body temperature	Normal body temperature

Fair-skinned people are at higher risk for sunburn, but even darker skin can be damaged by UV light, although the skin may not burn. Athletes must use sunscreen to protect their skin from harmful UV light and prevent sunburn.

Heat Loss and the Environment

The amount of body heat lost to the environment depends on the air temperature, humidity, radiation, body surface exposure, air currents, clothing, and equipment. **Evaporation** is the process that cools the body. When sweat evaporates, the amount of heat energy necessary to change liquid water (or sweat) to gas is removed from the skin, which cools the body. Thus, factors that affect the rate of evaporation also affect the body's ability to cool itself. These factors include air temperature, humidity, air movement, and radiation. If the humidity is low (that is, if the air is dry), the air can pick up and hold additional moisture, so sweat from a hot athlete will evaporate quickly and cool her effectively. If the humidity is high (that is, if the air is moist), the moist air cannot hold much additional moisture so the sweat does not evaporate. Air movement is helpful because a breeze tends to move moist air away and bring drier air to the skin, which aids sweat evaporation.

The **heat index** is a plot of air temperature and humidity. The AT uses a sling psychrometer to determine the relative humidity (see figure 21.1).

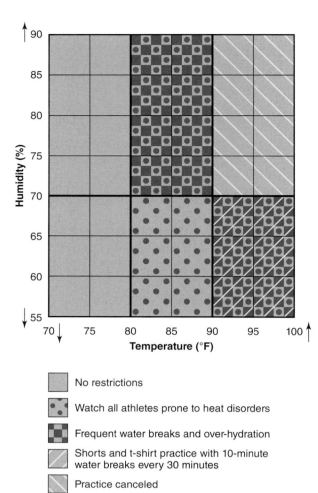

- No restrictions
- Watch all athletes prone to heat disorders
- Frequent water breaks and over-hydration
- Shorts and t-shirt practice with 10-minute water breaks every 30 minutes
- Practice canceled

Figure 21.2 Heat index training standards.

The heat index predicts the body's ability to dissipate heat and indicates how safe it is to participate in activities on a given day. For example, if the humidity is 90% and the temperature is 75° Fahrenheit (24 °C), it is safe to practice. However, if the humidity is 90% and the temperature is 90° Fahrenheit (32 °C), practice should be canceled (see figure 21.2).

In addition to evaporation, the body can lose heat in other ways, including conduction and convection. **Conduction** is the transfer of heat between two objects in contact with one another. Placing an ice pack on an athlete, for example, will cause the body heat to move to the ice pack. As heat is transferred in this way, the ice will start to melt. **Convection** is the transfer of heat from the movement of a medium. An example of a medium is water. If an athlete's legs are placed in a cold whirlpool, for example, heat is lost to the swirling water.

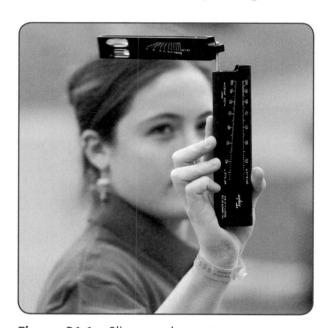

Figure 21.1   Sling psychrometer.

Preventing Heat-Related Illness

When preparing for athletic competition in hot weather, athletes must remember that the body needs time to get used to temperature extremes. In Steps to Prevent Heat-Related Illness, we present suggestions that will help athletes cope with heat. Rushing into athletic competition without proper conditioning and training can cause a heat-related injury.

Adjusting Clothing and Equipment

Clothing affects heat dissipation in several ways. Dark colors absorb heat, so light-colored clothes should be selected to reflect the sun. A layer of air between the clothing and the skin helps the process of evaporation, which subsequently cools the body. Air flowing through the clothing can improve evaporation, so jersey material in a loose weave is often desirable.

Choosing athletic clothing with wicking properties can aid in evaporation. Wicking means the sweat is pulled away from the body and efficiently evaporated. Cotton material will absorb sweat and can create difficulty with evaporation. Athletes should avoid heavy clothing, long sleeves, long socks, and additional taping or wraps. Rubber suits, such as those sometimes worn by high school wrestlers, are dangerous because they prevent cooling through evaporation and lock the heat around the body.

Equipment such as helmets, padding, and uniforms reduces the amount of body surface exposure, limiting the body's ability to evaporate moisture. Moreover, the athlete must work harder with the added weight of the equipment, which causes an increased energy expenditure that generates more heat. Coaches should modify practices so that some equipment does not have to be worn when there is a high heat index. During extremely hot and humid days, for example, if football players avoid contact, they can practice without shoulder pads and wear shorts instead of pants.

Other Preventive Measures

Heat-related illnesses can be prevented if athletes gradually acclimatize to the heat and humidity for 10 to 14 days, drink plenty of water or sport drinks, and take rest breaks as needed to keep cool. Ideally,

Steps to Prevent Heat-Related Illness

- Acclimatize.
- Wear lightweight uniforms.
- Take frequent water breaks.
- Change into dry clothing.
- Weigh in before and after practice.
- Check the humidity and temperature during each practice.
- Avoid staying in saunas and hot tubs for extended lengths of time.
- Eat properly.
- Get plenty of rest.
- Drink fluids after practice to replace fluid lost during practice.

if an athlete is physically fit and not overweight, is well nourished, and drinks plenty of fluids before, during, and after activity, she will be better able to prevent heat-related illnesses. Almost no one drinks enough fluids during activity to replace the water lost during participation, and most athletes drink enough to replace only half of the fluids they lose, so the AT should encourage athletes to drink more fluids. The NATA fluid replacement guidelines suggest that athletes ingest 17 to 20 ounces (503-591 ml) of fluid two to three hours before an activity and 7 to 10 ounces (207-296 ml) about 15 minutes before exercise. Also, they should drink approximately 10 ounces (296 ml) of water every 10 to 20 minutes during activity until they feel full. They will be able to drink more if the water temperature is about 50° to 60° Fahrenheit (10-15 °C).

We do not recommend fluids containing high amounts of sugar because they are absorbed more slowly than those without sugar. Drinking fluids with high salt content is usually unnecessary because most people get enough salt with a well-balanced diet. Sport drinks with some sodium and low levels of sugar work well for most athletes. Athletes should weigh themselves before and after practice—at least 2 cups of water should be consumed for every pound (.5 kg) of weight lost. If possible, workouts and practices should be scheduled in the morning or evening to avoid the hottest times of the day.

Heat Observation Technology

Heat-related deaths that have occurred in sports such as football have prompted some companies to develop technology to detect when an athlete is overheating. Schutt Sports, for example, has created the HotHead heat observation system, which consists of a sensor placed inside an athlete's football helmet. The sensor monitors the athlete's temperature and transmits the data to a PDA that is monitored by the athletic training staff.

COLD-RELATED PROBLEMS

In a cold environment, the body must conserve or generate more heat to maintain its normal core temperature. As mentioned earlier, the hypothalamus sends signals to reduce the size of blood vessels in the extremities to keep most of the blood in the chest, head, and abdomen. In addition, the body will metabolize some of its stores of fat and carbohydrate—think of it as burning fuel to generate heat. Thus, people with low energy supplies (little stored fat and carbohydrate) are more prone to cold-related injury.

To help retain body heat, the athlete must dress appropriately by wearing layered clothing, gloves, a hat, and warm footwear (see Dressing for Cold Weather and Preventing Cold-Related Injuries for additional ideas). Several light layers of clothing maintain more warmth for the body because warmed air is retained between each layer of clothing. However, the athlete should avoid wearing so many layers that she begins to sweat, because then

What Would You Do If...

After a rainy field hockey game, the coach tells you that one of the players is missing. You go back out to the field and find the player huddled in the corner next to the storage shed. He is cold and wet. His lips are blue, his skin is pale, and he is shivering uncontrollably. He is unable to walk.

Preventing Cold-Related Injuries

- Wear proper clothing.
- Cover the head, mouth, and extremities.
- Avoid use of alcohol or tobacco.
- Acclimatize.
- Avoid getting wet.
- Avoid sitting on cold objects (e.g., ice, aluminum benches).
- Stay indoors during extremely cold weather.
- If predisposed to being cold, stay indoors in cold weather.

she will lose heat by evaporation. As she warms up, she may be able to remove a layer or two so she can stay comfortable and dry. Clothing that is wind resistant prevents heat loss because it does not allow air flow over the body, which promotes evaporation.

Shivering is another mechanism the body uses to try to create heat. Shivering is uncontrolled muscular contractions—when muscles contract, they generate heat. If an athlete starts to shiver, he should be moved to a warm area. He can progress from a simple cold injury such as frostnip to hypothermia or death if care is not taken in extreme cold. If the extremities do not get enough blood flow to stay warm, the athlete will begin to get frostbite. If he gets so cold that his core body temperature begins to drop, he has **hypothermia**. Checking the windchill factor (table 21.1) can help an athlete prevent cold-related injuries.

Frostnip

Frostnip is caused from exposure to cold for an extended length of time. The exposure to cold causes the superficial skin tissue to begin freezing, but the deeper tissues are not affected. Signs and symptoms of this condition include pale, cold skin, and the athlete may report loss of sensation. Frostnip most commonly involves the ears, nose, and fingers, and it can be easily treated—rewarm the tissue using the athlete's warm breath or place the body parts near a heat source, such as the athlete's own body. For example, if the athlete's fingers are

Air temperature (°C)

Wind speed (km/h)	-10	-15	-20	-25	-30	-35	-40	-45	-50
5	-13	-19	-24	-30	-36	-41	-47	-53	-58
10	-15	-21	-27	-33	-39	-45	-51	-57	-63
15	-17	-23	-29	-35	-41	-48	-54	-60	-66
20	-18	-24	-30	-37	-43	-49	-56	-62	-68
25	-19	-25	-32	-38	-44	-51	-57	-64	-70
30	-20	-26	-33	-39	-46	-52	-59	-65	-72
35	-20	-27	-33	-40	-47	-53	-60	-66	-73
40	-21	-27	-34	-41	-48	-54	-61	-68	-74
45	-21	-28	35	-42	-48	-55	-62	-69	-75
50	-22	-29	-35	-42	-49	-56	-63	-69	-76
55	-22	-29	-36	-43	-50	-57	-63	-70	-77
60	-23	-30	-36	-43	-50	-57	-64	-71	-78
65	-23	-30	-37	-44	-51	-58	-65	-72	-79
70	-23	-30	-37	-44	-51	-58	-65	-72	-80
75	-24	-31	-38	-45	-52	-59	-66	-73	-80
80	-24	-31	-38	-45	-52	-60	-67	-74	-81

Very low	Freezing is possible, but unlikely	**High**	Freezing risk < 30 min
Likely	Freezing is likely > 30 min	**Severe**	Freezing risk < 10 min
		Extreme	Freezing risk < 3 min

Table 21.1 Windchill equivalent temperature chart showing various combinations of temperature and wind speed that result in the same cooling power as that seen with no wind.

Reprinted, by permission, from J.H. Wilmore, D.L. Costill, and W.L. Kenney, 2008, *Physiology of sport and exercise*, 4th ed. (Champaign, IL: Human Kinetics), 272.

Dressing for Cold Weather

When preparing to exercise in cold weather, remember these tips:

1. Protect yourself from wind and rain.
2. Insulate yourself to maintain body heat.
3. Allow the body to ventilate.
4. Use a base layer that wicks away moisture—polyester and nylon blends and silk are often used.
5. Use a middle layer consisting of fleece or brushed nylon to trap body heat.
6. Use a shell to protect you from the elements. Use a waterproof material such as Gore-Tex if the weather is rainy, use windproof material for windy conditions, or use a combination of wind- and waterproof materials.

affected, she should tuck them in her armpits inside her coat.

Frostbite

Frostbite is also caused from exposure to cold for a long period of time. The exposure causes the body part (usually nose, ears, fingers, toes, or penis) to freeze. The people most likely to get frostbite are those who fail to wear proper clothing, those who drink alcohol before or while outdoors, those who have diabetes, and those who have a heart condition. Symptoms of frostbite include numbness and a prickling sensation. Early signs of frostbite are redness of the skin and swelling; with continued exposure, the skin becomes pale, and eventually the tissue hardens.

Frostbite should be treated by gradually rewarming the affected body part in water heated to 102° Fahrenheit (38.5 °C). Once the body part is pink, gently dry it and wrap it in dry sterile dressings. Do not massage the affected body parts or ask the athlete to walk on frozen feet. Do not rub snow on the body part or apply any lotions or creams. The athlete must be referred to a physician.

Hypothermia

Hypothermia results from prolonged exposure to damp cold. The athlete's body temperature begins to drop, and at 95° Fahrenheit (34.6 °C), the first signs and symptoms of hypothermia occur. Symptoms include headache, a feeling of cold, numbness, dizziness, and slowed breathing and heart rates. Signs of hypothermia are pale skin, shivering, swelling, patches of discolored skin, decreased heart rate, change in consciousness, and low body temperature. One of the first signs of hypothermia is shivering—should it occur, send the athlete to a warm place. An athlete may be vulnerable to cold exposure if he has cardiovascular disease, alcoholism, or asthma; has had previous bouts of hypothermia; has poor nutrition; is exposed to water or rain; has inadequate protective clothing; or is fatigued.

An athlete who is not treated for hypothermia is at risk of death. Hypothermia is treated by getting the athlete near a heat source, such as placing her in a warm room and removing wet clothing. Warm the athlete with a dry blanket. Be careful not to place her too close to an open flame or a heater; this may cause the blood vessels to dilate rapidly, which causes ruptures. Remember that another person is a source of heat, so getting into a sleeping bag or a blanket with the chilled athlete will help to warm her. The AT will call 911—the athlete must be seen by a physician.

SEVERE WEATHER

Severe weather conditions increase the risk of injury to people who get caught outdoors. Thankfully, many cities support an early-warning weather system. When a severe storm is about to hit an area, a television and radio warning goes out, which may include a storm watch, storm warning, tornado watch, or tornado warning. The term *watch* indicates that conditions are right for severe weather or a tornado. A *warning* means that a storm or tornado has been sighted. In many communities, a tornado warn-

ing will activate sirens, telling people to take cover. During the severe weather season, the AT should have a battery-operated radio ready so that weather reports can be heard. The early-warning storm system will indicate when the storm has passed. Don't mess with Mother Nature. Take cover—she can be fierce!

Tornadoes

In the event of a tornado warning, athletes must move to safety immediately. The safest area during a tornado is a low, reinforced area such as a basement. If protection is not available indoors, the athletes should find a ditch or low-lying area and lie as flat as possible, which will allow the tornado to pass over and will protect them from flying debris. People should not seek shelter in a car or bus—although these vehicles appear to be safe, they are easily moved by a tornado.

Thunder and Lightning

The presence of thunder or lightning means that it is time to take cover inside. A lightning detector is the latest device to help the AT determine this (see figure 21.3). Many people either are not

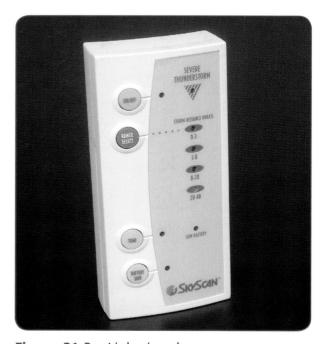

Figure 21.3 Lightning detector.

aware of the danger or do not want to appear to be afraid, so they stay outside in severe weather, sometimes with tragic consequences. Several years ago a group of people were walking to a high school football game in Michigan when they felt their hair stand on end, which is a sign that lightning is about to strike. They were hit and knocked to the ground, and many had no heartbeat. Luckily, several ATs were attending the game and administered CPR, and all of the injured survived. In another incident, three recreational soccer players tried waiting out a storm under a tree, hoping to resume a game. A bolt of lightning hit and traveled down the tree, knocking them to the ground. One of the players died when he could not be revived. Because these incidents are not unusual, the NATA created a position statement for lightning safety. The following suggestions are based on this policy statement.

Each school should have an established chain of command and make a well-trained and informed person responsible for stopping play and removing athletes, coaches, and spectators from the area. This person should be informed by a designated weather watcher who monitors signs of threatening weather. Lightning-safe locations close to each field should be identified.

The best policy regarding thunder and lightning is to take cover indoors immediately. The NATA position statement recommends that by the time the flash-to-bang count reaches 30 seconds (i.e., you can count to 30 seconds from the time you see lightning to the time you hear the associated thunder), athletes, coaching personnel, and spectators should already be in a lightning-safe location. A team can proceed with competition after thunder and lightning have not been heard or seen for 30 minutes after the last instance of thunder or lightning.

In the event that a team is caught by a sudden storm, the following hints may be helpful:

- Go inside.
- Stay away from all metal objects.
- Avoid electrical devices, including telephones, and avoid taking showers.

What Would You Do If...

There is a lightning storm, and you tell the lacrosse coach that you have been sent to ask the team to leave the field. The lacrosse coach responds, "We have a practice to get through today, and I'll decide what's in the best interest of this team."

- Do not stand under a tree or near a flagpole or light pole.
- Do not stand on a hilltop or near the highest point of a field.
- Remove all metal objects from your body (cleats, chains, money clips).
- Assume the lightning-safe position (crouching with legs and arms together).

If an athlete has been struck by lightning, the AT must be prepared to give CPR. An electrical charge may cause the heart to stop.

The facility you choose for shelter is important. Select a substantial structure that contains indoor plumbing and a phone. A concrete structure with a basement will protect you quite well.

BITES AND STINGS

We share our environment with an enormous number and variety of insects. Their bites may contain harmful venom or bacteria.

For most people, being stung by a bee or being bitten by some other insect is painful but not life threatening. However, a few people are so sensitive to the insect venom that bites or stings can result in shock and death. To treat an insect sting, the first thing an AT must do is remove the stinger. Many people try to remove the stinger by probing it with a needle or grasping it with tweezers. Any time the stinger is squeezed, it injects more poison into the athlete, so this should be avoided. It is best to use an object such as a knife or the edge of a credit card to scrape off the stinger. The AT can then apply ice, which will reduce the blood flow to and from the area and help control the pain and swelling. See figure 21.4 for a picture of an ant bite.

The affected athlete's breathing and heart rate should be monitored for an allergic reaction. If there are signs of breathing difficulty, wheezing, excessive swelling, or rapid heart rate, she should be taken by ambulance to the hospital. Athletes who have had previous severe reactions can be given medication to use in the event of a bite. The medication is already in a syringe, sometimes called an *EpiPen*, and the athlete just has to insert the needle and give herself the injection. The AT needs to be aware of athletes with this condition.

Insects are attracted to the sugar found on discarded candy wrappers and in empty soda cans. Keeping garbage cans emptied around playing fields will help reduce the numbers of insects present.

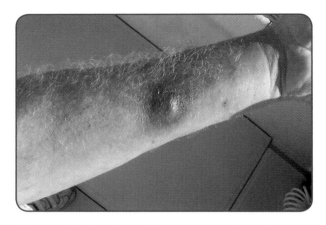

Figure 21.4 Not all stings involve stingers. These stings from a fire ant are the result of the ant biting and then injecting venom. There is no need to scrape out a stinger from this wound—just apply ice.
Photo courtesy of Bert Cartwright

The Real World

Most of us dislike bugs because they bite and sting, but they can cause unusual problems as well. I treated an athlete who reported having ear pain for a few days. We referred him to a physician, who was extremely surprised when he looked in the young man's ear with an otoscope and found a dead cockroach that had begun to decompose.

Phil Voorhis, MSEd, ATC

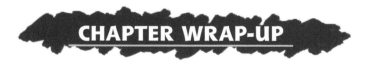

CHAPTER WRAP-UP

Summary

Many environmental athletic injuries can be prevented by following a few common-sense procedures—drink plenty of fluids, wear appropriate clothing, take cover from storms, and keep trash cans emptied. All of these measures increase athletes' safety. The role of the AT in preventing injuries is just as important as the part she plays in the evaluation and care of injuries. Athletes who are particularly sensitive to insect bites should be prepared to treat themselves for an allergic reaction in case they are bitten or stung, and the AT should be prepared to deal with an allergic reaction as well.

Key Terms

Define the following terms found in this chapter:

conduction	heat exhaustion	hyperthermia
convection	heat index	hyponatremia
evaporation	heatstroke	hypothermia
heat cramps	heat syncope	

Questions for Review

1. What is the difference between heatstroke and heat exhaustion? How are heat illnesses treated?
2. What is the difference between frostbite and frostnip?
3. How can heat- and cold-related injuries be prevented?
4. How does the body get overheated or too cold? How does the body rid itself of heat and warm itself when cold?
5. How are the various cold-related injuries treated?
6. What can an athlete do to avoid being bitten by insects?

Activities for Reinforcement

1. Design a policy for preventing heat-related injuries.
2. Design a policy for preventing cold-related injuries.
3. Using a computer, create a flowchart indicating an appropriate chain of command for lightning safety.
4. Find two Web sites that provide weather information and decide which would be most appropriate for use by a weather watcher at your school.
5. Visit the Schutt Web site and examine the HotHead system: www.schuttsports.com/aspx/Sport/ProductCatalog.aspx?id=953.
6. Visit the Running Warehouse Web site and watch their video on layering clothing for workouts in cold weather: www.runningwarehouse.com/LearningCenter/apparel.html.

Above and Beyond

1. Interview someone who has been struck by lightning, write an article, and print the story in the school newspaper.
2. Working with a local meteorologist, determine the number of days in the last year that could have caused a heat- or cold-related injury.
3. Design a severe-weather drill for athletes and coaches.
4. Examine the NATA position statement on lightning safety for athletics and recreation and create a lightning-safe drill for athletes and coaches at your school. The source for the position statement is as follows: Walsh, K.M, B. Bennett, M.A. Cooper, R.L. Holle, R. Kithil, and R.E. Lopez. 2000. NATA position statement: Lightning safety for athletics and recreation. *Journal of Athletic Training* 35(4): 471-477.
5. Examine the NATA position statement on exertional heat illness and write a report on a specific condition: Binkley, H.M., J. Beckett, D.J. Casa, D.K. Kleiner, and P.E. Plummer. 2002. NATA position statement: Exertional heat illnesses. *Journal of Athletic Training* 37(3): 329-343.

chapter 22

Stabilization and Transportation of Injured Athletes

Objectives

Upon completing this chapter, the student will be able to do the following:

- Understand why athletic equipment is sometimes removed.
- Explain how to remove an athlete from the field.
- Explain when a backboard is necessary.
- Explain when an athlete should walk or use an aid to get off the field or court.

Extrication involves removing injured athletes from a playing area or dangerous situation to get them care without causing additional harm. For instance, a tackler is carried off the field, an out-of-bounds skier is dug out of an avalanche and removed from the slope, or a diver is taken from the pool.

Once the athlete is accessible and out of immediate danger and the scene is safe to approach without risk of injury to rescuers, the athlete's injuries should be briefly assessed and primary or secondary care should be given. The steps of care for many musculoskeletal injuries involve stabilization of the victim's body. For example, a severe joint injury or fracture should be splinted before transporting the victim to a hospital for advanced care.

EQUIPMENT REMOVAL

Sometimes the athlete's equipment must be removed to treat the injury, but the team physician and local EMS may be comfortable treating a fully equipped injured athlete. The AT should check with them—in some cases, the equipment will not need to be removed. If there are too few trained personnel to help remove equipment, it should be left in place unless it is life threatening. A face mask must be removed in all breathing and cardiac emergencies, and shoulder pads must be removed for cardiac emergencies. The Inter-Association Task Force for Appropriate Care of the Spine-Injured Athlete recommends removing an athlete's face mask before transporting him, whether he has a respiratory problem or not.

Face Mask

An AT must remove the face mask to gain access to an athlete's airway. If the athlete has breathing problems, the trainer should always suspect a head or neck injury, so while she removes the face mask, a second person must hold the player's head and neck in line to prevent excessive movement.

A cutting tool or screwdriver is required to remove a face mask, depending on the helmet type or manufacturer. To remove a football face mask, the AT cuts the two side-mounting loops and flips the face mask up (see figure 22.1). This gives access to the athlete's face and mouth. In some instances the screws that hold the side-mounting loops to the helmet must be removed. Any time an athlete will be transported to medical care, his face mask and mouth guard should be removed, but his chin strap and helmet should be left in place because they hold the head and neck securely. The Inter-Association Task Force recommends that an athlete's helmet and chin strap be removed only if the athlete's airway cannot be accessed for rescue breathing after the

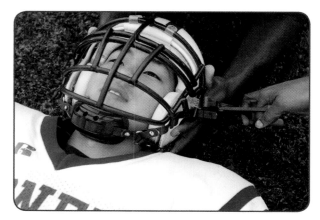

Figure 22.1 Football face mask removal: Cut the plastic retaining pieces located on each side of the helmet. Swinging the face mask up gives the rescuer access to the athlete's face.

face mask is removed, the helmet and chin strap do not keep the athlete's head secure, the helmet prevents the AT from properly positioning the athlete for immobilization and transportation, or the face mask cannot be removed from the helmet within a reasonable amount of time.

To remove a hockey player's face mask, the AT unsnaps the straps on each side of the mask and flips the mask up. A baseball helmet has a face mask that is held in place either by screws or loops similar to those on a football mask. If the face mask is secured with screws, they must be removed with a screwdriver, and the face mask can be lifted off. When loops are present, the two side loops are cut and the face mask flips away.

Jersey and Shoulder Pads

Shoulder pads can stay in place in most situations. When evaluating a shoulder, the AT can reach the injured area by sliding a hand up the sleeve or through the neck opening. If shoulder pads must be removed, however, first remove the jersey—it may need to be cut off to avoid excessive movement. The jersey can be cut at the seams to keep it for possible repair and reuse or else cut up the middle and up each sleeve to the neck. If the athlete is lying supine, unhook the chest straps and unlace or cut the laces in the front of the chest (or at the back of the pads if the athlete is lying prone). While one person holds the athlete's head and neck in line, a second person pulls the shoulder pads over the athlete's head, bends the pads backward around the first person's arms, and removes the pads (see figure 22.2).

To remove shoulder pads from an athlete who is lying on his side, remove the jersey, unhook the chest straps, and unlace or cut the laces or straps in the front and back of the pads. Someone must maintain the position of the head and neck while another person pulls the shoulder pads sideways and off. The shoulder pads on the side that is lying on the ground can be easily removed as the athlete is placed on the backboard.

Neck Roll

Removing the **neck roll** will depend on what type it is. If the neck roll is attached by string to the shoulder pads, the AT can cut the string. If the neck roll is attached by screws to the shoulder pads, the AT

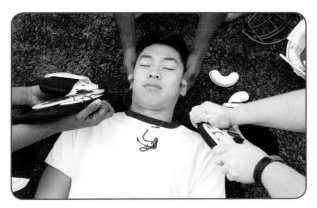

Figure 22.2   When an athlete is supine and the shoulder pads must be removed, cut the strings in the front and unhook the chest straps. Spread the shoulder pads apart and pull them over the athlete's head.

may decide to remove the shoulder pads with the neck roll still attached. When removing a neck roll that is screwed to the pads, someone must hold the athlete's head and neck in position while another person unscrews the neck roll.

A third type of neck roll is put on before the shoulder pads and is held in place by the downward pressure of the jersey. To remove this type of neck roll, remove the jersey and shoulder pads and then cut the laces on the front.

Helmet

Helmets should be left in place at all times unless they interfere with the AT's ability to give proper care. If she must remove a football helmet, the AT should enlist at least one trained first aider and proceed as follows:

1. The AT controls the head and keeps it in line (figure 22.3*a*).
2. The first aider removes the cheek pads (figure 22.3*b*).
3. The first aider controls the head from inside the helmet (figure 22.3*c*).
4. The AT unsnaps the chin strap.
5. The AT pulls the helmet up over the head while pulling the helmet opening apart (figure 22.3*d*).

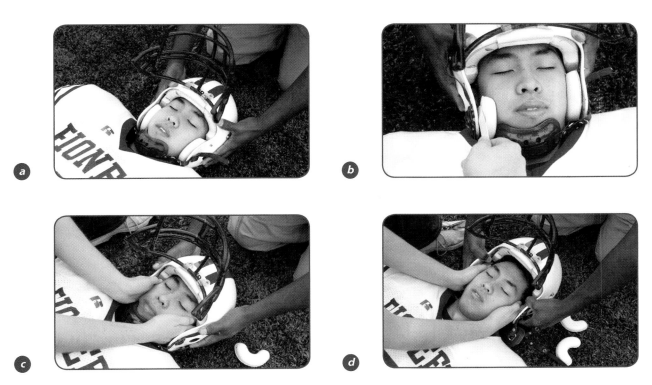

Figure 22.3   Football helmet removal. *(a)* The AT holds the exterior of the helmet, and *(b)* the cheek pads are loosened and removed. *(c)* The second rescuer controls the athlete's head from inside the helmet, and *(d)* from the top of the athlete's head, the AT grabs the helmet by the ear holes, widens the helmet as much as possible, and pulls it off.

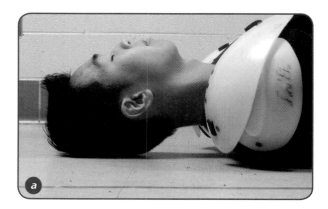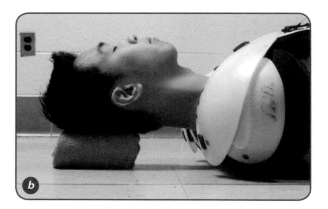

Figure 22.4　*(a)* If the helmet is removed while the shoulder pads are still on, the head will tip back to the floor at an angle. *(b)* Placing padding under the head or removing the shoulder pads maintains proper alignment of the head and neck with the body.

6. The AT fills the gap between the head and the ground with towels or other conforming cloth to keep the head and neck in line with the back (figure 22.4*b*).

7. The AT again takes control of the head as shown in figure 22.3*a*. If a helmet is removed, the shoulder pads and neck roll must also be removed; otherwise the athlete's neck will be placed in extension, which can aggravate head or neck injuries and cause further harm. See figure 22.4.

Uniform and Padding

If the AT needs to assess a nonserious injury, the athlete can remove her own uniform if she can do it without further harm to herself. If the injured part is a limb, it is generally best to first remove the uniform from the noninjured extremity. This will allow more room to manipulate the uniform around the injured body part. A sock can be removed from an injured leg or foot by widening the diameter of the sock while removing it. If that creates pain, cut the sock off.

Padding around an injured body part should be cut off—cautiously—to keep the injured body part from moving and causing unnecessary pain. Padding on the rest of the body can be removed in the normal fashion.

LIFTING AND MOVING AN ATHLETE

Once an athlete has been assessed, the AT will decide how she should be removed from the field. If the injury is minor, the athlete may be able to walk off on her own or with minimal help. However, if the injury is more serious, the AT can use devices such as straps, stretchers, and backboards to move the athlete from one location to another. When lifting an athlete, as when lifting any heavy weight, the AT must have a good base of support, keep his feet shoulder width apart, and always look up before and during the lifting. Once the athlete has been secured to a stretcher or backboard, she should be moved feetfirst rather than sideways so that she is less likely to become nauseated.

What Would You Do If...

At the football game, a player has injured his knee, which has been splinted. The AT indicates that she needs the golf cart to carry the injured player from the field. You try several times, but the golf cart will not start.

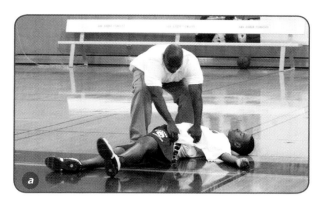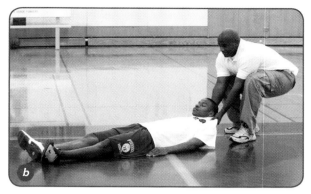

Figure 22.5   Emergency movement. *(a)* Moving an athlete sideways causes the extremities to move away from the direction of force. *(b)* Lengthwise movement is less likely to further injure the athlete. The AT must keep looking up to prevent personal back injury while lifting.

Under normal circumstances injured athletes are splinted and cared for before they are moved. However, in extreme emergencies an athlete may have to be moved before she can be splinted. If, for example, a wall is about to fall on the athlete, the AT must move her to prevent her death. If she is not splinted, move her lengthwise to keep her bones aligned (see figure 22.5).

Ambulatory Movement

Ideally, an athlete will be able to walk from the field without support; we can then say he is **ambulatory**. However, an athlete should not be allowed to get up and walk around before the AT or team physician has determined the extent of the injury. A serious injury should be immobilized before extrication, and an athlete with a suspected serious lower-extremity injury should not be allowed to walk without support. If two students are giving ambulatory aid, the athlete can place one arm over each assistant's shoulders, and the assistants can grasp the athlete's back or pants to give support. The athlete should not be allowed to apply pressure on the injured body part. If only one assistant is available to give aid, the assistant should be on the same side as the injury. The athlete's arm should be over the assistant's shoulder while the assistant holds the athlete's hip or pants (see figure 22.6).

An athlete who is not seriously injured and can cooperate may also be removed from the field using a seated carry. To perform the removal, two people

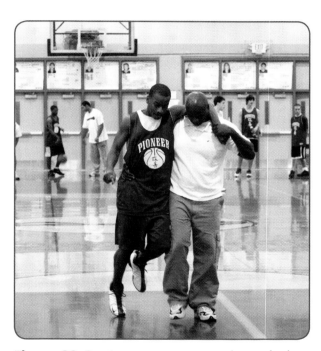

Figure 22.6   A one-person carry is used when the athlete is ill and needs support or when an injured lower extremity can support limited pressure. The injured lower extremity must be next to the rescuer.

face each other and lock their arms together as illustrated in figure 22.7. The athlete sits on one set of the locked arms while the other set supports his upper back. He places his arms around the shoulders of the assistants. The athlete is carried off in the direction he is facing (see figure 22.8).

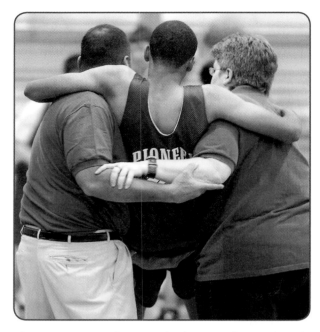

Figure 22.7 The arm lock is performed with the hand of one rescuer grasping the forearm of the other. If the hand slips off the forearm, there is still a hand to grasp, whereas if a hand-to-hand grip slips, only air is left.

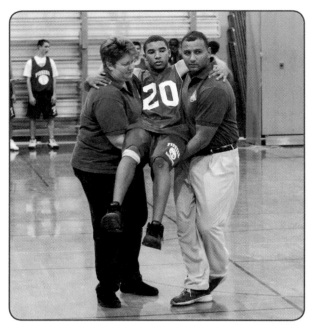

Figure 22.8 The two-person carry is used when the injured athlete cannot get off the field without help and should not apply pressure to the injured body part. All splinting should be done before moving the athlete.

The Real World

One of the basic rules in football is to keep your head up. When the athlete has his head up, he can see better, and his neck in a position where an impact is less likely to be harmful.

The running back was handed the ball; he dipped his head and was immediately hit by several opposing team players. He didn't get up at the end of the play. The AT assessed the player and asked him questions. His evaluation revealed that the injured player had a tingling sensation in both arms and legs. The AT decided not to move the player, and he called EMS. The paramedics evaluated the athlete and determined that he had suffered a life-threatening cervical spine injury. They called for a helicopter evacuation. It was a scary, sobering moment when the helicopter landed in the middle of the football field and evacuated the player to a local hospital.

Thankfully, the young man had suffered only muscle strains on both sides of his neck. He was kept overnight for observation and then sent home. His doctor ordered him to wear a neck brace and strengthen his neck muscles to rehabilitate the muscle strains before returning to football the following season.

His injury changed the behavior of every player on the team—they all paid more attention to their posture after that.

Anonymous

Stretcher

What is the difference between a stretcher and a backboard? A backboard is rigid and is used to immobilize spinal injuries, whereas a stretcher is made of canvas and is used to transport an athlete without spinal injuries.

A stretcher is used for an athlete suffering from a knee injury, an asthma attack, dizziness, a diabetic crisis, and so forth. After assessing the athlete and caring for all injuries, logroll the athlete onto the stretcher and secure her in place with three straps, one each at the chest, hips, and feet. The athlete may be able to slide onto the stretcher, which is fine as long as no pressure is placed on the injured body part.

As with a backboard, it takes at least four people to carry the stretcher—one on each end and two in the middle. The athlete should be moved feetfirst or headfirst.

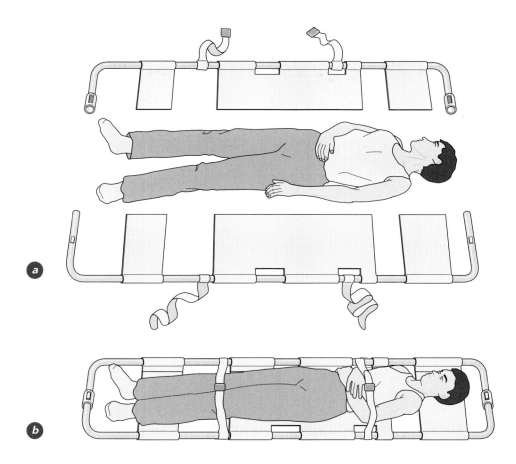

Figure 22.9 Scoop stretcher.

Scoop Stretcher

The scoop stretcher is made of metal and can be separated into two parts. One part provides a thin metal structure that slides under the athlete, and then the two parts are reattached at the head and feet (see figure 22.9). Presto, the athlete is on the stretcher and she has not been rolled or lifted. Athletes have one complaint about the scoop stretcher—on a cool night, the metal is cold to the touch.

Short Board

Short boards are used when an athlete reports spinal pain but is in a seated position. They should be used only by highly trained emergency personnel and ATs. Place an athlete on a short board (figure 22.10) according to the following procedure, with the person in charge controlling the head and neck of the injured person:

1. Control the head from behind.
2. Call 911.
3. Place a cervical collar on the injured athlete.
4. Prepare the short board:
   - Make sure all straps are in place.
   - Match the straps, buckle, and clip (usually these are color coded to avoid confusion).
5. With the person in charge maintaining tension on the head and neck, wedge the short board between the athlete and the chair.
6. Put the chest straps in place.
7. Control the head from the front and strap the head to the board.
8. Strap the legs with the hips flexed.
9. Place a long backboard perpendicular to the athlete's chair.

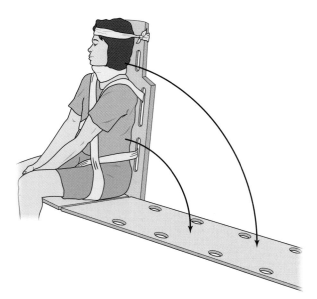

Figure 22.10   Short board. The injured person will be rotated onto her back on the long backboard.

10. Rotate the athlete onto the long backboard, keeping the knees drawn up toward the chest.

11. Release the leg straps so that the legs can lie flat on the backboard.

12. Place a strap across the chest (but not over the heart area).

13. Place a hip strap.

14. Place a foot strap.

Full-Body Vacuum Splint

More recently full-body vacuum splints have been used to stabilize an athlete with a spine injury. This splint is simply a larger version of the vacuum splints described in chapter 20. The athlete is surrounded by the nylon splint and the air is evacuated from it, creating a rigid encasement around the body.

Backboard

After an injured athlete receives an assessment and care, backboard him

- for any spinal or back injury,
- when the extent of injuries cannot be determined, or
- when there is not enough time to splint obvious fractures and the injury is serious.

Backboarding an athlete requires several trained emergency personnel and ATs. One person will be in charge and direct the others. Backboard an athlete according to the following procedure, with the person in charge controlling the head throughout the operation:

1. Control the head.

2. Call 911.

3. Place a cervical collar on the injured athlete to immobilize the spine.

4. Prepare the backboard:
- Make sure all straps are in place.
- Match the straps, buckle, and clip (usually these are color coded to avoid confusion).
- Remove the head block (or sandbags or rolled blanket) and keep it ready for placement.

5. Under the direction of the person in control of the head, roll the athlete 90° and position the board by sliding it just behind the him; once the board is in position, roll the athlete back onto the backboard so that his head is at the top and he is centered on the board.

6. Place both cross-chest straps over the collarbones and tighten.

7. Put the head block (or sandbags or rolled blanket) in place.

8. Tape the head to the board, one strip over the forehead and another over the chin. (Local EMS may or may not require a chin strap.)

9. Place a hip strap.

10. Place a foot strap.

What Would You Do If...

After successfully backboarding a wrestler, it is discovered that two of the straps are crossed and are not buckled to themselves but to another strap. The straps are then switched and buckled correctly. The AT directs you to make sure that the buckles and the clips are easily identified when backboarding.

At least four people are needed to carry the backboard—one on each end and two in the middle.

An alternative method for backboarding an athlete is the lift-and-slide technique. This technique requires five or more people and is used for an athlete who is already supine. As with the traditional logroll technique, the person controlling the athlete's head is in charge of the following procedure:

1. A cervical collar stabilizes the head, and the person directing the technique controls the head and neck.

2. The backboard is prepared the same as in the traditional spine-board technique explained earlier.

3. One assistant straddles the victim, facing the head, and is in charge of lifting the athlete's pelvis.

4. Two assistants are positioned on each side of the victim and are responsible for lifting his torso.

What Would You Do If...

An athlete goes down on the field. The AT has asked you to run out with her during such incidents today, but you are wearing clogs.

5. A fourth assistant straddles the victim and is responsible for lifting the athlete's legs. Under the direction of the person in control of the head, the team lifts the athlete, and a fifth assistant slides the spine board into position directly under the athlete.

6. On the leader's command, the team lowers the athlete onto the spine board.

7. As with the traditional logroll technique, the athlete is secured and strapped to the spine board.

After backboarding an athlete with a cervical spine injury, the head should be immobilized using foam blocks.

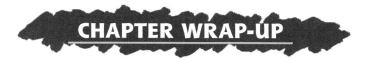

CHAPTER WRAP-UP

Summary

When an injured athlete must be examined or removed from the field, it is crucial that the injured body part be disturbed as little as possible. Movement of the body part causes pain and aggravation, and it may cause further injury. Athletes who are ambulatory may still need assistance. The AT must not be rushed into moving an athlete off the field before he is properly splinted or backboarded.

Key Terms

Define the following terms found in this chapter:

ambulatory   extrication
backboarding   neck roll

Questions for Review

1. When is it necessary to remove an athlete's equipment and uniform?

2. When should an athlete walk off the field without support?

3. An athlete who is standing indicates that he has neck pain and tingling sensations. What is the best way to remove him from the field?

4. List the ways a student assistant can help when the AT needs to backboard an athlete.

5. If an athlete has a suspected serious knee injury, list the ways she might be removed from the field.

6. Why is an injured athlete moved feetfirst when she is on a stretcher or a backboard?

Activities for Reinforcement

1. Make a list of the types of splints and other equipment necessary for removing an athlete from a game.

2. With the supervision of an AT, practice removing an athlete in the ways discussed in this chapter.

3. Prepare a checklist of items that are necessary for removing game equipment. Look for the equipment before two home games. Is it where it is supposed to be?

4. Invite EMS personnel to your school to provide an in-service on how to stabilize and backboard an athlete.

Above and Beyond

1. Using various tools, practice removing a helmet. Make a chart of any problems encountered with each tool. Determine which tool is the easiest to use.

2. Read one of the following articles and write a one-page report:

   Del Rossi, G., M. Horodyski, and M.E. Powers. 2003. A comparison of spine-board transfer techniques and the effect of training on performance. *Journal of Athletic Training* 38(3): 204-208.

   Gale, S., L. Decoster, and E. Swartz. 2008. The combined tool approach for face mask removal during on-field conditions. *Journal of Athletic Training* 43(1): 14-20.

   Greenstein, J.S., and D.M. Kleiner. 2000. Guidelines for the pre-hospital management of the spine-injured athlete. *Journal of Sports Chiropractic and Rehabilitation* 14(4): 105-110, 134-135.

   Luscombe, M.D., and J.L. Williams. 2003. Comparison of a long spinal board and vacuum mattress for spinal immobilization. *Emergency Medicine Journal* 20(5): 476-478.

   Swartz, E., S. Norkus, T. Cappaert, and L. Decoster. 2005. Football equipment design affects face mask removal efficiency. *American Journal of Sports Medicine* 33(8): 1210-1219.

   Tierney, R.T., C.G. Mattacola, M.R. Sitler, and C. Maldjian. 2002. Head position and football equipment influence cervical spine-cord space during immobilization. *Journal of Athletic Training* 37(2): 185-189.

3. Interview local EMS personnel. Determine the protocols used to remove an athlete by basic-level ambulance, advanced-level ambulance, and helicopter.

4. Compare and contrast the logroll technique versus the lift-and-slide technique for backboarding an athlete and present a report to your class.

UNIT VIII

Preventing Athletics-Related Injuries

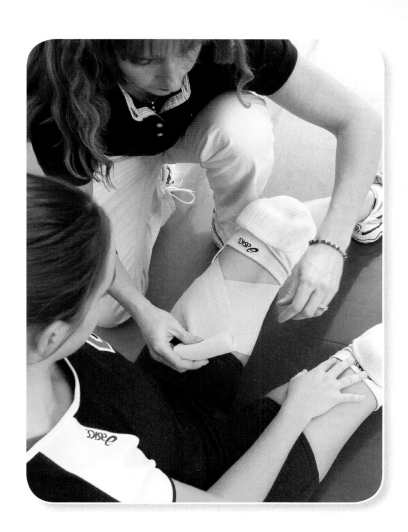

chapter 23

Protective Taping and Wrapping

Objectives

Upon completing this chapter, the student will be able to do the following:

- Understand why tape and wraps are applied to the body.
- Know what types of tape are available.
- Explain how to apply tape to the body by following the principles of tape handling, skin preparation, and taping techniques.
- Understand why and how elastic wraps are applied to the body for specific injuries.

Taping and wrapping have been the hallmark of practice for ATs. The techniques of selecting and applying protective tapes and wraps are skills that every AT must have. Although we discuss these skills in relation to injury prevention, they are integral parts of athletic injury care as well. We consider these skills to be as much art as they are science.

PRINCIPLES OF TAPING

Protective tape is used to prevent injuries and to keep existing injuries from getting worse, but it must be applied only if its use is indicated. An AT must understand the contraindications of applying tape as well as its proper use, which includes tape selection, tape handling, skin preparation, and taping techniques.

Indications for Applying Tape

Tape may be applied for the following reasons:

- *To provide support and stability.* After a joint injury, ligaments may be overstretched and somewhat loose. Taping the joint can improve stability and give the athlete a feeling of security.

- *To provide immediate first aid.* Taping as first aid is usually to hold a bandage in place. Some tape procedures, such as the open basket weave that we will discuss, can provide minimal compression to an injury if an elastic wrap is not available. In addition, applying tape to an area will reduce further movement.

• **To secure a pad or brace.** When treating an injury, an AT often applies tape to secure a brace or pad in place. If the AT needs to secure a foam pad to the skin to protect fresh bruises from another blow, he should cover it completely with tape. In other words, the AT will not be able to see the pad once he has taped it in place; otherwise, it will dislodge itself and fall off the body. If an athlete is required to wear a brace on her knee, she may simply want tape applied over any straps so that the brace does not loosen if she falls.

• **To prevent injury.** Tape is applied at specific joints to restrict certain motions. For example, the most common mechanism for ankle sprains is inversion. Therefore, tape is applied to the ankle to restrict that movement.

• **To restrict the angle of pull.** When tape is applied, it can be placed so that two bones are not allowed to move too far in a certain direction, thus limiting the range of motion. For example, if elbow extension is painful because of a biceps injury, tape can be applied to restrict the pulling on the biceps that occurs with elbow extension. When a muscle or tendon is strained, restricting the angle of pull can help reduce stress and prevent further injury.

• **To provide psychological assistance.** Although taping procedures are not intended to replace strong ligaments and muscles, they are sometimes used to give psychological assistance to athletes. Occasionally an athlete will feel more confident knowing she is protected with a specific tape job. Tape and wraps should not be used as a substitute for proper treatment, though. Many ATs do not tape or wrap an athlete unless he first takes the time to receive treatment.

Use of tape goes beyond understanding application techniques and procedures. It also includes tape selection, tape handling, skin preparation, and taping techniques.

Tape Selection

There are four types of tape from which to choose: linen, elastic, hybrid, and moleskin (see figure 23.1). An AT must understand the differences among the various tapes to select the best one for the goals she has in mind.

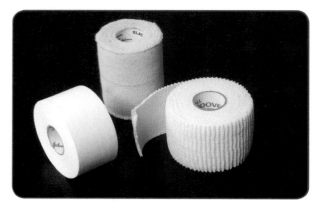

Figure 23.1 Types of tape include linen, elastic, and hybrid.

1. Linen tape is the most common type and can be torn by hand. It varies in width from .5 to 2 inches (1-2.5 cm), but 1.5 inches (4 cm) is the size most frequently used. Many manufacturers produce linen tape, and the quality of the products differs. Better tapes have more threads per square inch and come off the spool evenly. An AT must consider several factors when deciding what quality of tape to purchase. For example, if she tapes athletes often and frequently relies on taping procedures to prevent injury, purchasing a high-quality tape is warranted. However, if a school has a small budget, buying lots of expensive tape may leave little money to purchase other supplies, so she may choose a lower quality of tape.

2. Elastic tape, similar to an elastic wrap, can return to its original length after being stretched. Elastic tape has extra adhesive on one side and usually has to be cut with scissors. It is used when strong material is desired or when the tape ends need to pull toward one another. For example, if an athlete has a hyperextended elbow, the AT may not want the elbow to move into full extension, so he could apply elastic tape from the front of the forearm to the front of the upper arm. Because the tape is attempting to return to its original length, it pulls the elbow into a slight degree of flexion and subsequently prevents hyperextension.

3. Hybrid tape is a combination of linen and elastic—it is a linen-based tape with some elastic qualities. Hybrid tape can often be torn by hand.

Hybrid tape is used to surround strips of linen tape that have been applied to muscles and joints that must expand, contract, or bend. Covering the linen tape helps it stay in place. Hybrid tape is slightly more expensive than linen tape of a similar quality.

4. Moleskin is a thick tape with a lot of adhesive on one side. It sticks well to the skin and is very strong. Thus, it is often used when added strength is needed. It is rather expensive compared with other types of tape but is extremely useful when an athlete is returning to participation, such as after an ankle sprain when a great deal of reinforcement is needed so she does not reinjure her ankle.

Tape Handling

The smoothness and efficiency with which tape is applied depends on how proficient the AT is at tape handling. This involves proper tearing, winding, overlap, and contour.

Perhaps the hardest part of tape handling for beginners is tearing the tape. When tearing the tape, the roll is gripped in one hand and the strip of tape to be torn is held between the thumb and index finger of the other hand. A precise, quick movement must be used. The tape must not be pleated at the edge or the threads may not pull apart. Do not be discouraged if this is a difficult task. If at first you don't succeed, tear, tear again!

Winding involves applying individual strips of tape rather than a continuous length of tape off the roll, which builds tension quickly and is likely to cut off circulation. When tape is applied continuously around a joint, the AT must be careful to apply the tape at a proper tension without cutting off the athlete's circulation. Some athletes may like tape to be applied tightly, but until the AT becomes skilled at adjusting the tension, applying individual strips is most appropriate. A bluish skin color indicates a loss of circulation. The AT should ask the athlete if he can feel tingling or if it feels as if his foot or hand is falling asleep. She should also check circulation by examining the capillary refill of the nail bed. That is, if she is taping the athlete's wrist, she should pinch his thumbnail to squeeze the blood from it. If circulation is adequate, the nail bed should turn from white to pink in just a

few seconds when she stops pinching. She should do the same thing to a toenail if she has applied tape to the foot or ankle.

Overlap involves applying strips of tape so that half of the strip from one piece is covered by the next piece. If the AT does not apply the tape using an overlap method, he runs the risk of gapping the tape and creating areas of friction and irritation.

Tape must be applied so that it follows the natural contour of the body area. The AT will adapt the angle of application to the shape of the body area receiving the tape. He must be able to subtly alter the angle of application of the tape to get to the desired direction and subsequent support without affecting the body contour or disturbing the purpose of the procedure. If the AT forces the tape into a change of direction too abruptly, she may create areas of high pressure or wrinkles, which can cause blisters, cuts, and even contusions, not to mention an upset athlete.

Skin Preparation

Before applying tape to the body, the skin must be washed and dried, and hair around the body part must be removed by shaving with either an electric hair clipper with a guard or with a disposable razor. After the area is cleaned and shaved, a tape adhesive is applied. Tape adhesives come in spray cans or bottles and, once applied, they increase the stickiness of the skin, which allows the tape to be applied more securely.

When the tape adhesive has dried, a thin film of foamlike material is applied to the skin. This helps prevent skin irritation (and the tape from sticking to the athlete's hair if he has neglected to

What Would You Do If...

An athlete gets his ankle taped every day because he has a history of ankle sprains, and he is recovering from a recent ankle injury. He is required to perform a set of exercises before being taped, but he does not do them.

shave). Some body parts such as the front of the ankle and back of the heel are extremely sensitive because they rub against the shoe. Such areas are protected with thin foam pads to which the AT applies a petroleum-based lubricant—the pads minimize friction and improve comfort. After the practice or game, the athlete will remove the tape with special scissors or tape shears, which have a protective end so the athlete will not cut herself. Finally, she should clean the area with soap and water while in the shower.

TAPING TECHNIQUES

If you were to ask 10 ATs how to tape a body part, chances are you would get 10 different answers. Many taping techniques can be applied to various body areas. In this section we will explain and illustrate some of the basic procedures that we prefer to use.

Many taping procedures have a common foundation: They begin with anchor strips, which are single strips of tape placed around each end of the body part that will be taped. The anchor strips create borders to work within. Once the anchor strips are in place, support strips are applied. Support strips may be overlapped to create a fan shape, they may be pulled from one side of a joint to another, or they may be swirled around a joint. Support strips are deliberately placed based on the goals of the tape job. Closure strips, which are applied in the final step in most procedures, are placed over the sup-

port strips. They are vital to keeping the tape intact no matter how hard the athlete practices or plays. The AT cannot be stingy with closure strips. When you see the illustrations, you may wonder about the number of closure strips pictured for some of the procedures. We haven't gone crazy. Applying closure strips is not the time to try to save tape; you must be certain that your taping job won't fail when the athlete needs it most.

Turf Toe

The goal when taping for turf toe is to restrict the extension movement of the great toe. First place anchor strips of linen tape around the foot and around the base of the great toe (see figure 23.2a). Then place a minimum of three strips of 1-inch (2.5 cm) linen tape from the plantar aspect of the toe anchor strip to the plantar aspect of the arch on the anchor strip (see figure 23.2b). Apply closure strips over the loose ends to secure these strips in place (see figure 23.2c). Elastic tape may also be used for this procedure. Elastic tape is especially useful around the foot because it allows the foot to expand during the weight-bearing portion of the stride without binding the foot.

Bunion

A bunion can result in discomfort because of excess pressure on the medial aspect of the shoe. To alleviate the pressure, a bunion can be taped. First place an anchor strip around the great toe, just as with turf toe. The toe is moved in line with

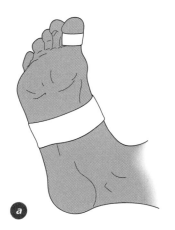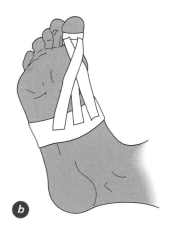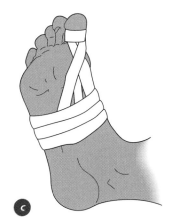

Figure 23.2 Turf-toe. (a) Apply anchors to the foot and great toe, (b) apply three strips of linen tape on the bottom of the foot between the anchor strips, and (c) cover the ends with closure strips.

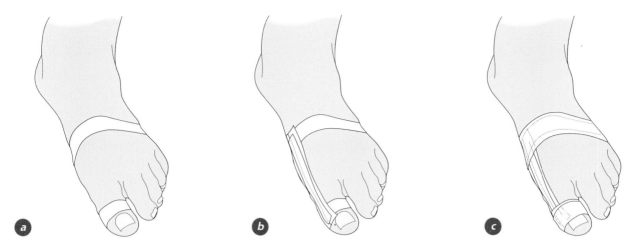

Figure 23.3 Bunion taping. (a) Place a small piece of foam rubber between the first and second toe, then place an anchor strip at the arch and toenail (1 and 2). (b) Place three tape strips medially on the toe (3, 4, and 5). (c) Lock all tape in place with anchor strips (5 and 6).

the first metatarsal, and strips are placed from the anchor strip along the medial aspect of the foot. Once in place, the medial strips are secured (see figure 23.3).

Longitudinal Arch

The purpose of the longitudinal arch procedure is to keep the medial foot from flattening. Start with one to three anchor strips around the ball of the foot. Start the first strip of 1-inch (2.5 cm) linen tape at the medial side of the anchor and go back toward and around the heel to the starting point at the anchor (see figure 23.4a). Start the second strip at the lateral side of the anchor, take it around the heel, and then return to the starting point (see figure 23.4b). Overlap the strips until four to six strips have been placed. Cover the loose ends with closure strips (see figure 23.4c). Many variations of this taping procedure exist.

Closed Basket Weave

The closed basket weave is used primarily to give support and help prevent inversion ankle sprains. We begin the closed basket weave with one anchor strip at the lower leg just below the bulky portion of the calf muscle and one at midfoot. With the anchors in place we begin placing support strips called *stirrups* and *horseshoes* on the ankle. The first stirrup is applied to the anchor strip on the medial aspect of the leg, pulled under the foot, and pulled up to the anchor strip on the lateral aspect of the leg

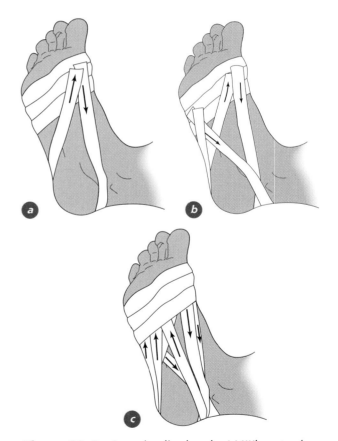

Figure 23.4 Longitudinal arch. (a) When taping an arch, begin with an anchor strip. Place the first strip of linen tape from the anchor back toward the heel and around to the other end of the strip at the anchor. (b) Overlap the strips until four to six strips have been placed. (c) Once the arch strips are situated, close the loose ends with closure strips.

(see figure 23.5a). Once a stirrup is applied, place a horseshoe strip at the distal aspect of the lower leg (around the ankle) from the lateral aspect to the medial aspect (see figure 23.5b). Apply these strips alternately, overlapping them until a minimum of three stirrups and three horseshoes are applied (see figure 23.5c).

Once this is completed, apply a figure eight around the ankle. Start the figure eight at the outer anklebone (lateral malleolus) and guide the tape across the top of the ankle down to the medial aspect of the foot. The figure-eight strip will then come up the lateral side of the foot just in front of the lateral malleolus and run a course to the medial malleolus and then around to the back of the lower leg, stopping at the lateral malleolus (see figure 23.5d). Once the figure-eight strip is in place,

apply two heel locks (one forward and one reverse). Start one heel lock just above the inside anklebone (medial malleolus) and angle the strip downward so that it crosses the outer aspect of the heel. Then the tape runs a course across the bottom of the foot and upward on the inside aspect, angling toward the outer anklebone (lateral malleolus), where it stops (see figure 23.5e). Start the next heel lock just above the lateral malleolus and angle it downward so that it crosses the medial aspect of the heel and runs across the bottom of the foot and upward on the lateral aspect, angling toward the medial malleolus, where it stops (see figure 23.5f). Heel locks can be done continuously once proficiency is developed with the angles and tape handling. After the heel locks are in place, apply closure strips to cover all loose ends.

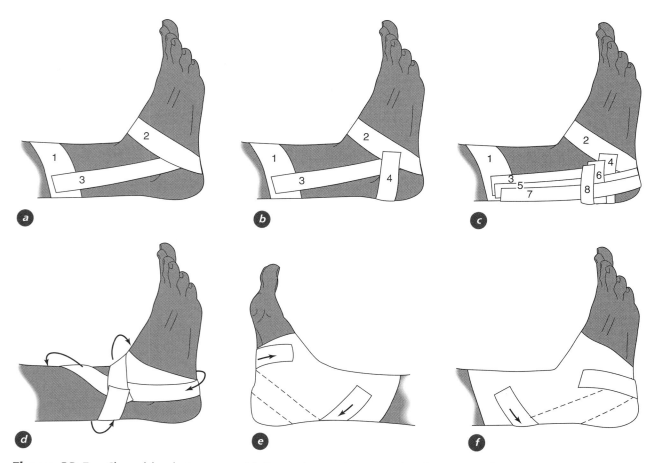

Figure 23.5 Closed basket weave. (a) Once the anchors are in place (1 and 2), a stirrup is applied (3), (b) and a horseshoe strip is applied (4). (c) Stirrup and horseshoe strips are applied in alternating fashion (5-8), (d) followed by the figure-eight strip. (e-f) Heel locks are applied after the figure eight from above the ankle, wrapping under the heel.

Open Basket Weave

The open basket weave (see figure 23.6) is used with acute ankle sprains to help prevent swelling if an elastic wrap is not available. It is applied in the same manner as a closed basket weave, with a few exceptions. The idea is to leave a gap down the front of the tape job in case too much swelling occurs. Thus, we leave the anchor strips open on the front of the leg and on top of the foot rather than circling the leg and foot with them, and we do not perform the figure-eight procedure. Do the heel locks, making sure they do not cross over the front of the ankle where a gap is to be left. The gap allows for expansion of the ankle caused by excessive swelling. This tape application is especially useful for an acute ankle sprain when an elastic wrap is not available and the ankle is expected to swell.

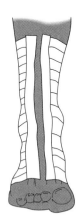

Figure 23.6 An open basket weave is helpful for supporting an ankle injury. The gap in the front of the tape job allows the ankle to swell.

Achilles Tendon

Achilles tendon taping restricts the amount of dorsiflexion at the ankle. When a person dorsiflexes her foot, the Achilles tendon is stretched. Therefore, when applying tape in an Achilles tendon procedure, the athlete lies facedown and points her injured foot into a few degrees of plantar flexion. Once the foot is in position, apply anchor strips midcalf, about 6 inches (15 cm) from the malleoli, and at the ball of the foot. Place a fan shape of three strips of elastic tape from the top anchor to the bottom anchor. These strips should cross over the back of the heel (see figure 23.7a). Once the strips of elastic tape are positioned, place linen closure strips over several inches at the ends to secure them in place (see figure 23.7b).

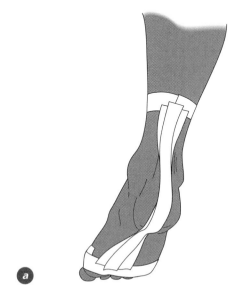
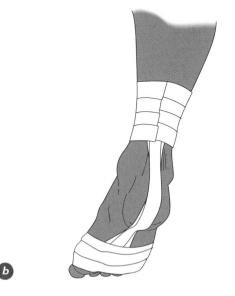

Figure 23.7 An Achilles tendon tape procedure. *(a)* Place a fan shape of three strips of elastic tape from the top anchor to the bottom anchor, and *(b)* secure the strips with closure strips.

Shin Splints

The term *shin splints* is sometimes used as a catchall for pain in the lower leg, because shin splints—formally called *medial tibial stress syndrome*—can be extremely painful. Tape application can help reduce the pain. When an athlete suffers from shin splints, place overlapping strips of tape around the lower leg from an inch (2.5 cm) above the ankle bones to the bottom of the calf. The strips should be applied one over the other from the Achilles tendon upward to the medial aspect of the lower leg (see figure 23.8). The small amount of compression that the tape provides can sometimes lessen the athlete's discomfort. This procedure should not be done if the athlete has compartment syndrome (see chapter 15), and the tape should be removed if symptoms worsen.

Collateral Knee Ligament Sprain

Injuries to the medial or lateral ligament of the knee are taped in the same manner on the appropriate side of the knee. Here we present an MCL tape procedure designed to reduce the amount of valgus movement. This type of movement opens the medial joint line of the knee, subsequently stretching or tearing the MCL (see chapter 14).

Begin taping the MCL by having the athlete stand, and put a block of wood about 2 inches (5 cm) high under the heel of the leg to be taped. This

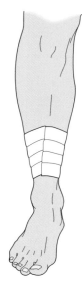

Figure 23.8   Taping for shin splints.

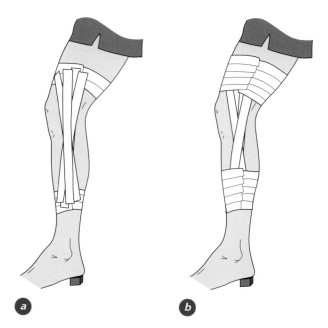

Figure 23.9   Collateral knee procedure. *(a)* Start by placing a block of wood under the heel of the leg being taped. Anchor strips and fan are placed across the joint line, and *(b)* closure strips are placed.

places the knee in flexion. Place three or four anchor strips around the midthigh and two or three anchor strips around the lower leg. Once the anchors are positioned, place a minimum of three strips of linen or elastic tape (2 in. [5 cm] wide) in the shape of a fan across the medial joint line of the knee (see figure 23.9a). Place closure strips over the ends of the tape at the top and bottom to secure them (see figure 23.9b).

Knee Hyperextension

Knee hyperextension is responsible for injuring the ACL. Taping a knee to prevent hyperextension also uses a fan technique. Begin by placing a block under the heel (figure 23.9) to put the knee into flexion, and place a lubricated foam pad at the back of the knee. Position three or four anchor strips at midthigh and two or three at the lower leg (see figure 23.10a). A minimum of five strips are placed in a fan shape between the anchors across the back of the knee (see figure 23.10b). Finish by placing closure strips across all tape ends (figure 23.10c).

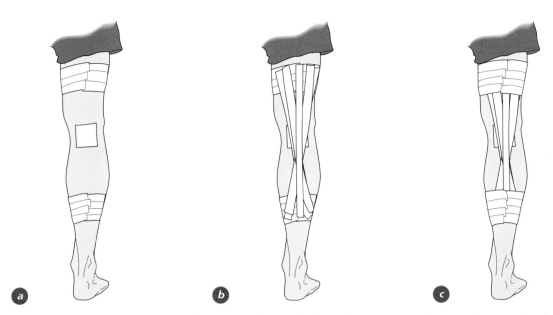

Figure 23.10 Knee hyperextension procedure. *(a)* Knee hyperextension anchors and a lubricated pad are applied, *(b)* five strips are placed in a fan shape, and *(c)* enough closure strips are applied to make sure the tape remains in place.

Elbow Hyperextension

One of the most common mechanisms for elbow injuries is falling on an outstretched arm, which makes the elbow vulnerable to hyperextension injuries. The goal of taping for an elbow hyperextension injury is to limit extension. Before taping, first place the elbow in a slight amount of flexion. Place anchor strips at the top of the biceps of the upper arm and at the mid- to lower forearm. Before applying the anchor strips, make sure the athlete is making the biceps muscle tight. When the anchor strips are in position, place three to five strips in a fan shape across the front of the elbow, running from anchor to anchor (see figure 23.11*a*). Elastic tape is preferred for these strips, but linen tape is also acceptable. Apply closure strips over the anchors at the upper arm and forearm to cover all tape ends (see figure 23.11*b*).

Wrist Hyperextension and Hyperflexion

Sprains and strains are common injuries to the wrist. Hyperflexion and hyperextension mechanisms cause most wrist sprains; therefore, the goal for wrist taping is usually to prevent excessive flexion or extension. Because most wrist injuries

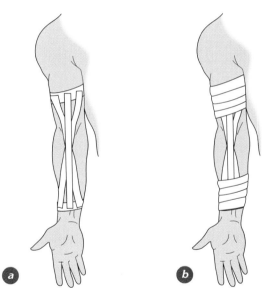

Figure 23.11 Elbow hyperextension taping procedure. *(a)* Elbow hyperextension anchor strips with tape placed in a fan shape over them, and *(b)* finished with closure strips.

are caused by hyperextension, we show a tape job to prevent it.

To prevent wrist hyperextension, start by placing an anchor strip around the distal aspect of the forearm and another around the hand just above the knuckles. With the anchors in place, position

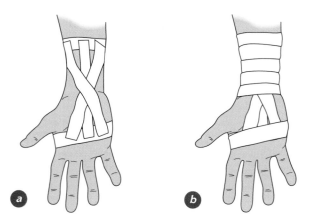

Figure 23.12   Wrist hyperextension tape procedure. (a) Wrist hyperextension anchor strips and fan strips and (b) closure strips.

the wrist into slight flexion and place a minimum of three strips of linen tape in a fan shape across the palmar aspect of the wrist (see figure 23.12a). Closure strips are placed over the tape ends to secure them (see figure 23.12b).

Thumb Hyperextension

Begin taping for a thumb hyperextension injury by placing anchors around the wrist, around the hand, and around the top of the thumb just above the nail. The thumb is then positioned into slight flexion and strips of 1-inch (2.5 cm) linen tape are applied over the back of the thumb in a fan shape between the anchors on the thumb and wrist (see figure 23.13a). Once these are in place, a tape wrap called a *spica* can be wound around the joint. Beginning at the palmar aspect of the wrist, guide the 1-inch (2.5 cm) tape toward the back aspect of the thumb, loop it around the thumb, and then guide the tape toward the dorsal aspect of the wrist and tear the tape (see figure 23.13b). Repeat this spica one more time and then apply closure strips around

FYI

Spica

A spica is a taping or wrapping procedure applied to joints such as the thumb, shoulder, or hip. It is a figure eight applied to an area so that the tape or wrap encircles the joint and gives support.

the wrist and around the hand to cover all tape ends. Also, to keep the thumb stable, a **checkrein** (see figure 23.13c) can be used to connect the index finger and the thumb.

Finger Sprain

Finger sprains are commonly treated using buddy taping; that is, the sprained finger is moved toward an adjacent noninjured finger and either the first and second or third and fourth fingers are taped together. Tape is applied between the joints of the fingers; rarely is it applied across the joint itself (see figure 23.14).

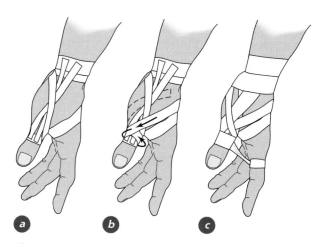

Figure 23.13   Thumb hyperextension procedure. (a) Thumb hyperextension taping begins with anchors on the wrist, hand, and thumb and strips of tape on the dorsal aspect of the thumb; (b) thumb taping complete with spica and (c) checkrein.

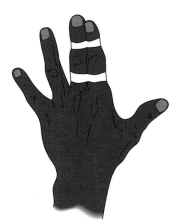

Figure 23.14   Buddy taping for a finger sprain.

ELASTIC WRAPPING TECHNIQUES

When an athlete suffers an injury, **elastic wraps** are often helpful for applying compression and support to the area. Elastic wraps come in various widths and lengths and are used for many musculoskeletal injuries, such as sprains and strains. Because elastic wraps can be washed and reused, they are less expensive than tape. Similar to tape, elastic wraps come in a variety of sizes. Common widths include 2, 3, 4, and 6 inches (5, 8, 10, and 15 cm). Two- and 3-inch (5 and 8 cm) elastic wraps are often used around the wrist or hand, 4-inch (10 cm) wraps are commonly used around the foot or ankle, and 6-inch (15 cm) elastic wraps are used around the thigh, hip, or shoulder.

The Real World

I worked with an athlete who had once sprained his finger, and he liked to have his fingers buddy taped. He also felt that elastic tape was better for him than linen, so I used elastic tape. On one occasion during practice, the athlete ran to the sideline and asked me to tape his fingers. He had a late class that day so he had not been taped before practice. I had some 1-inch (2.5 cm) elastic tape, and I began applying it to his hand, taping his fingers together. He was in a hurry to get back to practice and was practically dancing with impatience. He kept looking behind him to watch practice and his hand was moving all around. Although I warned him several times to keep his hand still while I cut the tape, he continued to fidget. Sure enough, when I was cutting the tape he moved his hand toward the scissors, and I snipped the webbing of skin between his fingers. Although the wound was minor, I felt bad. The moral of the story is this: Precut the lengths of elastic tape before applying them to the body unless you are in a controlled setting such as the athletic training room.

Anonymous

Ankle Sprain or Strain

When applying an elastic wrap, we make sure to leave the toes exposed so we can check circulation (see figure 23.15). Begin at the bottom of the foot close to the toes and wrap to above the ankle. Overlap the wrap by one-half of the width each time while working up over the ankle, and use a wrap at least 4 inches (10 cm) wide so that the finished wrap does not roll up on the edges and become too restrictive. Begin with moderate pressure, and as the wrap is applied toward and above the ankle, decrease the amount of pressure. Always check the athlete's circulation after the wrap has been applied.

Thigh Injury

When wrapping the thigh for hamstring or quadriceps injuries, we use a double-length, 6-inch (15 cm) elastic wrap and begin just above the knee. Overlap the wrap as it is applied upward toward the hip. While applying the wrap in a spiral around the leg, use subtle upward and downward angles to contour the wrap appropriately. The finished product will look as though there are Xs up the front of the wrap. Secure the wrap in place with elastic tape (see figure 23.16).

Groin (Adductor) Strain

Begin by having the athlete put on compression shorts, spandex shorts, or other shorts over which the wrap can be applied comfortably. When wrapping adductor strains, place the hip in a slight amount of flexion and adduction by placing a small block of wood under the heel or using a small step.

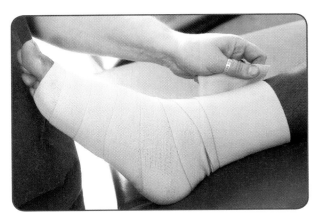

Figure 23.15 Elastic wraps are applied to joints to prevent swelling.

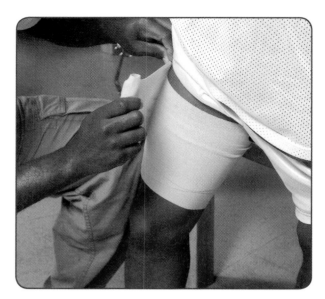

Figure 23.16 Thigh wrap. Wrap the thigh from above the knee toward the hip.

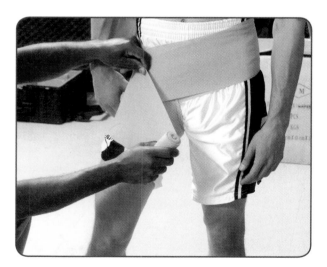

Figure 23.17 Adductor strain wrap. Note the slightly flexed and adducted position of the thigh.

Secure the wrap around the proximal thigh, continue by moving the wrap around the waist above the iliac crest and then down around the upper thigh, and repeat. Secure the wrap with elastic tape (see figure 23.17).

Hip Flexor Strain

Begin by having the athlete put on compression shorts, spandex shorts, or other shorts over which the wrap can be applied comfortably. When wrap-

ping hip flexor strains, place the hip into flexion and slight adduction by using a small block or step under the heel. Secure the wrap around the proximal thigh and apply the wrap in a counterclockwise direction. Progress by moving the wrap around the waist above the iliac crest and down around the upper thigh, and then repeat. Secure the wrap in place by taping over it with elastic tape (see figure 23.18).

Shoulder Dislocation

Elastic wraps are often applied to the shoulder to restrict motion that causes shoulder dislocations (see figure 23.19). To begin, have the athlete place

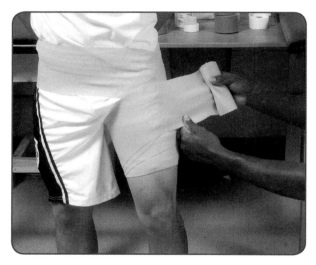

Figure 23.18 Hip flexor strain wrap. Note the flexed position of the hip and leg.

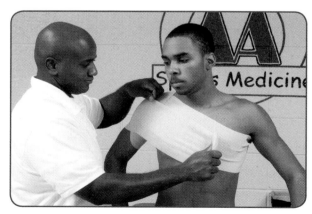

Figure 23.19 Shoulder spica. The athlete's arm is on the hip with the shoulder spica applied using an elastic wrap. This position puts the upper arm in an internally rotated position.

Protective Taping and Wrapping

the arm to be wrapped on her hip and the other arm straight out, like a teapot. Secure the wrap around the upper arm, applying the wrap in a clockwise direction. Once the wrap is secured to the upper arm, pull the wrap from the posterior aspect of the shoulder around the front of the chest, under the opposite arm, and across the back to the shoulder. Loop the wrap around the upper arm (clockwise) and repeat. Secure the wrap by taping over it with elastic tape. This wrapping of the shoulder is known as a spica.

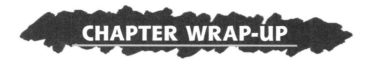

CHAPTER WRAP-UP

Summary

Taping and wrapping have become essential skills for any AT. Tape and wraps are commonly used for immediate injury care, such as to secure a dressing, pad, or ice, as well as for injury prevention. Tape application relies on understanding tape selection, tape handling, skin preparation, and taping techniques. Linen, elastic, and hybrid tape are used for different reasons, and a variety of application techniques exist.

Key Terms

Define the following terms found in this chapter:

checkrein   hybrid tape

elastic tape   linen tape

elastic wraps   moleskin

Questions for Review

1. List the reasons why ATs use tape and elastic wraps.
2. What types of tape are available, and what are the advantages of each?
3. What do we mean by the term *winding tension*? Is it helpful or harmful?
4. Why should tape be overlapped on a previous strip when applying it?

Activities for Reinforcement

1. Take a roll of tape home and practice tearing it.
2. Under the supervision of an AT, work with a partner and prepare the skin for taping. Practice the techniques included in this chapter.
3. Practice applying elastic wraps to your partner under the supervision of an AT.
4. Have an AT demonstrate alternative taping techniques and compare them with those in this text.
5. At the end of the year, have a tournament to identify the fastest and best tape job to an ankle.
6. Visit the following Web sites and find alternative ways of taping and wrapping the body areas discussed in this chapter:

    www.mindef.gov.sg/life/indexsp.htm

    www.nismat.org/traincor/ankle_tape.html
7. With a partner, practice taping continuous heel locks.

Above and Beyond

1. Examine the following Web site about a relatively new procedure called *Kinesio Taping* and give a brief report: www.ahealthyway.net/kinesiotape/what-is-kinesiotape.

2. Examine one of the following articles and write a brief report.

   Abián-Vicén, J., L. Alegre, J. Fernández-Rodríguez, and X. Aguado. 2009. Prophylactic ankle taping: elastic versus inelastic taping. *Foot and Ankle International* 30(3): 218-225.

   Bradley, T., C. Baldwick, D. Fischer, and G. Murrell, G. 2009. Effect of taping on the shoulders of Australian football players. *British Journal of Sports Medicine* 43(10): 735-738.

   Delahunt, E., J. O'Driscoll, and K. Moran. 2009. Effects of taping and exercise on ankle joint movement in subjects with chronic ankle instability: a preliminary investigation. *Archives of Physical Medicine and Rehabilitation* 90(8): 1418-1422.

   Gross, M.T., and H. Liu. 2003. The role of ankle bracing for prevention of ankle sprain injuries. *Journal of Orthopaedic and Sports Physical Therapy* 33(10): 572-577.

   Meana, M., L.M. Alegre, J.L. Elvira, and X. Aguado. 2008. Kinematics of ankle taping after a training session. *International Journal of Sports Medicine* 29(1): 70-76.3.

   Wilkerson, G.B. 2002. Biomechanical and neuromuscular effects of ankle taping and bracing. *Journal of Athletic Training* 37(4): 436-444.

3. Examine a taping technique from the following text, and compare and contrast it with the technique identified in this text: Macdonald, R. 2003. *Taping techniques: principles and practice.* 2nd ed. Los Angeles: Butterworth Heinemann.

24

Protective Equipment Used in Athletics

Objectives

Upon completing this chapter, the student will be able to do the following:

- Explain the principles of protection.
- Describe guidelines of protective equipment use.
- Explain what protective equipment is necessary for various sports.
- Describe proper equipment application.

Protective equipment is specialized equipment that has been designed to prevent athletic injuries. All athletes should use equipment that provides protection to the body parts most often injured in their sport.

Each sport has its common injuries and thus requires specialized equipment to prevent them. Equipment is designed to dissipate forces away from the area it is protecting. It must be durable yet allow enough movement to enable the athlete to play the sport. Players should never use anything but certified equipment. Two primary agencies test and certify athletic equipment. The **National Operating Committee on Standards for Athletic Equipment (NOCSAE)** sets the standards for football, baseball, and softball helmets, and the **Canadian Standards Association (CSA)** sets the standards for eye guards and ice hockey helmets.

PROTECTIVE EQUIPMENT FOR THE HEAD AND FACE

Equipment to protect the head and face falls into two main categories: helmets and face masks. Unfortunately, it takes years to get athletes to accept new safety equipment. Usually younger athletes follow the example of the professionals and use it if the pros do. Today, for example, there are helmets to protect soccer players who are making headers (hitting the ball with the head to make a pass or shot), but they are not used with any regularity by professional athletes, and thus they are relatively unknown among younger players.

Other Protection for the Head and Face

Outside of the main categories, several other pieces of supplementary equipment are used in various sports for head and face protection.

● *Nose guards.* In recent years a clear face mask designed to protect an athlete's fractured nose has made an appearance. The nose guard fits against the face so that no pressure is applied to the nasal bones. If the athlete is hit on the nose, the pressure is borne by the areas of the face under the nose guard rather than by the nose, and the force is dissipated. These nose guards are made of white or clear plastic. Most athletes prefer the clear plastic because the white color is distracting and the athlete tends to notice it from the corner of his eye.

● *Mouth guards.* Mouth guards are worn to protect the teeth and head from injury. They come in two types: custom and dip (see figure 24.1). A custom mouth guard is made by the athlete's dentist to fit her teeth. A dip mouth guard is purchased as a blank, placed in hot water for 30 seconds, and then put in the athlete's mouth to mold to her teeth. Mouth guards must fit over the molars so those teeth can be protected. Studies have shown that mouth guards offer significant protection from oral and facial injuries (Woodmansey 1999), so mouth guards are commonly recommended (Collins and Comstock 2008).

● *Eye protection.* The CSA sets standards for eye guards. For example, sunglasses that are not certified by the CSA may shatter, and if a shard enters an athlete's eye it could cause blindness. A certified pair of sunglasses will not shatter upon impact. Athletes should not be fooled into believing that any pair of glasses or sunglasses will automatically protect them from eye injuries. The glasses must be certified by the CSA.

● *Throat and neck protection.* Throat protectors are used in softball and baseball and by lacrosse and field hockey goalkeepers. The throat protector is attached by string to the face mask of a helmet, which allows the throat protector to shift back and forth with the athlete's movement. The protectors work well as long as they are in place.

● *Neck rolls.* An athlete in ice hockey or football uses a neck roll, which is a pad that fits tightly around the neck and prevents excessive head motion. An athlete will often use a neck roll after he has suffered a neck or shoulder injury such as a burner (a cervical nerve injury)—the neck roll restricts head movement and thus prevents stretching the nerve. Neck rolls are attached directly to shoulder pads.

● *Earplugs.* Only two types of equipment protect the ear: earplugs and helmets or headgear. Earplugs are used to prevent ear infections. They can be rubber or wax, but wax provides better resistance because it molds itself into the curves of the ear.

● *Headgear.* Wrestlers and water polo players wear headgear that is made of a piece of aluminum covered by a quarter-inch (.5 cm) of padding with earpieces to protect the ears (see figure 24.2). The padded aluminum earpieces are held together by

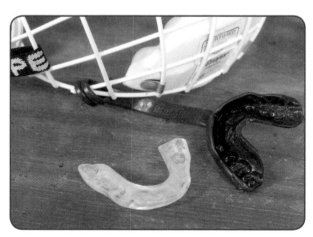

Figure 24.1 A custom-made mouth guard and a dip mouth guard are shown from left to right.

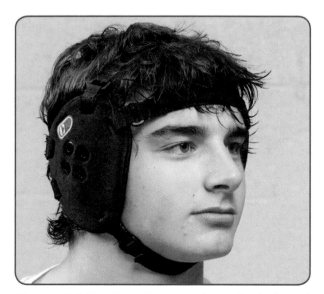

Figure 24.2 Wrestling headgear is designed to protect the athlete's ears.

What Would You Do If...

A lacrosse player has a laceration on the bridge of his nose. You notice blood inside the front of the helmet. When you ask the athlete how the injury occurred, he says, "Some guy hit me and the helmet shifted down." You tell him you would like to have the equipment manager look at the helmet. He says, "This happens every year. I just get stitches and that's it."

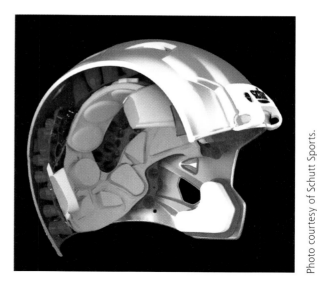

Figure 24.3   Football helmet interior.

either cloth or straps. The straps need to be fastened tightly to hold the headgear in place.

Helmets

Injuries to the head and brain are a leading cause of time loss in sport. Moreover, such injuries can create a great deal of disability in both sport and everyday life. It is necessary, therefore, to protect the head and brain to the fullest extent possible. Various helmets have been created to meet the demands of sport while protecting the head.

Football

In 1939, colleges began to require that players wear football helmets; until that time, the head had been

uncovered. Before helmets were invented, football players let their hair grow long as a way of protecting their heads. Helmets have changed dramatically over the years. The first helmets were close-fitting leather caps, and today's helmet has a hard outer shell with either an air bladder or a fluid-filled cell liner designed to disperse the force of impact over a wide area or away from the skull (see figure 24.3). Figure 24.4 illustrates proper helmet fit. Helmets

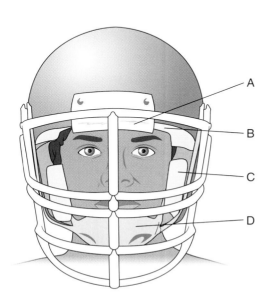

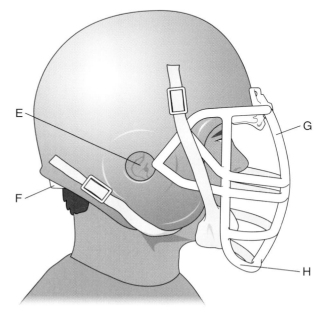

Figure 24.4   *(a)* The interior of the helmet must be one finger-width above the eyebrow, *(b)* the forehead pad must fit snugly against the forehead, *(c)* the cheek pads must fit snugly against the cheeks, *(d)* the chin strap must be snug and square on the chin, *(e)* the ear hole must line up with the ear canal, *(f)* the neck pad must be snug to the head, *(g)* the face mask must be three finger-widths from the nose, and *(h)* the face mask must be lower than the chin.

Photo courtesy of Schutt Sports.

should never be thrown or sat on, because this can crack the shell. Several manufacturers produce football helmets, including Schutt and Riddell. Helmets from each manufacturer provide unique features. For example, Schutt football helmets are as round as possible to deflect as much energy as possible and the helmet surface has no raised edges. The Riddell Revolution helmet has a shell that extends over the side of the face and has a special pad to protect the athlete's jaw and absorb shock from blows to the side of the head.

Ice Hockey

Ice hockey helmets are manufactured by several companies, but each one is tested and must meet the standards of the CSA. They do not, however, need to be retested annually. The interior of the helmet is made of foam that conforms to the helmet shell. A hockey helmet should fit snugly. If it is too loose, it will not protect the head under significant impact. The last helmetless professional hockey player retired in 1997. Now all players in the National Hockey League wear helmets. Ice hockey helmets are also used in sports such as lacrosse and field hockey. Goalkeepers in many sports wear ice hockey helmets because they are lightweight yet effective (see figure 24.5a).

Lacrosse

Similar to hockey helmets, lacrosse helmets have a protective plastic shell with interior foam. The helmet has a four-point chin strap to stabilize it on the head. Lacrosse helmets are required for male players, and helmets must meet NOCSAE standards (see figure 24.5b). Only the goalie wears a helmet in women's lacrosse.

Baseball and Softball

All batting helmets are required to have the NOCSAE inspection seal, but they need not be tested annually. Batting helmets for players from Little League through college are required to have earflaps on both sides (see figure 24.5c). Professional baseball players are required to wear helmets, but earflaps are not required. However, most professionals wear a helmet with an earflap on the side closest to the pitcher when they are batting. The interior of the helmet is lined with hard foam, which distorts slightly on impact. Depending on the league, a chin strap or even a face mask might be required. Batting helmets with face masks are required for all fielders in Little League games.

Face Guards

Many sports involve a great deal of contact and ball movement that put an athlete at risk for facial

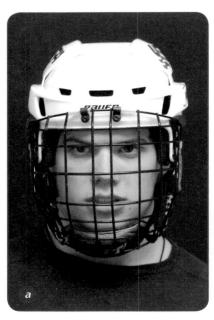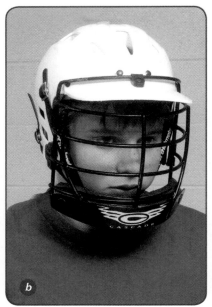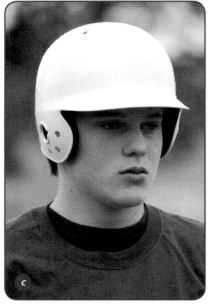

Figure 24.5 *(a)* Ice hockey helmet, *(b)* lacrosse helmet, and *(c)* batting helmet.

injuries. Several sports have implemented the use of face guards to protect an athlete's face from contusions and lacerations.

Football

In football, the face mask is made either of rubber-covered metal or plastic. The face mask must be appropriate for the position the athlete will be playing. Quarterbacks and receivers wear face masks without a center bar so that they can see better. Running backs and defensive backs wear face masks with center bars. Linemen, defensive ends, and linebackers wear extended masks with center bars to keep fingers away from their face and throat. Properly fitted, the face mask must be three finger-widths from the nose.

Ice Hockey

There are three types of face masks for hockey helmets: full wire, full plastic (see figure 24.6), and half plastic. The wire face mask has small (1 in. or 2.5 cm) square openings that prevent a puck or stick from entering. The full plastic face mask is clear,

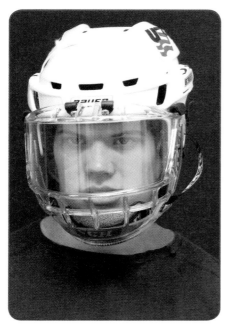

Figure 24.6 Ice hockey helmet with a clear face shield.

but sometimes the mask gets foggy during play. College-aged and younger athletes are required to wear full face masks, either wire or plastic. Referees and professional hockey players use the half mask.

Lacrosse

Lacrosse face masks are connected to the helmet and provide full-face wire protection. The wire mask has small openings to prevent a stick or ball from entering. A large, thick chin pad is placed at the base of the face mask to protect the athlete's chin. Lacrosse goalies are required to attach throat protectors to their face masks. A properly fitting lacrosse helmet will not shift positions when the athlete rotates his head.

Baseball and Softball

A catcher wears a face mask that attaches to a protective helmet. The face mask has a padded interior surface that rests against the face and elastic straps to hold it in place. It allows the catcher to see while protecting the face from errant balls.

PROTECTIVE EQUIPMENT FOR THE UPPER BODY

Protective equipment for the upper body must allow the athlete to move yet also absorb shock. Designers are challenged to make devices that can take impact in a variety of positions. Most equipment is made of a hard exterior plastic shell with padding close to the body.

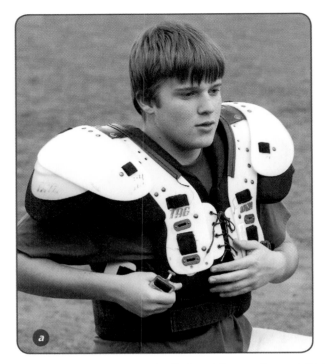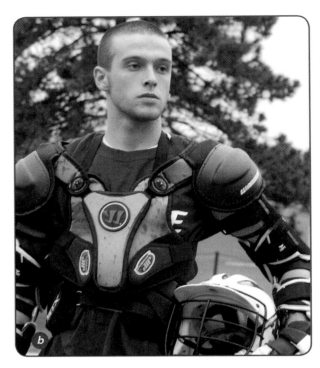

Figure 24.7   *(a)* Football shoulder pads and *(b)* lacrosse shoulder pads.

Shoulder and Upper Arm

Shoulder pads are the main protection for the shoulders in hockey, football, and lacrosse. All shoulder pads are designed similarly—a plastic exterior with soft padding next to the skin.

Football shoulder pads are designed for the position the athlete plays (see figure 24.7*a*). Regular shoulder pads cover the chest and shoulders. A quarterback wears pads that are smaller and allow for more shoulder movement; a lineman's pads are larger and longer. The pads lace in the front and have straps that run from the back and lock in the front. The soft padding is covered with a sweat-resistant material.

Compared with football pads, ice hockey and lacrosse shoulder pads are made of thin padding (see figure 24.7*b*). They lace and have a hook-and-loop closure in the front so that they are easily removed. These pads can be cleaned in a regular washing machine.

Shoulder lifts are thin (.5 in. or 1 cm) pieces of padding that are worn under shoulder pads. Lifts provide additional padding, and they are sometimes used after an injury. The lifts lace in the front and have underarm straps from back to front. Athletes who hit or who get hit the most often wear lifts—

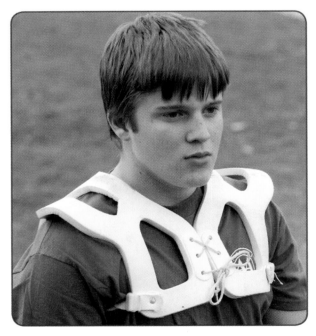

Figure 24.8   Shoulder lifts.

these include quarterbacks, running backs, and linebackers (see figure 24.8).

A restrictive harness for the glenohumeral joint is worn when an athlete has had a dislocation or subluxation of the shoulder joint. The harness is tightened to keep the arm from being lifted up and

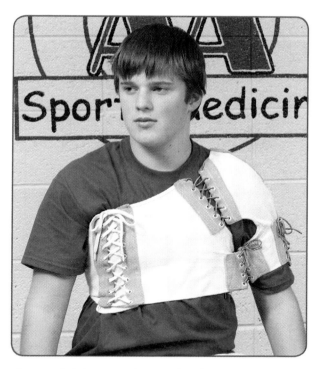

Figure 24.9   Restrictive shoulder harness.

abducted, because this is the position in which the shoulder is injured. The harness is made of straps and laces that can be adjusted to limit motion (see figure 24.9).

Elbow, Wrist, and Hand

Elbow pads are worn most often by football and ice hockey players (see figure 24.10a). Football players wear pull-on elbow pads, which are soft pads enclosed in elastic material. Hockey players wear pads with plastic exteriors that are fastened in place

with hook-and-loop closures. The newest hockey pads are made of thick, soft padding covered with sweat-resistant material. They are very protective. An elbow sleeve is made of either elastic or neoprene for warmth. The sleeve lacks padding so it does not offer protection from impact, but it is supportive and can prevent abrasions.

Gloves are used by soccer and field hockey goalies as well as by ice hockey, football, and lacrosse players. The glove style varies by sport. Soccer goalies wear a glove that has a tacky leather palm. A field hockey goalkeeper wears a leather glove that is padded on both sides for protection because she is not allowed to use a closed hand on the ball. Ice hockey goalies wear a different glove on each hand. The glove that is used to catch pucks consists of a large leather mitt that is strapped tightly around the hand and extends up to the middle of the forearm. The other hand wears a glove attached to a large pad called a *blocker*. It has a leather palm and a big chunk of padding over the top of the hand and fingers. A football lineman wears a fingerless glove with padding for the back of the hand, which is used during blocking. As an alternative to the glove, the lineman may wear a pad that can be pulled on over the back of the hand to protect it (see figure 24.10b). Wide receivers use gloves made of neoprene, which is tacky and good for catching the ball, to protect the hands from cold and abrasions.

Ribs, Sternum, and Abdomen

Football shoulder pads offer some chest protection but only for the uppermost ribs and the sternum, and a specific pad is often necessary to protect the

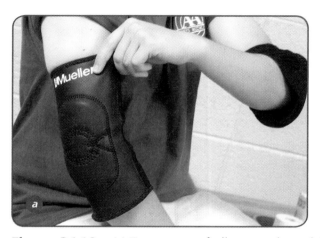
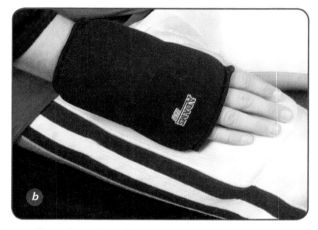

Figure 24.10   (a) Two types of elbow pads and (b) a pull-on hand pad.

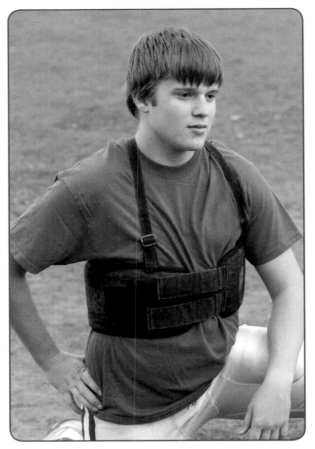

Figure 24.11   Rib protector.

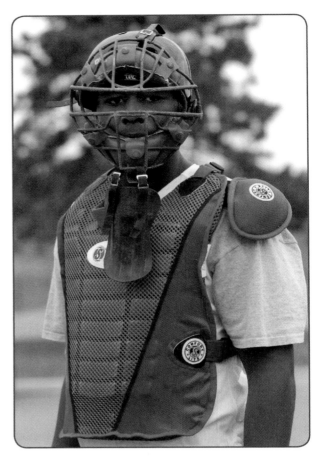

Figure 24.12   Chest protector for baseball.

ribs (see figure 24.11). No other shoulder pads offer chest protection. Football equipment manufacturers have also designed a sternum protection pad that is not standard equipment but can be worn if an athlete requires extra protection.

Specific equipment has been designed to protect the chest and abdomen in various sport activities. Chest protectors, for example, are designed to protect both the abdomen and the chest.

In field hockey, baseball, and women's lacrosse, players wear a standard chest protector designed specifically for baseball and softball. It is made of soft padding inside a durable cloth cover and uses elastic straps to hold it tightly against the body. Little League baseball players use a similar type of chest protector while batting. A word of caution—chest protectors are not safety rated. This means anyone can design a chest protector and claim that it works.

A catcher wears a chest protector that is .75 inch (2 cm) thick to prevent baseball impacts against the body. The protector is made of padding that covers the chest and abdominal areas. It is big and cumbersome yet very effective in preventing injury as well as deadening the ball (see figure 24.12).

Athletes who have been or are likely to be injured and those who receive the most impacts, such as quarterbacks, running backs, and wide receivers in football, are equipped with rib protectors. Participants in impact sports such as men's lacrosse, football, and ice hockey are likely to need this equipment.

Low Back

Back braces are designed to keep the athlete warm and to limit motion. Most back braces are made of neoprene or elastic and are fastened tightly in the front with a hook-and-loop closure. Back braces

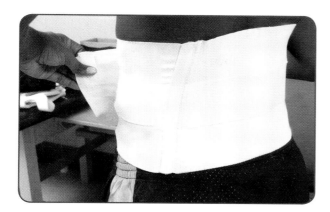

Figure 24.13 Back brace.

have small metal wires inside to provide a more stable brace (see figure 24.13).

PROTECTIVE EQUIPMENT FOR THE LOWER BODY

Protection for the lower body must not hinder the athlete's movement. If you watch professional football, you will notice that many of the players do not wear all of the pads or standard sized pads required by the rules in high school or college. Players at the professional level are paid to play and be fast; they believe that lower-body protective padding slows them down and may cost them their jobs.

Thigh, Hip, and Tailbone

Thigh pads are used in four sports: football, field hockey, women's lacrosse, and ice hockey. Thigh pads must be big enough to cover the quadriceps musculature. They must fit properly, and the pants that cover them must be snug. Football and hockey pants are designed to hold the pads tight against the bony areas they are designed to protect (see figure 24.14). Ice hockey pads go inside a pair of fitted shorts. These shorts hold thigh, hip, and lower-abdomen pads and lace up in the front. Ice hockey pads are very effective, and field hockey and women's lacrosse goalkeepers thus wear ice hockey pads for protection.

Soccer goalkeepers wear shorts or long pants with hip pads in them. The padding is lightweight to allow maximum movement and provides limited protection. Compression shorts were originally designed to hold football pads in place over the

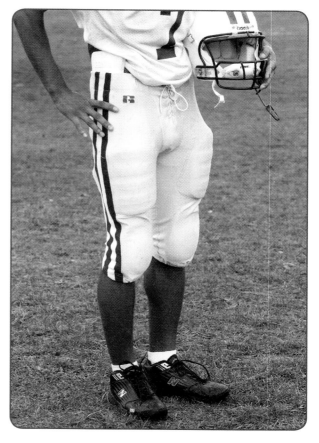

Figure 24.14 Football pants are designed to hold a variety of pads in place to protect the thigh, iliac crest, and knee.

muscles, but they are now used to provide support and warmth to the muscles without padding. In baseball and softball, a thin fiber pad that covers the hip is added to prevent sliding abrasions.

Knee

Repetitive bruises to the knee can limit an athlete's ability to play. Thus, knee pads are designed to cover the anterior aspect of the knee. The pads, which are made of foam and covered with an elastic material, are sewn into an elastic sleeve that is pulled on over the foot and up to the knee.

A variety of neoprene sleeves provide warmth and support, including patellar and shin sleeves, hinged sleeves, and sleeves with stays. A patella brace has a horseshoe-shaped pad that fits around the patella to prevent it from slipping out of alignment.

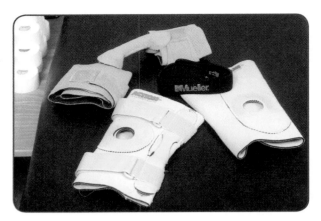

Figure 24.15 Knee braces.

A football player may wear a hinged knee brace, which is a metal or plastic bar with a hinge that protects the joint but allows flexion and extension of the knee (see figure 24.15). Some players, especially linemen and quarterbacks, think the brace prevents knee sprains. The braces are worn laterally because most blows come from that side and stretch the medial ligament. Athletes claim that these braces slow them down, but the effect is insignificant. An athlete who has bowlegs or knock-knees should not wear this type of brace because it tends to straighten the knee and cause soreness. Instead, he should have his knees taped, even though taping takes more time. Currently there is conflicting research on the effectiveness of wearing the brace, so the athlete's parents should decide if their child will use it.

Lower Leg

In some sports, a shin guard and knee pad are combined into one protective pad, which is usually a hard outer plastic shell with a padded interior. A catcher in baseball or softball and an ice hockey player wear such protection. Straps hold the shin guard in place (see figure 24.16).

A catcher's shin guard has an extension that covers the ankle. In ice hockey, field hockey, and soccer, the ankle is not covered and is vulnerable to injury from blows. For ice hockey, a special pad that covers both malleoli and the front part of the ankle is used only after a player has suffered a contusion of the anterior ankle.

Field hockey and ice hockey goalkeepers wear goalie pads that cover the foot, shin, thigh, and knee. The thick padding is made of foam, cotton,

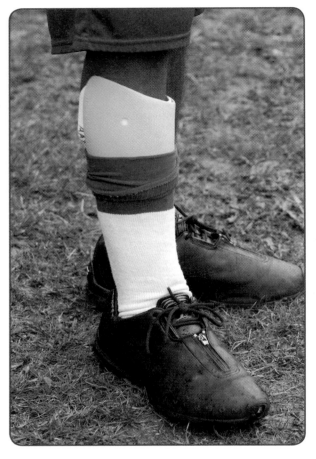

Figure 24.16 Shin guard.

and plastic and is covered with canvas or leather, with flaps around the sides of the legs and the feet. The pads are designed for protection and for deadening the ball upon impact. The pads come in various sizes based on the distance between the instep and the groin (the inseam) to ensure proper fit. They are held in place with buckled straps. The goalie pads are very effective for preventing injury.

What Would You Do If...

The best baseball player on your team slides into second base and sprains an ankle. You notice that there is not enough tape to apply a protective support. Thinking quickly, you remember that one of the bench sitters has an ankle brace.

Foot and Ankle

In many sports, athletes' feet are stepped on and injured. The top of the foot can swell so much that the athlete is unable to wear a shoe. The AT may have to design a special pad to protect the top of the foot when an injury occurs.

Heel cups are designed to prevent heel bruises. There are two types of cups: a rubberized padded cup and a rigid plastic cup (see figure 24.17). The rubberized cup has an elevated heel that can compress downward so that the heel never makes contact with the interior of the shoe. This type of heel cup is good for athletes who have been injured. A plastic heel cup fits snugly and does not allow the fat tissue to flatten, thus protecting the heel.

A heel pad is a soft cushion made of rubber, foam, or felt that is placed between the heel and the shoe. Heel pads are used to prevent bruises and to equalize the length of an athlete's legs if they are different. Unless it is being used to lengthen one leg, a pad should be used in each shoe.

What Would You Do If...

You are taping an athlete's ankle. Your nail scratches her shin, causing a minimal amount of bleeding. You notice that your nails are about .75 inch (2 cm) long. You just had an expensive manicure.

Arch supports are soft foam, rubber, or leather pieces. The foot flattens during every step, and an arch support keeps the foot from flattening too much. Most athletic shoes have built-in arch supports. The athlete must be sure to purchase a shoe with an arch support that fits her foot.

Ankle braces come in elastic, lace-up, and hinged versions. The elastic pull-on ankle brace provides support but only minimally; however, it does give the athlete an awareness of her ankle, thus possibly preventing an injury. The lace-up ankle brace is similar to a shoe without a toe (see figure 24.18). The

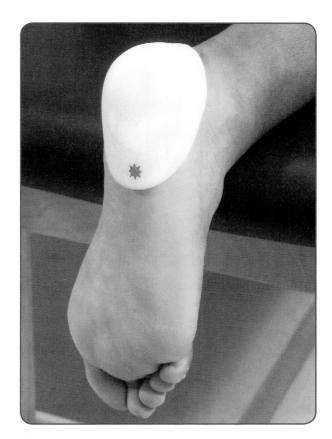

Figure 24.17 Heel cup.

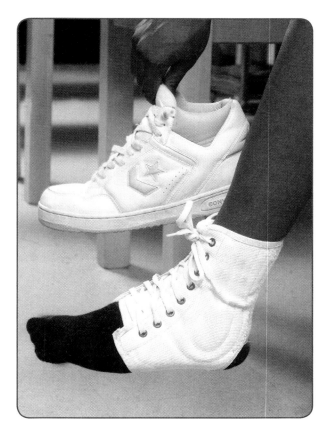

Figure 24.18 Ankle brace.

brace is laced up tightly, especially over the ankle, to limit movement. Some lace-up braces have pockets in which to insert plastic pieces that prevent inversion and eversion. In other lace-up braces, a figure-eight elastic strip can be pulled tightly around the ankle to prevent inversion or eversion.

ATs have become accustomed to designing special equipment to meet athletes' needs. In some cases foam and plastic pads provide needed protection, and other times taping and supportive wrapping will be the most effective. Padding and equipment are the first line of protection from impact.

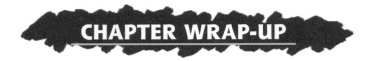

CHAPTER WRAP-UP

Summary

Equipment exists to protect athletes from injury when participating in athletic activity. Athletes must be educated about the purpose and use of equipment because, although no equipment will totally prevent injury, it can decrease the severity of injury. Properly fitted and certified equipment is essential—old or noncertified equipment should be discarded.

Key Terms

Define the following terms found in this chapter:

> Canadian Standards Association (CSA)
>
> National Operating Committee on Standards for Athletic Equipment (NOCSAE)

Questions for Review

1. What are the principles of padding and equipment?
2. How does equipment vary by position on a team?
3. What is the purpose of NOCSAE and the CSA?
4. What types of equipment are available to prevent head and facial injuries?
5. What equipment is recommended for arch pain?

Activities for Reinforcement

1. Assist the equipment manager in fitting football helmets and shoulder pads.
2. Have your AT bring in a variety of equipment for the class to inspect.
3. Work with a team dentist who is making fitted mouth guards.
4. Try on a full set of pads and equipment for a sport you do not play. What does it feel like? What limitations does the equipment impose?
5. Ask the AT to make a list of common injuries, and design a new pad to prevent one of the injuries.

Above and Beyond

1. If you could change the rules of a game, speculate what kinds of padding and equipment might be needed or eliminated as a result. An example might be playing football without tackling a person. Another example is a bike race with only three wheeled bikes.

2. Examine the information at the following Web sites and compare and contrast the helmets made by these companies:

    www.schuttsports.com/aspx/Sport/ProductListing.aspx?sp=3&id=89

    www.sportsdepot.com/footballhelmets.html

    www.riddell1.com/newsite/football.php

3. Visit the Consumer Products Safety Commission Web site and learn about bicycle helmet use: www.cpsc.gov/cpscpub/pubs/bike.html.

4. Examine one of the following articles and give a brief report.

    Caswell, S.V., and R.G. Deivert. 2002. Lacrosse helmet designs and the effects of impact forces. *Journal of Athletic Training* 37(2): 164-171.

    Chew, K., H. Lew, E. Date, and M. Fredericson. 2007. Current evidence and clinical applications of therapeutic knee braces. *American Journal of Physical Medicine and Rehabilitation* 86(8): 678-686.

    Knapik, J., S. Marshall, R. Lee, S. Darakjy, S. Jones, T. Mitchener, et al. 2007. Mouthguards in sport activities: history, physical properties and injury prevention effectiveness. *Sports Medicine* 37(2): 117-144.

    Miller, M., D. Berry, G. Gariepy, and J. Tittler. 2006. Attitudes of high school ice hockey players toward mouthguard usage. *Internet Journal of Allied Health Sciences and Practice* 4(4).

    Nicholls, R.L., B.C. Elliott, and K. Miller. 2004. Impact injuries in baseball: prevalence, aetiology and the role of equipment performance. *Sports Medicine* 34(1): 17-25.

    Rodriguez, J.O., A.M. Lavina, and A. Agarwal. 2003. Prevention and treatment of common eye injuries in sports. *American Family Physician* 67(7): 1433-1435, 1481-1488, 1494-1496.

    Ubell, M.L., J.P. Boylan, J.A. Ashton-Miller, and E.M. Wojtys. 2003. The effect of ankle braces on the prevention of dynamic forced ankle inversion. *American Journal of Sports Medicine* 31(6): 935-940.

5. Examine the NOCSAE Web site and learn about their recent activities: http://nocsae.org.

6. Read the following text and write a report on a piece of athletic equipment: Street, S.A., and D. Runkle. 2000. *Athletic protective equipment: care, selection, and fitting.* Boston: McGraw-Hill.

UNIT IX

Other Athletic Conditions and Concerns

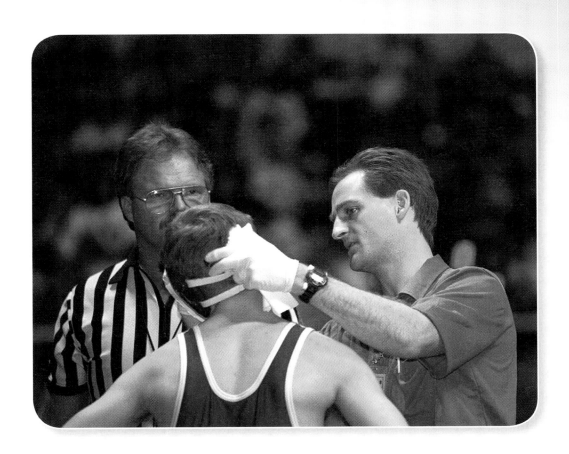

Conditions and Illnesses

Objectives

Upon completing this chapter, the student will be able to do the following:

- Describe conditions that cause illnesses.
- Understand how to prevent conditions and illnesses from occurring.
- Know that many of the signs and symptoms are similar among conditions.
- Describe various conditions that affect athletes.

An athlete may have a preexisting condition that can reduce the ability to perform normally. The AT and team physician will attempt to discover all such conditions during the preparticipation physical. Knowing of a condition and preparing to care for it before a crisis occurs can make everyone more comfortable, and some conditions require limited activity. In this chapter, we discuss conditions of the respiratory, circulatory, and gastrointestinal systems as well as diabetes, epilepsy, arthritis, and the female athlete triad.

RESPIRATORY CONDITIONS

Conditions of the respiratory tract generally affect the lungs. Any condition that reduces an athlete's ability to get air into the body will make it difficult to perform at a high level. The most common respiratory condition is asthma.

Bronchial **asthma** is a condition in which certain triggers may cause the sufferer's air passages (bronchial tubes) to narrow, which obstructs breathing. The triggers vary from person to person but include allergies, emotional distress, exercise, and body chemistry responses. In some cases there may be a genetic component. An athlete with bronchial asthma describes it as running the 100-yard (91 m) dash and then trying to catch her breath while breathing through a straw. Coughing that does not bring up phlegm is common. The athlete will wheeze on exhalation and will be in obvious respiratory distress. Asthmatic athletes will have medication, often in the form of an inhaler, to open the air passage; their use obviously should be permitted.

In 2005, NATA produced a position statement on the management of asthma in athletes (see the highlight box on this page. According to the position statement, many signs and symptoms may indicate asthma. The major signs and symptoms include the following:

- Tightness in the chest
- Coughing or wheezing, even if induced by exercise
- Shortness of breath, lack of full breath
- Diminished physical ability due to breathing difficulty
- History of family asthma

An asthma attack can be a scary experience for the athlete and the AT. The AT needs to remain calm because exciting the athlete will only make the asthma more uncontrollable. He should ask the athlete to relax and breathe in through the nose and out through the mouth. By concentrating on her breathing pattern, the athlete can focus on something constructive. The athlete will be more comfortable sitting up than lying down. If she is not getting better, the AT should call for an ambulance and get medical attention immediately. If the athlete stops breathing, the AT should attempt to perform mouth-to-mouth resuscitation, but he may not be successful because air cannot get to the lungs through the closed-off bronchial passages. An athlete who has had an asthma attack for the first time needs to be seen by a physician for evaluation.

Athletes who are known asthmatics are often required to give their inhalers to their coaches before practice so the medication is available. Athletes should provide these to the coach or AT to hold during practice or game. Athletes who fail to provide an inhaler that day are not allowed to practice. As a backup measure, some ATs carry the athlete's second rescue inhaler. An athlete should not use another athlete's medication because asthma medications vary. Each state and school district has rules about school personnel dispensing medication, so the AT should check the rules before handling someone else's medication.

The NATA position statement recommends checking the environment for allergens to prevent an asthma attack in athletes known to have asthma. These procedures can be done by accessing Web-based resources to check the pollen level in a specific geographical area.

Asthma in Athletes

The NATA position statement classifies the severity of asthma as follows:

Step 1: Mild intermittent—symptoms occur two or fewer times per week (with two or fewer nighttime symptoms per month), and the athlete has brief attacks lasting between a few hours to a few days.

Step 2: Mild persistent—symptoms occur more than two times per week but less than once per day, and an event may negatively affect physical activity level. Nighttime symptoms occur fewer than two times per month.

Step 3: Moderate persistent—symptoms occur daily, daily use of medication is needed, and an event will negatively affect physical activity level. Nighttime symptoms occur more than once per week.

Step 4: Severe persistent—Continual symptoms, frequent attacks, and limited physical ability occur; nighttime symptoms are frequent.

VASCULAR CONDITIONS

If there is a problem with the blood, heart, or blood vessels, an athlete can become ill. The AT should know about hypertension, hypotension, and anemia.

Hypertension

Hypertension is blood pressure above normal levels. (See chapter 20 for more information about blood pressure.) If blood pressure is taken on several occasions and the systolic pressure is above 140 mmHg at rest or the diastolic pressure is above 90 mmHg at rest, hypertension is present. Hypertension has several causes, including poor diet, stress, overexercising, and severe vascular damage, such as constriction, or narrowing, of the blood vessels as a result of disease. Hypertension can also cause vascular damage. Athletes with high blood pressure may report frequent headaches. They should be referred to a physician to determine the severity of the disease and treatment. Hypertension can usually be controlled with medication.

Hypotension

Hypotension is abnormally low blood pressure. Some medications cause hypotension, and an athlete taking such medications may pass out as blood pressure decreases. An athlete who has been bedridden may experience hypotension and may even pass out when she sits up or walks for the first time because her vascular system is no longer used to responding to changes in body position. After she moves around for a few days, the hypotension subsides. An athlete who is in shock or losing blood will also experience hypotension. It is important to know the cause of hypotension so it can be treated. To get the athlete's blood pressure back to normal, she may have to be treated for shock, bleeding may need to be stopped, or her medication may have to be changed.

Anemia

Anemia is the lack of red blood cells necessary to provide oxygen to the body tissues. Anemia occurs from blood loss, insufficient iron, improper functioning of cells, medication, or malfunction in the construction of cells. Anemia caused by surgery is corrected by blood transfusions. Menstrual anemia corrects itself in a couple of days.

Iron-Deficiency Anemia

Red blood cells must have iron to carry oxygen. When iron is insufficient, the condition is known as iron-deficiency anemia. The athlete may not be eating enough iron-rich foods to meet the average person's needs, or he may have an unusually high need for iron. This condition can be resolved by eating liver, beef, oysters, and iron-enriched cereals. An athlete with iron-deficiency anemia will have pale skin, fatigue, dizziness, decreased capillary refill, and tiredness. The signs and symptoms are not unlike the characteristics of cross country runners at the finish of a race. The best way to identify this type of anemia is through a blood test.

Sickle Cell Anemia

Sickle cell anemia is a chronic inherited disease. Although it is often thought of as an illness found in African Americans, it also occurs in people of other races; for example, people of Eastern European descent are also at high risk for sickle cell anemia.

The normal red blood cell is round and has a large surface area for carrying oxygen. The red blood cells of an athlete with sickle cell anemia look like sickles or crescents (see figure 25.1). The sickling of the cells causes them to hook onto the sides of the blood vessels, producing a logjam of cells in the capillaries. Also, the sickle cell is not capable of carrying as much oxygen as a normal red blood cell. The result is that oxygen is not carried efficiently to all parts of the body. The athlete with sickle cell anemia who is in crisis may have a blue skin tone, feel nauseated and weak, and have abdominal pain. Most often the athlete can be treated with high-flow oxygen from an oxygen tank; therefore, some ATs and team physicians have oxygen tanks available for the athlete. However, if signs of shock or respiratory distress are evident, the athlete should be transported to the emergency room. Athletes with sickle cell anemia have problems at high altitudes, and it may be best to restrict playing time or not allow the athlete to travel to these places. Preventing a sickle cell crisis includes taking in fluids, avoiding high altitudes (above 4,000 ft or 1,220 m), warming up well, and avoiding short bursts of activity.

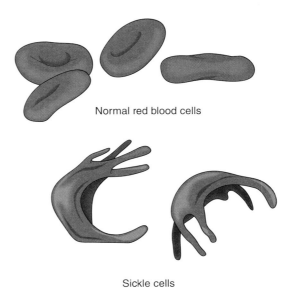

Normal red blood cells

Sickle cells

Figure 25.1 Normal red blood cells and sickle cells.

Hemophilia

Hemophilia is a blood disorder that delays blood clotting with consequent difficulty in controlling bleeding even after minor injuries. Hemophilia is a sex-linked inherited blood condition that is carried by females but occurs in males. An athlete with hemophilia may not be able to return to action after an injury, and bleeding may continue to the point that a blood transfusion is necessary. An athlete can be taught to self-administer shots to improve clotting time. Hemophilia cannot be cured, but it can be controlled. An athlete with hemophilia should play noncontact sports to help avoid unnecessary bleeding episodes.

GASTROINTESTINAL CONDITIONS

The gastrointestinal tract includes the organs that are involved in processing food, such as the stomach and large and small intestines. Here we discuss common conditions that affect the gastrointestinal tract.

Indigestion

When an athlete eats a food that the body has difficulty digesting, she has indigestion. The stomach has a high acid content to break down food. When acid levels are excessive, the acid may go up into the esophagus, causing a burning sensation called *heartburn*. The athlete may burp, have excessive gas, feel nauseated, and even vomit. She may experience pain around the heart that mimics the sensations of a heart attack. Serious cases of indigestion cause anxiety, sweating, pale skin, and nausea. Such cases must be referred to a physician. The athlete should avoid overeating and eating foods that cause

What Would You Do If...

A good friend of yours is dying to tell you a secret, and you promise not to tell anyone. He is trying out for the football team and has told only you that he is a hemophiliac.

indigestion. A physician can recommend over-the-counter medications to control the stomach acid. However, if used excessively, these medications may mask a more serious problem. If problems persist, a physician should be consulted to rule out a more serious condition such as ulcers.

Food Poisoning (Gastroenteritis)

Food poisoning is a common cause of diarrhea or upset stomach. Recently, there have been many incidents of poisoning from foods (including fruits, meats, dairy products, and vegetables) contaminated with *E. coli* (*Escherichia coli*). Preventing food poisoning requires careful food handling and preparation—washing hands and utensils, cooking foods thoroughly, and bleaching countertops, dishrags, and cutting surfaces. An athlete with food poisoning will complain of abdominal pain, tiredness, vomiting, nausea, diarrhea, and possibly a high temperature. The athlete should rest, drink plenty of fluids, and be referred to a physician.

Appendicitis

An athlete with appendicitis will feel pain over the right lower quadrant of the abdomen. Common signs and symptoms include diarrhea or constipation, nausea, vomiting, and increased temperature, all within a couple of hours. He will find that bringing the knees to the chest is the most comfortable position. The athlete needs to be referred to a physician for care because the appendix must often be surgically removed. He will be sidelined for at least four weeks. In severe cases the appendix can rupture and spread the infection throughout the abdominal cavity, which can result in death.

DIABETES

Diabetes occurs when the pancreas does not secrete insulin effectively or when the body is resistant to insulin. Insulin is a key hormone that is responsible for glucose (a form of sugar) entering cells and fueling them. An athlete with untreated diabetes may lose weight, become unusually thirsty, urinate more often, get tired faster than usual, and have a high level of sugar in the blood. After a diabetic athlete eats, her blood sugar level rises, and the pancreas releases insulin so that the body can control the blood sugar. If the blood sugar level gets too high, it is called **hyperglycemia**; if it gets too low, it is called **hypoglycemia**. If a diabetic athlete who uses insulin forgets to eat, her blood sugar level may fall below normal, causing her to pass out (figure 25.2). Something similar may happen due to exercise. An exercising athlete requires energy from the bloodstream (blood glycogen). If a diabetic athlete exercises excessively, she may use additional sugar for energy, and if she also takes insulin, this situation can cause dangerously low blood sugar levels. Many athletes can control their diabetes by eating foods that take time to digest, such as meats and vegetables. Avoiding sugary foods and drinks will also help prevent a diabetic emergency.

> ### Understanding Diversity

Haitians and Mexicans are more likely to suffer from diabetes.

Diabetes is divided into four forms, including type 1, type 2, gestational, and prediabetes. With type 1 diabetes, the body simply is unable to produce insulin. With type 2 diabetes, the body produces insulin but the cells are resistant to it and

> ### Understanding Diversity

Some American Indians have traditionally used blueberries to treat diabetes (Yehieli and Grey 2005).

---

fail to utilize it properly so that glucose gets into the cells. The majority of Americans diagnosed with diabetes have type 2.

Gestational diabetes occurs in pregnant women. People with prediabetes have high blood sugar levels but not so much that they are diagnosed with type 2 diabetes.

Insulin Shock

An athlete who needs injections of insulin to survive is insulin dependent. An insulin-dependent athlete usually takes insulin several times a day, especially near meals. Like anyone, an insulin-dependent athlete may not always eat regularly. If he takes insulin and then fails to eat, he may go into **insulin shock** because he gave himself medication to lower his blood sugar when it was not high. Insulin shock can also happen if he eats a food with a high sugar content that is absorbed before the insulin has returned to the standard level.

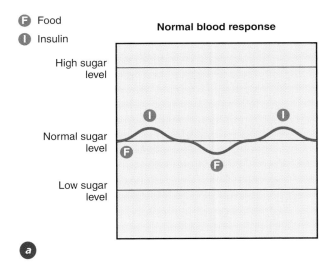
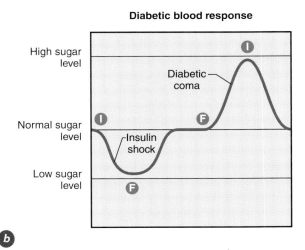

Figure 25.2 Insulin response. *(a)* An athlete with normal blood sugar response: The athlete eats food, insulin is released, and the blood sugar level returns to normal. *(b)* Insulin shock occurs in a diabetic when the blood sugar is very low. The athlete may have taken insulin but failed to eat enough food. A diabetic coma occurs when the blood sugar is very high. The athlete may have forgotten to take insulin just before or after eating.

Table 25.1 Comparisons Between Diabetic Coma and Insulin Shock

Diabetic coma	Insulin shock
Conscious but confused	Unconscious
No seizures	Seizures possible
Breath smells fruity	Breath smells normal
Low blood pressure	Normal blood pressure
Thirsty	Not thirsty
Rapid breathing	Normal breathing
Dry skin	Sweating
Possible fever	Normal body temperature
No body sensations	Tingling in hands and feet
Gradual onset	Rapid onset
Normal food intake	Little food intake
No headache	Headache
No response to food	Quick response to food

When insulin shock occurs, the athlete will feel lightheaded and weak and have an ashen skin tone and rapid pulse. In many cases the athlete will appear to be intoxicated. The AT should give the conscious athlete juice or candy so that the insulin will be temporarily counteracted, and then the athlete should consume a meal to level off the insulin. Table 25.1 presents the signs and symptoms of insulin shock and diabetic coma. If the athlete is unconscious, liquid glucose (sugar) can be placed under the tongue.

The AT should never place hard candy or food into the mouth of an unconscious athlete—this action may cause an airway obstruction. Whenever a diabetic athlete is unconscious, the AT should call EMS and get him to the nearest hospital. If the AT cannot remember the treatments for diabetic emergencies, she should give the athlete a sugar-based food—it will help the athlete in insulin shock, and it will not make a diabetic coma any worse

What Would You Do If...

A diabetic ice hockey player has forgotten to bring his juice box with him for a snack. He tells you he can get along without a snack this time.

Diabetes Care Plan

According to the NATA position statement for management of diabetes in athletes (Jimenez et al. 2007), each athlete should have a care plan that includes the following:

- Monitoring of blood sugar levels and identification of a level that would exclude the athlete from participation
- Documentation of the type of insulin the athlete uses and dosages and adjustments in the amount of insulin that may be necessary for planned activities, plus insulin dosages if the blood sugar level is found to be high
- Documentation of any other medications used to control blood sugar
- A guide for recognizing and treating hypoglycemia
- A guide for recognizing and treating hyperglycemia
- Documented emergency contact information for the athlete
- Use of a medical alert tag stating the athlete has diabetes

Adapted from: Jimenez, C.C. Corcoran, M.H., Crawley, J.T., Hornsby, W.G. Peer, K., Philbin, R.D. & Riddell, M.C. (2007). National Athletic Trainers' Association Position Statement: Management of the Athlete With Type 1 Diabetes Mellitus. *Journal of Athletic Training* 2007;42(4):536–545.

In 2007, NATA published a position statement for the management of athletes with type 2 diabetes (see the highlight box on the previous page). The position statement suggests that each athlete should have a diabetes care plan for all practices and games. Based on the content of this care plan, an AT must have a blood sugar monitoring kit available as well as the appropriate items to care for an athlete in the event of hyper- or hypoglycemia.

Diabetic Coma

A **diabetic coma** may occur when there is not enough insulin to control the amount of sugar in the blood. A diabetic coma may be preceded by an illness that alters the amount and availability of insulin. The coma comes on gradually with signs of vomiting and high temperature. The symptoms experienced by the athlete are thirst, abdominal pain, nausea, and confusion. The athlete approaching a coma will present labored breathing, sweet-smelling breath, and low blood pressure. A diabetic coma may be prevented by helping the athlete administer her insulin. Some athletes carry premade insulin shots, and if conscious they can inject themselves. Rush an unconscious athlete to a hospital emergency room.

The Real World

One afternoon, a student-athlete rushed into the training room shouting that a student had seriously injured herself while running in the hall. I grabbed my bag and ran from one end of the school to the other. Upon reaching the injured girl, I found her lying facedown and unconscious, with her glasses ajar. She was breathing and had a normal heartbeat. Saliva was dribbling from her mouth, but she had no visible wounds. No one could tell me what had happened, and no one knew her name. Furthermore, she was not wearing identification or medical alert tags. Other ATs who arrived on the scene performed a head-to-toe assessment and checked for a medical alert tag while I held her head to keep her neck in alignment. Because she was unconscious, we immediately called 911. She was eventually backboarded and taken to the hospital, still unconsciousness. Had she accidentally run into the wall and knocked herself out because she wasn't watching where she was going? Did she have a previous condition that caused her to faint? We had no idea. The mystery was solved when it was determined that she had experienced her first seizure.

Lorin Cartwright, MS, ATC

EPILEPSY

When the brain does not work properly, the entire body can malfunction. **Epilepsy** is the general term given to various disorders marked by disturbed electrical rhythms of the central nervous system.

The cause of epilepsy can be chemical, neurological (brain defect), infectious, or traumatic. A sign that an athlete has epilepsy can be a grand mal **seizure**—she may shake, drool, lose bladder control, or lose consciousness. The athlete who is about to have a grand mal seizure may hear a sound or see an aura, warning her to move to a safe area before the seizure begins. If the seizures are controlled by medication, exercising will not cause her to experience more problems. There is no reason to keep an athlete from participating because of epilepsy. Care for an athlete having a grand mal seizure includes moving items out of her way, loosening her clothing, padding her head, and allowing the seizure to end on its own. Because the tongue may fall back and block the airway, the athlete should be monitored for breath sounds. If an athlete experiences a first-time seizure, the AT should call EMS for immediate emergency care.

ARTHRITIS

Arthritis is the inflammation of a joint. In athletes, arthritis may result from an injury, repetitive trauma, or surgical intervention on a joint. Arthritis is a degeneration of the joint surfaces. Typical signs and symptoms are swelling, joint deformity, pain, grating during movement, and stiffness.

Gout is a form of arthritis that is inherited. It generally stays in one joint of the lower extremities. Uric acid buildup in the joint is the cause.

Rheumatoid arthritis may be found in some high school athletes. An overgrowth of the connective tissue occurs within a synovial joint. The extra tissue attaches to the articular surface of a joint, causing degradation of the joint surface. The most common joints for rheumatoid arthritis are in the feet and hands.

FEMALE ATHLETE TRIAD

Some athletes who are worried about how they look in a uniform may end up with an eating disorder as they try to attain a certain weight or to look a certain way. Eating disorders often appear in sports such as swimming, cross country, track, gymnastics, and wrestling. Officials who give scores based on a look, image, or smile push athletes in the wrong direction. Athletic associations and coaches could help by being more accepting of baggy shorts, shirts, or skirts—but do not count on that happening.

Disordered eating is an umbrella term that covers many problematic eating behaviors. Abnormal eating behaviors include **anorexia nervosa**, whereby an athlete restricts food intake, and **bulimia nervosa**, characterized by high caloric intake followed by self-induced vomiting. Both conditions are complex and need to be treated not only from a nutritional standpoint but also from psychological, sociological, and physiological standpoints. Anorexia and bulimia are most often thought of as eating disorders that occur chiefly in white females, but they also are common among males and athletes of color. Anorexia nervosa and bulimia have a death rate of 22%. The AT should check with the athlete's physician for advice on the athlete's ability to participate safely if he has an eating disorder. In 2008, NATA published a position statement for preventing, detecting, and managing disordered eating (see the highlight box on this page).

Disordered eating, amenorrhea, and osteoporosis are associated with one another: If an athlete restricts caloric intake and exercises heavily, her menstrual cycle may stop and her bone health will be compromised. These three conditions are collectively known as **female athlete triad syndrome**. This triad is common among female athletes who are driven or pressured to achieve high-level sport-related goals. Prevention of the triad is critical, and athletes, parents, coaches, and administrators should be educated about each of the three conditions as well as preventive strategies.

Amenorrhea is a condition whereby an athlete's menstrual cycle stops or an athlete fails to have a menstrual cycle by the age of 16. Some causes of amenorrhea are low body weight; endurance activi-

Preventing, Detecting, and Managing Disordered Eating

The 2008 NATA position statement written by Bonci and colleagues (2008) contains many recommendations as well as signs, symptoms, and screening materials for disordered eating.

Highlights of the recommendations include the following:

1. A multidisciplinary team of caregivers from medicine, psychology, nutrition, and counseling should be organized to intervene and care for a person with disordered eating. This health care team should create a protocol that identifies everyone's role. The group should work with legal counsel to make sure standards of care are followed.

2. The multidisciplinary team should create an educational program to inform athletes, coaches, administrators, and others about preventing disordered eating.

3. Detect disordered eating problems as early as possible by recognizing warning signs and symptoms.

4. Understand that the female athlete's menstrual cycle is sensitive to calorie restriction. When the menstrual cycle stops, efforts must be made to restore it to normal to prevent bone loss.

5. If disordered eating is suspected, an authority figure who has good rapport with the athlete should approach the athlete and express concern. This person should focus on specific behaviors of the athlete and be ready with a timely referral to a physician for an initial physical examination.

6. ATs must recognize that physician and psychotherapeutic intervention are needed along with a multidisciplinary team approach.

From: Bonci, C.M., Bonci, L.J., Granger, L.R., Johnson, C.L., Malina, R.M., Milne, L.W., Ryan, R.R., Vanderbunt, E.M., (2008). National Athletic Trainers' Association Position Statement: Preventing, Detecting, and Managing Disordered Eating in Athletes. Journal of Athletic Training, 43(1), 80–108.

ties such as distance running, cycling, or swimming; high stress levels; and disordered eating. **Dysmenorrhea** is a painful menstrual cycle. Both amenorrhea and dysmenorrhea can be caused by hormonal imbalances, among other things, and a full evaluation by a physician is warranted to rule out serious conditions. One key issue with both conditions is that the athlete's bone health can be compromised, leading to fractures and osteoporosis.

Osteoporosis is a loss of bone density. It occurs due to hormonal imbalances, poor or inadequate nutrition, and lack of exercise. Genetic factors also play a role in whether one is at risk of developing osteoporosis. A lack of bone density results in frailty and high risk of fractures. As you might imagine, if an athlete has an eating disorder, it can put her at risk for osteoporosis.

CHAPTER WRAP-UP

Summary

Certain medical conditions affect an athlete's ability to participate in sport. The AT must be prepared to respond to emergencies because an incorrect evaluation can result in serious consequences if the athlete has a condition such as appendicitis, asthma, or diabetes. Regular physical exams can help find certain conditions early. Conditions that are not preventable, such as asthma, diabetes, or epilepsy, may be controlled by medication and careful monitoring. The AT should know if an athlete is in a high-risk category for certain conditions so she can assist the athlete in taking preventive measures such as selecting the proper sport, using protective equipment, making sure medication is available, and knowing first aid.

Key Terms

Define the following terms found in this chapter:

amenorrhea	disordered eating	hypoglycemia
anemia	dysmenorrhea	hypotension
anorexia nervosa	epilepsy	insulin shock
asthma	female athlete triad syndrome	osteoporosis
bulimia nervosa	hemophilia	seizure
diabetes	hyperglycemia	sickle cell anemia
diabetic coma	hypertension	

Questions for Review

1. What is diabetes? How can it be treated?
2. What does an AT need to know to ensure safe participation of athletes with asthma?
3. What is the treatment for hypertension?
4. What is the difference between iron-deficiency anemia and sickle cell anemia?
5. In which sports should a hemophiliac participate?
6. What is the care for an athlete who is suffering an epileptic grand mal seizure?
7. What is the relationship between ammenhorrea and osteoporosis?
8. What pressures in athletics may push an athlete toward disordered eating patterns?

Activities for Reinforcement

1. Make a list of common signs and symptoms discussed in this chapter and indicate the conditions with which they are associated.
2. Invite someone with asthma, diabetes, or another condition to talk to the class about it.
3. Learn how to take someone's blood pressure.

Above and Beyond

1. Make a poster about one of the conditions discussed in this chapter; include causes, prevention, and treatment of the condition and who is most likely to have it. Display the poster in the classroom.
2. Visit the following Web site and click on Diseases and Conditions to learn more about selected conditions discussed in this text: www.intelihealth.com/IH/ihtIH/WSIHW000/408/408.html.
3. Examine one of the following articles and write a one-page report.

   McGavock, J.M., N.D. Eves, S. Mandic, and N.M. Glenn. 2004. The role of exercise in the treatment of cardiovascular disease associated with type 2 diabetes mellitus. *Sports Medicine* 34(1): 27-48.

   Mickleborough, T.D., and R.W. Gotshall. 2003. Dietary components with demonstrated effectiveness in decreasing the severity of exercise-induced asthma. *Sports Medicine* 33(9): 671-681.

   Niedfeldt, M.W. 2001. Managing hypertension in athletes and physically active patients. *American Family Physician* 66(3): 445-452, 457-458.

   Papanek, P.E. 2003. The female athlete triad: an emerging role for physical therapy. *Journal of Orthopaedic and Sports Physical Therapy* 33(10): 594-614.

   Stopka, C. 2003. Disability and special needs. Athletic therapy for athletes with disabilities, part 2: special conditions. *Athletic Therapy Today* 8(3): 23-25.

   Storms, W.W. 2003. Review of exercise-induced asthma. *Medicine and Science in Sports and Exercise* 35(9): 1464-1470.

   Vinci, D.M. 2002. Nutrition notes: athletes and type 1 diabetes mellitus. *Athletic Therapy Today* 7(6): 48-49.

4. Visit the CDC Web site (www.cdc.gov) for information related to the conditions and illnesses described in this chapter. Give a five-minute presentation to your peers.
5. Visit the Web site for the American Academy of Allergy, Asthma, and Immunology and access brochures related to allergens, pollen counts, and asthma: www.aaaai.org/nab/index.cfm.
6. Visit the Web site for the American Diabetes Association to learn more about the disease: www.diabetes.org.
7. Visit the Web site for the National Center for Physical Activity and Disability to learn more about disabilities and conditions: www.ncpad.org.
8. Visit the Web site of the National Osteoporosis Foundation and examine various brochures related to bone health: www.nof.org.
9. For a catalog listing free and low-cost government publications, write to the following address: Superintendent of Documents, U.S. Government Printing Office, 732 North Capitol Street, NW, Washington, DC 20401-0001 Or go to the web site: www.gpo.gov/.

chapter 26

Communicable Diseases

Objectives

Upon completing this chapter, the student will be able to do the following:

- Explain how contagious diseases affect athletic competition.
- Describe how to control and prevent contagious diseases.
- Describe the common signs and symptoms of contagious diseases.

Our environment contains microorganisms that cause infectious diseases. The immune system helps defend the body from foreign cells and substances, but when the immune system is low or the invader is strong, the body will become ill. Many of these illnesses can be transferred from one person to another through the air, bodily contact, using each other's personal items, or unsanitary conditions. The student assistant and AT will come in contact with illnesses on a daily basis. To help prevent the spread of communicable diseases, the AT (and students) can keep vaccinations current, clean the training room daily, avoid bodily fluids and sick athletes, use protective barriers, exercise, screen athletes during physical examinations, maintain healthy nutrition and hydration, and get enough sleep. In this chapter we discuss various communicable diseases.

DEFENDING AGAINST MICROORGANISMS

Microorganisms are the microscopic and submicroscopic bacteria and viruses that are everywhere in the environment, including on and in everyone's body. If the microorganism is one the body has never encountered before, it might create an infection.

Infectious microorganisms that manage to get into the body are attacked by the lymphocytes of the **immune system**. Lymphocytes are specialized leukocytes, the white blood cells that attack invaders.

When physicians draw blood, it is easy to check the number of leukocytes. Elevated numbers of leukocytes may mean the body is fighting an infection. Low numbers of leukocytes are an indication that the immune system is deficient and thus the athlete may be susceptible to infectious microorganisms.

Some microorganisms are effectively fought with **vaccinations**—preparations of tiny amounts of the microorganism (sometimes live and sometimes dead) that are injected into the body. Once the microorganism has entered, the body begins to fight and build immunity against it. There are vaccinations against many diseases, including the following: tetanus, measles, flu, hepatitis B, mumps, and polio. Viruses cause all of these diseases except tetanus, which is caused by bacteria.

Medical science has done an outstanding job of increasing public awareness of communicable diseases. People are more careful than they used to be around others who appear to be ill. People who are coughing and sneezing cover their mouths and wipe their noses. We can all do our part to prevent the spread of disease by getting vaccinations, washing our hands, using sterile techniques, and staying at home when early signs and symptoms of illness appear. Sharing food, water, or clothing should be avoided. Daily cleaning of clothing, training tables, and doorknobs will reduce the possibility of infection through contact with these items.

When the AT notices an athlete with cold and flu symptoms—sneezing; itchy, watery eyes; low-grade fever; runny nose; sore throat; headache; tiredness—or signs of a rash, the athlete should be referred immediately to a physician for care. Many of the early signs and symptoms of life-threatening illnesses mimic those of mild contagious illnesses. Neither the AT nor the athlete should risk spreading a contagious disease among teammates and classmates. There have been several outbreaks of measles (rubeola) among athletes when, unknowingly, an infected athlete was allowed to participate in a tournament—the illness can devastate every

What Would You Do If...

You notice that thirsty athletes are unwilling to wait in line while the water cooler distributes water slowly. The athletes take the lid off the cooler and dip their cups in, drink, and dip some more.

team attending. The physician should indicate when it is safe for the athlete to return to play.

Viral Diseases

Many viral illnesses are considered childhood diseases because they once caused misery and even death for millions of children. Though these diseases still thrive in many underdeveloped countries, most have become rare in the developed world because of childhood vaccination programs. They are occasionally seen even in the United States in both children and adults, however, and ATs and their assistants should be aware of them. Of the viral diseases listed next, aseptic meningitis and plantar warts are not childhood diseases.

Plantar Warts (Human Papillomavirus)

Plantar warts occur when human papillomavirus (HPV) enters a small cut or lesion in the skin. At the feet, this usually occurs at pressure areas such as the balls or the heel. Plantar warts are characterized by hard, slightly raised areas with brown or black pinpoint-sized dots. Plantar warts can be painful, especially as they enlarge. Athletes should see a dermatologist if the warts persist—they will likely need to be treated.

Chicken Pox (Varicella)

A virus causes **chicken pox**, which is characterized by a polka-dot body rash, a low-grade fever, tiredness, itching, and headache. The rash will leave small, craterlike scars if bumps are broken open. The athlete who gets this rash is able to spread it to others on the team through nose or mouth secretions and fluids from broken blisters. She needs to be referred to a physician for treatment. After about one week, when the athlete has dried scabs, she will be able to return to school and competition. A vaccination against chicken pox is now available.

Mumps

A virus causes **mumps**. The athlete will feel tired and have a headache. The distinguishing feature of mumps is swelling of the glands below and in front of the ear, which causes a fullness of the face and difficulty talking and swallowing. The swelling subsides in about a week. The athlete must be referred to a physician, who will recommend isolation, rest,

What Would You Do If...

The AT evaluates an athlete and is puzzled by the signs and symptoms of a rash. You recognize the signs and symptoms as being similar to those of measles, which you had as a child.

fluids, aspirin, and soft foods. Prevention includes vaccination or avoiding those who do not feel well or who are known to have the mumps.

Measles (Rubeola)

There are two types of measles: rubeola and rubella (German measles). Viruses cause both. **Rubeola** causes cold symptoms, with a cough and high temperature in the early stages. As the disease progresses, the body becomes covered with a rash, including inside the mouth. The athlete will be tired, his eyes will be sensitive to bright light, and he will have a headache. The AT should refer the athlete to a physician, who will treat the symptoms. Rubeola is prevented through vaccination.

German Measles (Rubella)

Rubella causes a rash that starts at the head and covers the body within a day's time. The rash will stay for about three days, but the athlete remains contagious for about five. She is treated for pain or itching. Rubella is prevented through vaccination.

Aseptic Meningitis

Aseptic meningitis is characterized by a viral inflammation of the coverings of the brain. The virus will cause the athlete to have flulike symptoms: headache, stiff neck, fever, and vision problems. If healthy, the athlete can survive, and the virus runs its course in about two weeks. Outbreaks of the virus have caused several athletes to be hospitalized, however, and some have even died from this virus.

Some ATs tolerate two practices that can contribute to aseptic meningitis—they allow players to dip cups into water coolers, and they allow players to touch their lips to cooler spigots. Prevention is simple—every player uses his own cup, no one dips a cup into the cooler, and no lips touch the

watercooler spigot. Water coolers and bottles must be cleaned after each use with a bleach solution.

Infectious Mononucleosis

Infectious mononucleosis is a viral infection that causes extreme fatigue, fever, body ache, and an enlarged spleen. The enlargement of the spleen means that athletes are at risk for splenic ruptures if they are allowed to participate with this condition. Also called *mono*, infectious mononucleosis is caused by the Epstein-Barr virus that is transmitted to others through saliva. For this reason, the disease is often referred to as the *kissing disease*. An athlete with mono must rest, and a physician must monitor her condition. The physician will allow the athlete to return to play as long as her spleen is a normal size, her signs and symptoms have resolved, and her liver function is normal.

Respiratory Conditions

The respiratory tract includes the nose, sinuses, trachea, bronchial tubes, and lungs, any of which can be affected by viruses or bacteria. Conditions of the respiratory tract include colds, sinusitis, pneumonia, influenza, asthma, and bronchitis.

Common Cold (Coryza)

The **common cold** is caused by a virus. Signs and symptoms of a cold include sore throat, coughing, sneezing, runny nose, loss of voice, and tiredness. To prevent a cold, athletes must maintain a good diet, wash their hands frequently, avoid others who have colds, avoid being in crowds, and avoid sharing cups. A viral illness can only be treated symptomatically, which means treating the signs and symptoms of the illness. An athlete with a sore throat or cough may use throat lozenges, and tissues should be used to cover coughs and dab runny noses. An athlete who is tired should rest. A rundown athlete who does not treat the cold may become more susceptible to other illnesses.

Understanding Diversity

According to Spector (2004), some Germans believe that wearing warm clothes and sleeping with the windows open will prevent illness.

Laryngitis

An inflammation of the larynx is called **laryngitis**. Laryngitis can be caused by an infection of the upper-respiratory tract or from talking too much or too loudly. The athlete with laryngitis will have a sore throat and no voice. The infection may also involve the rest of the body, so he may have a fever. Drinking water will help humidify the throat and keep the athlete more comfortable. He will need to refrain from talking until the infection subsides. He should treat the symptoms, but if he has a fever, a physician's services should be sought.

Bronchitis

Inflammation of the bronchial passages, called **bronchitis**, can be caused by an infection or an allergy. The athlete will have a fever, sore throat, tiredness, chills, a deep cough, and even wheezing. Bronchitis mimics colds, flu, and other respiratory conditions. It is best for the AT to refer athletes to a physician if they have persistent coughing and wheezing.

Flu (Influenza)

An athlete with **influenza** will report headaches, nausea, vomiting, dizziness, tiredness, stomach upset, chills, and possibly fever. The flu is communicable, and the sick athlete should stay away from her teammates. She is treated symptomatically and should get plenty of rest. Generally the team physician cannot do much to comfort the athlete once she has the flu. Some over-the-counter medications decrease nausea, headache, and body aches. The athlete can avoid getting the flu by getting a flu shot and avoiding those who are ill.

Skin Infections

The skin is a primary protector against disease—it keeps microorganisms from entering the body. It is critical to wash microorganisms off the skin to prevent the spread of disease (see the highlight box on the next page). Even so, some microorganisms directly infect the skin and then enter the body (see table 26.1). As another way of preventing the spread of skin infections, high school wrestling rules require that any wrestler with open sores be kept from wrestling. A physician's note indicating that the wrestler's rash is not communicable can permit participation, but the wrestling official can overrule the note.

Some skin rashes are the result of an invader that attacks the whole body, such as measles. In other cases the invader attacks a localized area of the skin. Some skin areas become irritated by padding or athletic equipment and then the infection occurs. It is important to recognize skin irritations early to prevent them from spreading to other athletes. A referral to a physician can keep a skin condition under control.

Acne

Acne is a skin condition that is common among adolescents. It involves clogging of the sebaceous glands at the site of hair follicles. The clogging can be the result of bacteria entering the pores of the skin and creating an infection. Acne is characterized by redness, swelling, and the formation of white pustules. Prevention often takes the form of cleansing the skin to prevent clogging of the pores. Referral to a dermatologist may be needed.

Table 26.1   Types of Skin Lesions

Type	Characteristics
Crusts	Dried accumulations of pus, often thought of as scabs. Often associated with impetigo and cold sores.
Pustules	Collections of pus from infection. Often associated with wounds, folliculitis, furuncles, and acne.
Ulcers	Open weeping wounds. Often associated with burns or trauma.
Vesicles	Collections of clear fluids under the skin. The vesicles may be singular or in bunches. The contagion is in the fluid, so breaking a vesicle causes the disease to spread. Some vesicles are of no consequence, such as a blister. When vesicles break they are prone to infection.

Hand Washing

1. If you will dry your hands on a paper towel, first unroll the towel from the dispenser without touching the paper towel.
2. Use the automatic liquid soap dispenser—if you do not have one, get one.
3. Turn on the water with your forearm.
4. Lather your hands and wrists, scrubbing under the fingernails and any jewelry.
5. Say your ABCs twice—this is a long enough scrubbing time.
6. Rinse your hands.
7. Tear off the paper towel and dry your hands.
8. Using the wet paper towel, dispense another clean paper towel.
9. Throw out the used wet towel.
10. Turn off the water with the paper towel.
11. Open the bathroom door with the same paper towel.
12. Discard the paper towel.

Blisters

Blisters are wounds that result from stress on the skin. They are commonly caused by friction and pressure on weight-bearing regions of the skin, such as the balls of the feet. When the skin is compressed and rubbed repeatedly, the layers of skin will begin pulling apart and swelling under the outer layer of skin will result. Prevention strategies include wearing two layers of socks and properly fitting footwear. Some athletes apply lubrication to their skin to reduce friction. Once a blister forms, it can be treated by padding around it to relieve pressure. If the blister breaks, the wound must be cleaned and a sterile dressing applied. Some ATs use a sterile needle to drain a large blister. After this draining, the area is cleaned with an antiseptic and dressed with antibacterial cream and a sterile dressing.

Folliculitis

Folliculitis is an inflammation of a hair follicle. The athlete will need antibiotics to cure the infection, which is caused by bacteria, but he can participate with proper covering of the follicles. Wet hot packs can open the follicle, which may look like a pus-filled sore, and help reduce the infection faster. African Americans and athletes who wear protective equipment such as shoulder pads are more prone to folliculitis. These athletes should wear an additional layer of lightweight clothing to help decrease the pressure on the follicles.

Boils (Furuncles)

Furuncles, or boils, are bacterial infections in skin glands. The boil will be bright red with a hard central core that is painful to the touch. The furuncle will give the appearance of a large pimple, and the athlete may want to squeeze it. Instead, he should apply warm packs several times a day to draw the infection outward. The AT must use caution to prevent the bacteria from getting on the hot packs; it is helpful to assign a towel to the infected athlete that is then sent to the wash daily. All parts of the body that have contact with protective equipment are prone to this infection, and it needs to be treated by a physician.

Athlete's Foot (Tinea Pedis)

Tinea pedis, commonly called *athlete's foot*, is caused by a fungal infection. Athlete's foot results in red, dry, scaly, itchy skin. Over-the-counter anti-fungal medication is often effective in resolving the condition. The athlete can help prevent tinea pedis by cleaning and drying her feet.

Ringworm (Tinea Corporis)

Tinea corporis, commonly called *ringworm*, is caused by a fungal infection. A red, scaly, ring-shaped abnormality appears on the skin. Anti-fungal creams are frequently prescribed to resolve the condition. This condition is commonly spread from contact with infected clothing, equipment, or another person's body.

Molluscum Contagiosum

Molluscum contagiosum is caused by a virus that raises pink lumps in the area of contact. A physician removes the lumps surgically and applies a medication. They usually heal without scarring.

Impetigo

Impetigo is caused by a staphylococcus or streptococcus infection. There will be clusters of blisters that break open and develop a crusted yellow

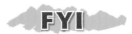

Cold Sore

A cold sore is a group of blisters around or in the mouth caused by the herpes simplex virus.

---

exterior. The athlete will need antibiotics to stop the spread of impetigo. Washing playing surfaces and not sharing towels or clothing will help prevent the spread of impetigo.

Herpes

Herpes simplex is a virus that causes an infection of the skin or mucus membranes. Herpes simplex is categorized as type 1 or type 2. The virus stays in the body, and when the immune system weakens, a cold sore can appear. The athlete needs to get enough sleep, good nutrition, and exercise.

Signs of **herpes** include a weeping open blister with a red base and a yellow crust, swollen glands, and possibly a fever. Herpes simplex is spread by skin-to-skin contact. In sports characterized by considerable contact, such as wrestling and rugby, herpes simplex can spread rapidly. This is often referred to as *herpes gladiatorum*. Prevention involves showering after practice; covering all open wounds; excusing athletes with open wounds from practice; making sure that athletes do not share towels, toothbrushes, or clothes; and washing mats before and after each use with a bleach and water solution or commercial product. Herpes runs its course in about two weeks. Three things will help a person who is subject to cold sores: eating properly (well-balanced meals), getting enough rest, and, most important, managing stress.

BLOODBORNE CONDITIONS

Two contagious bloodborne diseases are HIV and hepatitis B. These diseases are transmitted especially by contact with infected blood. Say a trainer treating an athlete's bleeding wound gets blood in a cut on her hand. Microorganisms in the blood can easily enter the cut. Needles or razors shared by more than one athlete may also transfer blood

from one person to another. The best way to prevent transmittal is to place a barrier between the infected athlete and others. The universal precautions discussed in chapter 20 should be employed in these situations.

Hepatitis B

Hepatitis B virus (HBV) causes an infection of the liver. The virus tends to persist in the blood of the infected athlete and can be transmitted by contact with infected blood, including dried blood. Those who are infected with HBV have it for life and are more prone to cirrhosis (liver disease)—they may feel tired and nauseated and experience a lack of appetite. Some infected people may be carriers of the disease but are not themselves ill. The signs and symptoms of hepatitis B are not unlike those of a cold or flu. The athlete will have signs of jaundice—yellowing of the skin and sclera. He needs immediate medical attention to control the damage from hepatitis B. It is possible that he will have chronic problems and may even die. The good news is that hepatitis B is preventable through a series of shots. Because ATs and student assistants are in contact with blood on a regular basis, they should consider receiving the shots. Exposure to this condition can be limited by observing universal precautions (see chapter 20).

HIV and AIDS

HIV (human immunodeficiency virus) causes a disorder of the immune system and is acquired through the transfer of bodily fluids: Blood, semen, vaginal secretions, and breast milk can all transfer the virus to another person. Transmittal of HIV through saliva and tears is highly unlikely since it

What Would You Do If...

While cleaning up after an athlete who was bleeding profusely, you notice a drop of blood on a recent abrasion on your forearm. You know the athlete and trust that she does not have any communicable diseases.

takes about 1 gallon (4 L) of saliva or tears to transfer enough of the virus to infect someone.

Because an infected athlete's immune system is suppressed, the AT may notice that contusions or sores take longer to heal than normal. The athlete will lose weight, have a sore throat, and become tired. A series of blood tests over a six-month period will confirm HIV. The physician will prescribe medication to boost the athlete's immune system and reduce her susceptibility to infections.

There has been dramatic progress in increasing the strength of the infected person's immune system.

AIDS (acquired immunodeficiency syndrome) is a disease caused by infection with HIV. The drug AZT inhibits replication of the virus and is used to slow the progress of AIDS. The athlete will report fatigue, night sweating, sores that will not heal, coughing, and diarrhea. The disease is fatal, so the best thing to do is to prevent it. For the AT, this means using the universal precautions outlined in chapter 20.

The Real World

As a second-year AT intern, I ventured to New Zealand for a year of studying abroad. I found a position working as a physio (a name used outside of the United States that is often synonymous with *AT*) for a men's semiprofessional rugby team. At the first game I was getting an idea about the rules of the game from the equipment manager. At halftime I grabbed my kit to meet with the team. The equipment manager grabbed a bucket of water with a few sponges soaking in it. I worked my way around the team, checking on all the wounded. I watched as a player removed a sponge and placed it on his sweaty head, wringing water on himself. He threw the sponge back in the bucket. Next, a player picked up a sponge, wiped some blood off his leg, and threw the sponge back in the bucket. Finally, a player rinsed his mouth guard in the bucket.

Being the outspoken American that I am, I asked the equipment manager, "Have you ever heard of bloodborne pathogens?" He responded, "Oh, we don't have those here."

After speaking to a few members of the sports medicine community, I learned that it was taking time to institute a commitment to hygiene in the rugby community. My job as the team physio was to expedite the sanitation and hygiene process with my rugby club. The coach, manager, equipment manager, and I got together to discuss changes that would be necessary to control disease. I left the team after the season knowing that their risk of disease and infection had been reduced.

Tracey Gropper, ATC

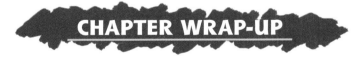

CHAPTER WRAP-UP

Summary

Microorganisms may cause an illness when a person's immune system is low. Ideally, those who are ill will stay at home to avoid infecting others. Maintaining a healthy lifestyle will keep the immune system high and keep the microorganisms at a distance. Avoiding contact with bodily fluids and using universal precautions will also prevent the transfer of some diseases. Athletic competition places athletes in close proximity and thus more at risk for contacting communicable diseases. Rules now force the removal of a bleeding athlete from a game to protect other competitors. Signs and symptoms of many communicable diseases are the same. The only way to diagnose the offending microorganism is to be seen by a physician. Because athletes hide their illnesses, and many illnesses mimic each other, it is critical that the members of the athletic training team have up-to-date immunizations.

Key Terms

Define the following terms found in this chapter:

acne

aseptic meningitis

blisters

bronchitis

chicken pox (varicella)

common cold (coryza)

folliculitis

furuncles

hepatitis B virus (HBV)

herpes

human immunodeficiency
  virus (HIV)

immune system

impetigo

infectious mononucleosis

influenza

laryngitis

microorganisms

molluscum contagiosum

mumps

plantar warts

rubella

rubeola

tinea corporis

tinea pedis

vaccinations

Questions for Review

1. How can student assistants protect themselves from getting a communicable disease?
2. How are communicable diseases transmitted?
3. What is the general treatment for communicable diseases?
4. How can communicable diseases be distinguished from one another?
5. What sport rules were designed to prevent the spread of communicable diseases?
6. Why does the AT recommend seeing a physician for communicable diseases that seem to be mild?

Activities for Reinforcement

1. Investigate how vaccinations work.
2. Make a list of the signs and symptoms of each communicable disease discussed in the chapter.
3. Make a list of the ways to prevent each contagious disease.
4. Practice proper hand washing in public places.
5. Develop a presentation about the importance of hand washing and, with the direction of your AT, present it to various groups such as elementary classes or Boys and Girls Clubs.
6. Volunteer your time at a walk-in clinic. What communicable diseases are commonly seen at this clinic? Investigate whether the communicable disease rate changes depending on the type and location of the clinic or the economic status of the community.
7. Design a plan for cleaning the training room daily. What types of solutions and protective attire should be worn while cleaning?
8. Visit the CDC Web site and learn more about the forms of hepatitis: www.cdc.gov/hepatitis/.
9. Visit the Web site of the Ohio High School Athletic Association (OHSAA) to learn more about its policy for preventing the spread of communicable diseases: www.ohsaa.org/medicine/disease.htm.
10. Visit KidsHealth.org to learn more about bronchitis: http://kidshealth.org/parent/infections/bacterial_viral/bronchiolitis.html.
11. Examine the position statement for controlling herpes gladiatorum from the NFHS Sports Medicine Advisory Committee: www.nsaahome.org/textfile/spmeds/Herpes.pdf.
12. Visit the Web site of the National Institutes of Health and learn more about various skin conditions: http://health.nih.gov/category/SkinHairandNails.

Above and Beyond

Read one of the following articles and present a summary of the information to your classmates.

Adams, B.B. 2002. Dermatologic disorders of the athlete. *Sports Medicine* 32(5): 309-321.

Bechtel, M., A. Bechtel, and M. Zirwas. 2009. Skin infections in wrestlers and other athletes. *Emergency Medicine* 41(1): 25-29.

Dougherty, T.M. 2003. Physician perspective. Sports dermatology: what certified athletic trainers and therapists need to know. *Athletic Therapy Today* 8(3): 46-48.

Luke, A., and P. d'Hemecourt. 2007. Prevention of infectious diseases in athletes. *Clinical in Sports Medicine* 26(3): 321-344.

Midgley, A.W., L.R. McNaughton, and M. Sleap. 2003. Infection and the elite athlete: a review. *Research in Sports Medicine* 11(4): 235-259.

Velasquez, B.J. 2002. When is a skin rash more than just a rash? Sexually transmitted diseases: a dermatological perspective. *Athletic Therapy Today* 7(3): 16-23, 38-39, 64.

Weber, T.S. 2003. Environmental and infectious conditions in sports. *Clinics in Sports Medicine* 22(1): 181-196.

Winokur, R., and W. Dexter. 2004. Fungal infections and parasitic infestations in sports: expedient identification and treatment. *Physician and Sportsmedicine* 32(10): 23.

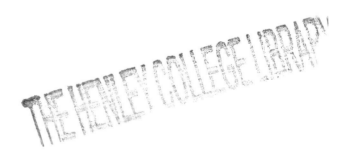

chapter 27

Common Drugs Used in Athletics

Objectives

Upon completing this chapter, the student will be able to do the following:

- Understand the difference between therapeutic and recreational drugs.
- Know the medications commonly used for various conditions.
- Have a basic knowledge of how medications work.
- Understand why athletes use substances to improve their performance.
- Understand the signs and symptoms of substance abuse.
- Have a basic knowledge of performance-enhancing aids commonly used in athletics.
- Define *addiction*.

Drugs have long been thought capable of giving athletes a competitive advantage. When certain drugs were found to give an advantage, the governing bodies of athletics banned their use. In this chapter we discuss drugs that enhance or are perceived to enhance athletic performance.

A **drug** is any substance other than food or water that changes the body's chemistry when it is either ingested or applied topically. Athletes use drugs for therapeutic purposes, performance improvement, and recreation.

THERAPEUTIC DRUGS

Therapeutic drugs have a medical purpose. They are often prescribed or recommended by the team physician. A therapeutic drug is used to treat a disease, an infection, or a disorder such as diabetes and is used to relieve pain or swelling and the like.

Nonsteroidal Anti-Inflammatory Drugs

Nonsteroidal anti-inflammatory drugs (NSAIDs) reduce the amount of tissue swelling after an injury.

They include aspirin and ibuprofen, which are over-the-counter drugs, meaning they can be legally purchased without a prescription.

After an injury, aspirin can be used to reduce pain. Aspirin is a blood thinner and can cause more swelling in an area initially. An athlete who is anemic may want to avoid aspirin because of its blood-thinning ability; it will be counterproductive to resolving the anemia.

Ibuprofen reduces pain and swelling, and it is commonly used for strains and sprains. In large amounts it often causes an upset stomach and, therefore, should be taken with food. Regularly taking ibuprofen in large doses can cause liver and kidney damage.

Local Steroids

A **local steroid** is applied to the skin or injected in a joint to reduce swelling and pain; it should not be confused with anabolic steroids. Local steroids are used mainly for allergies, skin disorders, or joint pain. Injected local steroids can weaken tendons. The team physician prescribes them and will also monitor their use.

Beta-Adrenergic Drugs

Beta-adrenergic drugs maintain the airway during an asthma attack by controlling the release of chemicals. These medications are available by prescription only and can be administered via injections, inhalation, or pills. It is common to see athletes with inhalers. However, sometimes athletes are not allowed to use the inhaler during competition. Of course if the athlete needs the inhaler to save her life, she must use it regardless of the activity. The rules regarding use of medication change constantly. The AT should check the rules of each sport annually to determine which drugs are acceptable.

Antibiotics

A physician prescribes antibiotics for bacterial infections. There are many antibiotics, the most famous of which is penicillin and its derivatives. The drug

Understanding Diversity

Many cultures use acupuncture to help relieve pain. Acupuncture originated in China and involves the insertion of thin needles in specific areas of the body to illicit a physical response.

What Would You Do If...

Before the start of every hockey game, the players have a ritual of inhaling from ammonia capsules. They say it makes them more aware of what's going on in the game.

enters the bloodstream and assists white blood cells. Using an antibiotic improperly can cause bacteria to change and become resistant to the drug; thus, the drug must be taken as prescribed and until it is gone so that the infection will not flare up again. When bacteria become resistant to antibiotics, the infection can take over.

RECREATIONAL DRUGS

Drugs that have no medical purpose are called **recreational drugs**. Many recreational drugs such as alcohol and tobacco are legal for some age groups and illegal for others. Other recreational drugs, such as cocaine, are illegal for everyone. Use of illegal drugs can present at least three major problems:

1. Negative side effects ranging from lack of motivation to death
2. Unknown impurities in the drugs, which result from the lack of legal control over their manufacture and sales and can have unexpected side effects, including death
3. Involvement with criminal elements, which can result in legal and personal problems

Caffeine

Caffeine is a drug found in coffee, tea, and chocolate as well as in some brands of aspirin, cold medications, weight-loss products, and soda. Caffeine is a stimulant, meaning it increases heart and breathing rates. It is also a diuretic, meaning it flushes fluids from the body. But recently it has been found that acute intake of medium to low levels of caffeine does not dehydrate the body (Armstrong, Casa, Maresh and Ganio 2007). Athletes in endurance events such as marathons have used caffeine because they thought it would improve their endurance; however, you can't take bathroom breaks when you're running a marathon, so most runners avoid its use.

The amount of caffeine in products varies. Some athletes may have difficulty sleeping after ingesting caffeine. An athlete with a headache may take an aspirin to help the pain without checking to see if it contains caffeine and then lie awake all night. Athletes who become addicted to caffeine may have headaches, nausea, and tiredness when they go through withdrawal.

Tobacco

Tobacco may be used in two forms: smoked and smokeless. Tobacco is smoked in cigarettes, cigars, or pipes. It is well known that cigarette smoking is highly addictive. It lowers stamina, and it has many negative long-term side effects. It greatly increases a person's chances of developing lung cancer, heart disease, emphysema and other breathing disorders, and blindness from macular degeneration. Some people are under the impression that cigar and pipe smoking are not as damaging as cigarettes, but this idea is incorrect.

Smokeless tobacco—snuff or chewing tobacco—is placed against the gums, and nicotine is absorbed into the bloodstream. Athletes use this form of tobacco because they have seen professional athletes use it, especially baseball players. Nicotine increases heart and breathing rates. All forms of smokeless tobacco contain cancer-causing substances.

Smokeless tobacco is regulated by the laws applying to all tobacco, so sale to a minor is illegal. High school and college association regulations state that smokeless tobacco is not to be used. In the professional ranks, use of smokeless tobacco is currently not regulated.

People who use smokeless tobacco can develop precancerous cells of the cheek, tongue, and gum within two years of use. These cells, called **leukoplakia**, develop quickly because of the frequency with which the smokeless tobacco is held in the

What Would You Do If...

A baseball player pulls back his lip and asks you what the blisters on the inside of his cheek and gum indicate. He reveals that he chews tobacco when his family is not around.

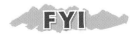

Emphysema

Emphysema is an incurable lung disease characterized by the inability to breathe deeply. It is progressive and will eventually destroy the sufferer's ability to take in enough oxygen to sustain life.

cheek. The precancerous cells are white and some have blisters. If a cancerous growth occurs, surgery may involve removal of the jaw and possibly the tongue. If the cancer has spread throughout the body and the warning signs are overlooked, the athlete may die. In addition, smokeless tobacco can cause serious dental complications—gum disease, bad breath, and cavities are more common among smokeless tobacco users than among others.

Tobacco candy, or tobacco mints, another form of smokeless tobacco, has become a popular way to obtain nicotine. This type of smokeless tobacco takes the form of dissolvable strips or pellets that are flavored and packaged to look like candy. Unfortunately, this form of tobacco has been linked to accidental tobacco ingestion in children (Aleccia 2010).

Alcohol

Alcohol is produced by fermentation, which occurs when yeast breaks down the carbohydrate in grains or fruits. Alcohol is consumed as beer, wine, and hard liquor.

The alcohol content in a can of beer, a glass of wine, and a shot of hard liquor—all of which are considered one drink—is roughly equivalent. The difference in the volume is the amount of water present with the alcohol. Beer has the most water, and liquor has the least.

Alcohol causes the heart rate, breathing rate, and reaction time to slow; thus, it is a depressant. The slowing of bodily processes is not what an athlete needs during competition—imagine the runner who runs slower, loses balance, loses concentration, and forgets what she is doing. Alcohol also slows reaction time, which makes it unsafe for the drinker to drive. The body treats alcohol as a poison, and it is sent to the liver for detoxification. It takes about an hour and 20 minutes for the liver to detoxify one drink. If the body cannot remove the alcohol fast enough, the person will become

Understanding Diversity

Alcohol is metabolized more slowly in people of Vietnamese descent (Purnell and Paulanka 2005).

intoxicated and perhaps vomit the poison from the body. If the drinking continues, the person may lose consciousness, go into a coma, or die. Loss of consciousness occurs when the blood alcohol content is .4%, and death occurs shortly thereafter.

Those who use alcohol persistently and excessively are prone to liver disorders, nutrition problems, illnesses, brain disorders, stomach ulcers, and early death. Some studies have indicated that red wine used in moderation is helpful in the prevention of heart disease. However, before anyone decides to start drinking based on those studies, he needs to give careful consideration to his overall health. No one should drink when harm could come to oneself or someone else.

Cocaine

Cocaine is a white powder that can be inhaled to give the user a feeling of euphoria, or a feeling of well-being. The euphoric effects are short in duration. The more cocaine one uses, the more cocaine is required to achieve euphoria. Athletes will be restless after use.

Side effects of cocaine use include death from heart problems, suppression of the immune system, poor nutrition, loss of money, and cocaine bugs—the hallucination that insects are crawling under the skin. There are no benefits to be derived from the use of cocaine.

What Would You Do If...

The golf team has just won the state title. You are invited to a party at a local hotel. At the hotel the entire team is drinking and smoking cigars. Your ride home stumbles up to you and says it's time to go.

MDMA

MDMA is short for methylenedioxymethamphetamine and it goes by the slang term *ecstasy*. This drug can enhance sensory perception, mental stimulation, and physical energy. It is addictive for some people and can cause muscle cramping, blurred vision, nausea, and chills (www.drugabuse.gov/drugpages/mdma.html).

PERFORMANCE-ENHANCING DRUGS

A performance-enhancing drug is one that an athlete believes will make her play better. An athlete may choose to use alcohol to calm down before a game. Some athletes may use cocaine to get fired up. Other athletes use steroids to increase muscle bulk. Regardless of the drug used to improve performance, its use is illegal, and most often it does not work and may even cause death.

DMSO

After research on animals showed that **dimethyl sulfoxide (DMSO)** decreased healing time and wound swelling, veterinarians began using DMSO as an anti-inflammatory agent. Some athletes have considered using DMSO to speed their return to participation after an injury. The DMSO is absorbed quickly through the skin and leaves a garlic taste in the mouth. It has never been approved for human use, but athletes have found ways of obtaining it. There are no human studies showing that DMSO actually works, and the long-term side effects are unknown.

Ephedra

Ephedra was used for quite some time as a weight-loss drug. In sports where thinness and body weight needed to be controlled, it was sometimes used by athletes. Ephedra can cause health problems such as high blood pressure, heart attack, and strokes, and in 2004 the Food and Drug Administration (FDA) banned the sale of supplements containing the drug.

Blood Doping

An athlete participating in an endurance event can benefit from having extra oxygen-carrying blood cells, and the more red blood cells he has, the better his oxygen-carrying ability. On the basis of that theory, an athlete may have his blood drawn and stored while his body replaces the lost blood cells. He then injects the stored blood just before the event so that he has more red blood cells than usual. However, placing additional blood into an athlete's system can result in shock.

Anabolic Steroids

Anabolic steroids are hormones such as testosterone, the male hormone that is responsible for creating and maintaining male secondary sex characteristics. Physicians prescribe anabolic steroids to treat asthma, severe muscle injuries, and arthritis. Steroids have been used to combat the side effects of cancer, which may cause the whole body to atrophy. Athletes use anabolic steroids for the purpose of building muscle.

Androstenedione, often referred to as *andro*, is a steroid hormone that is used by some athletes looking for a competitive edge. Androstenedione increases testosterone production in men over a short time frame, usually an 8-hour period.

When athletes discovered that greater muscle mass could be obtained artificially, they began taking steroids to increase strength. Steroids are injected and ingested by a method called *stacking*, which means the athlete uses a combination of pills and injections to try to avoid the side effects caused by taking a single high dose all at once. However, side effects cannot be avoided. A male using anabolic steroids will experience the following side effects: acne, decreased testicular output, heart problems, cancer, addiction, enlarged breast tissue, mental illness, hair loss, weakened ligaments, decreased growth, violent behavior ('roid rage), vascular problems, and impotence. In females who use anabolic steroids, side effects include deepening of the voice, addiction, cessation of the menstrual cycle, increased body and facial hair, and decreased body fat—they are turning themselves into males without changing their anatomy.

Use of steroids is illegal in all competitions, including professional and Olympic competitions. Gold medals have been taken away from athletes who have used steroids. Asthmatics are allowed to

What Would You Do If...

Just before the start of an all-day wrestling tournament, a wrestler shows you the latest rage from the health food store. He drinks the green frothy substance before you have a chance to ask him what it is.

use their inhalers, but drug-testing boards regulate the amount of steroids allowed.

Human growth hormone (HGH) is a protein-based hormone used by some athletes to facilitate muscle growth. HGH is sometimes prescribed by physicians when a child has a growth disorder. Sport organizations have banned HGH.

Gamma hydroxybutyrate (GHB) is often referred to as a *club drug* because it is a central nervous system depressant. When used with alcohol, it can incapacitate victims and prevent them from resisting sexual assault. There are also anabolic effects associated with GHB because it can help synthesize protein and thus facilitate muscle building. A side effect of GHB use is seizure or coma (www.drugabuse.gov/Infofacts/clubdrugs. html).

DRUG ABUSE

It is well known that people are living longer, partly because of the medications available to us. Unfortunately, many have the false notion that medications can solve any problem. Physicians are prescribing more medications, and recreational drugs are readily available. Some athletes choose to use drugs because they think their athletic performance will improve. Students pressure other students to use so they are not alone, and many students and athletes see professionals or their parents using drugs and copy that behavior. Athletes who use drugs may appear to enjoy themselves and seem more relaxed because the drugs reduce inhibitions. Ultimately, however, teenagers who use drugs can develop long-term health problems. Remember, there are more students and athletes who choose not to use drugs and for better reasons than those who choose to use.

DRUG TESTING

Few high schools test for drugs, but drug testing is becoming common in professional, international, and college settings. In school settings, a panel of drugs is often investigated. A panel can consist of tests for marijuana, cocaine, opioids, amphetamines, and PCP. Other drugs can also be screened. For example, many schools also screen athletes for MDMA, GHB, or steroids.

To test for illegal drugs, a urine sample is collected. After competition, the winning athlete is tested along with other competitors who are selected at random. To ensure that the sample is from the athlete, not someone else, the athlete must give the sample in a secured room while a drug-testing supervisor watches. The sample is sealed, signed by the athlete, and sent for testing to determine if the types of drugs used by the athlete are illegal. If a sample is found to have illegal substances, the results are given to the drug-testing governing board. The board determines the penalty for the illegal drug use. In some instances the penalty means the athlete will be banned from competition for a certain amount of time, and in others it means the athlete will lose medals. Questions about drugs and their use in athletics can be answered by the United States Olympic Committee using the toll-free hotline at 800-233-0393.

For high school athletics, the banned drugs may differ, but prohibition tends to revolve around the following classifications:

1. Stimulants—used to heighten alertness and enhance reaction time
2. Anabolic agents (anabolic steroids)—used to build muscle
3. Diuretics—used to excrete fluids to lose weight
4. Peptide hormones—used to gain strength and build muscle

These drug classifications are banned because they give one athlete an unfair advantage over another or because negative health-related side effects. Usually they are banned for both of these reasons.

The Real World

I was working with an impressionable athlete who made a habit of jumping from fad to fad looking for the most up-to-date methods for improving his fitness. He indicated that he had constant diarrhea but could not pinpoint a reason. I had him write down everything that he ate and all the supplements that he took. I compared all the foods and supplements and found that he was overdosing on vitamin C. Once he stopped taking large doses, his diarrhea went away. I recommended that he see a dietitian to help him develop a proper diet, but unfortunately, he did not heed my advice. He decided to simply try another new dietary fad.

Anonymous

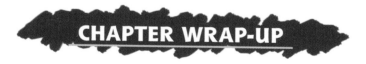

CHAPTER WRAP-UP

Summary

Athletes use drugs, which may be therapeutic or recreational, for a variety of reasons. Therapeutic drugs are used to assist an athlete returning from an injury or recovering from an illness or to prevent illness during competition. Over-the-counter drugs can be purchased to treat problems such as headaches and colds. Recreational drugs have no real value—they are used during social occasions and for the feelings they create.

Some athletes believe that a drug will improve their performance only to find out that the improvement is a myth. Caffeine, anabolic steroids, and oxygen are commonly used as performance-enhancing substances. Athletes who use performance-enhancing drugs may see an improvement in their performance, but the side effects and long-term problems outweigh any benefits.

The side effects of all drugs must be considered. The team physician should be consulted to determine proper use and dosage of a drug. Drugs can become habit forming, and addiction can be dealt with through various programs depending on the type of drug involved. Drug testing is commonplace among elite athletes. Olympic and international competitors are tested for banned drugs on a regular basis.

Key Terms

Define the following terms found in this chapter:

anabolic steroids	human growth hormone (HGH)
androstenedione	leukoplakia
beta-adrenergic drugs	local steroid
dimethyl sulfoxide (DMSO)	nonsteroidal anti-inflammatory drug (NSAID)
drug	recreational drugs
ephedra	therapeutic drugs
gamma hydroxybutyrate (GHB)	

Questions for Review

1. Describe the difference between therapeutic and recreational drugs.
2. What are the reasons why athletes use various drugs?
3. What are the myths behind the use of recreational drugs in athletics versus the reality?
4. Why is drug testing done?

Activities for Reinforcement

1. List the types of helpful drugs and their common uses in athletics.
2. Write to the Olympic training center and get a copy of the list of banned drugs.

   Olympic Training Center
   1750 E. Boulder St
   Colorado Springs, CO 80909

3. Visit a substance-abuse center and determine which drugs substance abusers were most likely to use when first starting to experiment with drugs.
4. Make a list of positive reasons why athletes choose not to use drugs.
5. Go online to review the NCAA list of banned substances:
   http://grfx.cstv.com/photos/schools/domi/genrel/auto_pdf/ncaa-banned-substance-list.pdf.
6. Visit the NCAA Web site and explore its drug-testing protocol:
   www.ncaapublications.com/productdownloads/DT11.pdf.

Above and Beyond

1. Attend an open meeting on substance abuse, and write a report describing various experiences people have had with drugs. Discuss why some people choose not to use drugs and why people have stopped using.

2. Interview a local dentist concerning the long-term effects of chewing tobacco and give a presentation to your peers.

3. Obtain brochures from the following web addresses. Design your own brochure, website or podcast on one of the drugs discussed in this chapter.

   http://ncadi.samhsa.gov/

   http://aacap.org/page.ww?name=Teens:+Alcohol+and+Other+Drugs&section=Facts+for+Families

   www.nida.nih.gov/scienceofaddiction/

   www.nida.nih.gov/MarijBroch/Marijteens.html

4. Read one of the following articles and write a one-page report:

   Beduschi, G. 2003. Current popular ergogenic aids used in sports: a critical review. *Nutrition and Dietetics* 60(2): 104-118.

   Cooper, J., J.A. Ellison, and M.M. Walsh. 2003. Spit (smokeless)-tobacco use by baseball players entering the professional ranks. *Journal of Athletic Training* 38(2): 126-132.

   Gaudard, A., E. Varlet-Marie, F. Bressolle, and M. Audran. 2003. Drugs for increasing oxygen transport and their potential use in doping: a review. *Sports Medicine* 33(3): 187-192.

5. Visit the Web site of the National Institute on Drug Abuse and learn more about drug testing in schools:

   www.drugabuse.gov/DrugPages/testingfaqs.html.

6. Visit the NIDA Web site and learn more about steroid use:

   www.drugabuse.gov/drugpages/steroids.html.

7. Examine the Illinois High School Association sports medicine link and find information about the state's drug testing policy and list of banned drugs: www.ihsa.org/initiatives/sportsMedicine/.

8. Visit www.mayoclinic.com/health/acupuncture-for-back-pain/AN02055 to learn more about the effects of acupuncture on back pain.

chapter
28

Nutrition and Weight Control

Objectives

Upon completing this chapter, the student will be able to do the following:

- Understand metabolism.
- Understand the basic food groups.
- Understand the role that nutrition plays in a healthy body.
- Design a diet for an athlete.
- Understand that food myths are common among athletes.

The body's fuel is food, and its energy system is known as **metabolism**. Food that can be broken down by the body for use consists mainly of carbohydrate, protein, and fat. Other nutrients include vitamins, minerals, and water. The heat-producing, or energy-producing, value of food is measured in calories, and if the body does not require all of the metabolized calories for growth, maintenance, or heat, it stores them, yielding weight gain. If the number of calories brought in is less than what the body needs, the athlete will lose weight. When the body needs energy, it uses carbohydrate first, then fat, and finally protein or the body's muscles—people who are starving lose muscle because the body needs it for fuel.

Metabolism is the sum of the chemical changes that take place as the body functions. The body's metabolism can change depending on activity level and sex. Males and teenagers normally have higher metabolisms, as do people who exercise. An athlete's metabolism slows as she gets older.

MAJOR NUTRIENTS

Nutrients are substances that the body uses in metabolism. They include water, vitamins, minerals, carbohydrate, fat, and protein.

Water

Water is an essential component of the diet and makes up about 57% of the total body weight. Water is necessary for proper body functioning. It is beneficial to kidney function, excretion, chemical reactions throughout the body, sweating, blood flow, and joint lubrication. Water comes from the faucet, in bottles, or in various products such as soda, sport drinks, juice drinks, coffee, and tea. When an athlete is competing, the AT must remember that most athletes do not drink enough water to replace what they lose in sweat. Also, an athlete's thirst level is a poor indicator of how much water is needed to replace sweat.

When an athlete fails to replace the fluids lost through sweating or other normal body processes, he can become dehydrated. Signs and symptoms of dehydration include headache, dry mouth, dizziness, fatigue, and thirst. Another indicator that a person is dehydrated is the color of his urine. The urine should be clear; a bright yellow color indicates dehydration. Mild dehydration occurs when an athlete loses 2% of his body weight or more. Even this small amount of dehydration can result in poor athletic performance.

Generally, an athlete should drink at least eight 8-ounce glasses of water a day. According to NATA, proper preexercise hydration involves drinking 17 to 20 ounces (500-600 ml) of sport drink or water two to three hours before activity and 7 to 10 ounces (200-300 ml) 10 to 20 minutes before exercise. The ACSM has slightly different recommendations that take into consideration an athlete's weight (see the highlight box on this page). Fluid should be replaced at the rate of 7 to 10 ounces (200-300 ml) every 10 to 20 minutes. To adequately rehydrate after exercise, an athlete should drink about 20 ounces (600 ml) of sport drink for every pound (.5 kg) of weight lost through exercise. Those trying to lose weight will find that drinking

What Would You Do If...

You are hauling a 10-gallon (38 L) watercooler out to football practice. The head coach stops you, removes the lid, and pours in a container of creatine. You are shocked. The coach responds by saying, "If we are going to win a state title, we need a little extra advantage." He insists that you bring him the watercoolers every day.

Fluid Replacement

According to the 2007 ACSM position stand for exercise and fluid replacements proper preexercise hydration involves the following:

- Slowly drink beverages four or more hours before exercise. The ACSM recommends ingesting 5 to 7 milliliters for every kilogram of body weight. For example, a 150-pound athlete (68.2 kg) would need to drink between 341 and 477 milliliters at least four hours ahead of the exercise session.

- An athlete who does not urinate or whose urine is not clear should drink an additional 3 to 5 milliliters for every kilogram of body weight. Using the same example as before, the athlete would drink an additional 205 to 341 milliliters.

- Eating snacks or drinking beverages with a small amount of sodium will make an athlete thirsty and encourage drinking. This will also help retain fluids.

Adapted From: Michael N. Sawka, M.N., Burke, L.M., Eichner, E.R. Maughan, R.J., Montain, S.J., & Stachenfeld, N.S. American College of Sports Medicine. (2007). Exercise and Fluid Replacement. Medicine & Science in Sports & Exercise, 39(2):377-390.

this much water will cleanse their system of waste products and make them feel full.

Wrestlers are notorious for cutting weight to get into a particular weight class. Unfortunately, most often they cut the weight over a short time, losing only water weight and becoming dehydrated. This restriction of water and the water-weight loss will cause the wrestler to be fatigued and much less effective. Wrestlers who want to lose weight need to be supervised by a dietitian, and they must still drink eight glasses of water per day.

Vitamins

Vitamins are substances that help the body perform specific functions by regulating metabolic processes. Vitamins are found in all foods, so people who eat a balanced diet get all of the vitamins they need. An athlete who eats improperly,

Table 28.1 Vitamin Overview

Vitamin	Type	Food source	Deficiency
A	Fat soluble	Butter, cheese, carrots, green leafy vegetables	Impaired vision, eye inflammation, blindness
B1	Water soluble	Whole grains, legumes, meat products	Weakness, confusion, muscle atrophy
B2	Water soluble	Green vegetables, milk, eggs, whole grains	Dry, cracking skin; skin irritation
B6	Water soluble	Meat, whole grains, legumes, green leafy vegetables	Dry, cracking skin; skin irritation; anemia
B12	Water soluble	Meat, fish, eggs, milk	Anemia, neurological disorders
C	Water soluble	Fruits, green vegetables, potatoes, tomatoes	Immune system deficiencies, bleeding gums, dry skin
D	Fat soluble	Dairy products, fish oils, sunlight	Bone loss, rickets,
E	Fat soluble	Nuts, vegetable oil, whole grains, butter, green leafy vegetables	Neurological disorders (deficiencies are very rare)
K	Fat soluble	Green leafy vegetables	Bleeding

however, will need to obtain vitamins through supplements to meet the daily needs for proper body functioning.

Vitamins are either fat soluble or water soluble. Fat-soluble vitamins include A, D, E, and K. Water-soluble vitamins include B complex (B_1, B_2, B_{12}) and C. Fat-soluble vitamins dissolve in fat before being used by the body, whereas water-soluble vitamins dissolve in water before being used by the body. Excess fat-soluble vitamins are stored in the liver, and excess water-soluble vitamins are urinated out of the body.

Minerals

Minerals are inorganic chemical elements that are necessary for building bones and muscles, conducting nerve impulses, and maintaining normal metabolism and heart function. Minerals are found in all foods, and the athlete does not require a supplement unless her diet is not balanced. The incidence of some diseases has been reduced after scientists added minerals to commonly used products. For example, fluoride is added to water to prevent tooth decay, and calcium is added to orange juice to help bolster its intake for those who do not like dairy products. Bone strength is improved by

the added calcium for growing athletes as well as the prevention of osteoporosis as athletes age. See table 28.2 for a list of common minerals and their sources.

Carbohydrate

Carbohydrate is the main fuel source for the body. The digestion of carbohydrate begins in the mouth when it is mixed with saliva secreted by the salivary glands. Nutritionists recommend that carbohydrate make up 40% to 50% of the daily diet and that athletes get 55% to 60% of their calories from carbohydrate. See examples of carbohydrate foods in the following highlight box.

What Would You Do If...

The latest fad diet is eating a single food—cabbage. The athletes mention that they can eat cabbage any way they want but nothing else is on the menu. They rave about how much weight they have lost and you begin to think, "Maybe I should try this diet."

Table 28.2   Mineral Overview

Mineral	Food source	Deficiency
Calcium	Dairy products, spinach, almonds	Decreased bone density, tooth formation
Iron	Beef, eggs, broccoli	Anemia
Magnesium	Nuts, beans, seeds, legumes	Muscle weakness, fatigue, cramping
Phosphorus	Dairy products, meats	Anemia
Potassium	Raisins, bananas, pees, beef	Muscle cramping, heart problems
Selenium	Nuts (Brazil), tuna, beef, eggs	Heart disease, hypothyroidism, weakened immune system
Sodium	Salt	Hyponatremia (with endurance events over 4 hours coupled with high volume of water intake)
Zinc	Oysters, fortified breakfast cereal, almonds, cheese	Growth retardation, loss of appetite, impaired immune function

Carbohydrates

Simple	Complex
Honey	Bread
Fruit	Potatoes
Soda	Bagels
Sport drinks	Cereal
Candy and sweets	Beans
	Vegetables
	Nuts and seeds
	Pasta

High-Fiber Carbohydrates

Beans	Kidney beans
Vegetables	Corn
Nuts and seeds	Sunflower seeds
Fruits	Apples
Lima beans	Broccoli
Peas	Bananas
Almonds	Coconuts
Prunes	

Fiber is the indigestible material found in foods high in carbohydrate. Fiber stimulates the intestines, so diets high in fiber reduce constipation and colon disease. A list of high-fiber carbohydrate is found in the following highlight box.

Many people, including athletes, restrict their carbohydrate intake in order to lose weight. According to the American Heart Association, much of the weight loss from low-carbohydrate diets is due to a loss of body fluids. Also, many foods that are high in carbohydrate have extremely high nutritional value, and greatly reducing them in a diet may lead to other health problems. Most

people get plenty of protein if they eat a balanced diet. There is speculation that decreasing the intake of carbohydrate and increasing the intake of protein and fat may increase cholesterol and the risk of heart disease.

Fat

Fat is a necessary component of a healthy diet. For example, the female reproductive system cannot function properly without a certain amount of fat, and the body cannot support a pregnancy without enough body fat. In addition to being a source of energy, fat helps cells function, is required for the metabolism of some vitamins, and helps maintain normal body shape. Dietary fat can be classified as saturated or unsaturated.

Saturated fat is found primarily in animal products such as meat, chicken skin, lard, milk, cheese, cream, butter, some oils (e.g., coconut), and chocolate. Unsaturated fat is generally found in plant products such as soybeans, nuts, and some oils (e.g., olive, canola, peanut). Although fat can make food taste better, too much may contribute to an unhealthy lifestyle and lead to illness. Heart disease, high blood pressure, diabetes, some cancers, and obesity have all been linked to excessive fat intake, especially saturated fat. An athlete needs to review the amount and kinds of fat he is eating and determine if he can improve his diet.

Cholesterol is a fatlike substance produced within the body to perform essential cellular functions. Some cholesterol is not essential for life and is stored in the blood vessels. Cholesterol accumulation on a vessel wall can close off the vessel over time and lead to a heart attack.

Cholesterol levels in the body increase when more saturated fat is consumed. Many people avoid foods with cholesterol as a way of decreasing cholesterol in the blood vessels, so many food manufacturers label foods as *cholesterol free*. Cholesterol occurs in all products containing animal fat—it is found in egg yolks, milk, cream, cheese, butter, and all red meats. See the preceding box for examples of foods that are sources of fat.

Cholesterol is divided into two types, good and bad. The bad cholesterol (low density) can clog your arteries and cause heart disease. Good cholesterol (high density) can be helpful to your body. When bad cholesterol levels are high and good cholesterols levels are low, you are at serious risk for heart conditions.

Trans fat, or trans-fatty acid, is fat that is created when hydrogen is added to vegetable oil so it is more solid. Many foods are fried in trans fat, but the consequences are harmful. Trans fat raises bad cholesterol levels and lowers good cholesterol levels. Ingesting trans fats also increases the risk of developing type 2 diabetes. There is no safe level of trans fat to ingest.

Protein

The basic components of protein are **amino acids**. The body uses amino acids to form new tissues and

---

Examples of Fat

Unsaturated fat	Saturated fat	High cholesterol
Fish	Meat	Brains
Margarine	Chicken skin	Kidneys
Vegetable oil	Lard	Liver
Olive oil	Whole milk	Egg yolk
Fish oil	Cheese	Cheese
Peanut oil	Some oils (coconut and palm)	Lobster
Nuts	Chocolate	Dark turkey meat
	Butter	Butter
	Processed cheese	Pork
	Ice cream	Ice cream
	Cream cheese	Lamb
	Cocoa butter	Veal
		Cream
		Salmon
		Shrimp

Examples of Protein

High amount	Medium amount
Beef	Yogurt
Chicken	Milk
Fish	Beans
Turkey	Dried peas
Veal	Lentils
	Eggs

fruits, vegetables, meat and beans, milk, and oils (see the highlight box on this page). The quantities of the food groups are identified in MyPyramid (figure 28.1); note that a higher intake of grains, fruits, and vegetables is recommended. Because different cultures place varying emphases on food intake, other food guidelines exist. The CANFit organization has designed an example of the Native American food pyramid which can be found online by searching that topic or visiting the Department of Agriculture Web site.

repair damaged tissues. Teenagers are growing and must make sure they are getting enough protein so that their growth is not slowed; they require more protein than adults do. Protein is found in meat, beans, nuts, dairy products, fish, and eggs. Protein is the last source of energy used by the body. Anywhere from 15% to 20% of an athlete's daily diet should be protein. A list of protein sources is found in the box on this page.

Protein supplements are sold for those who may not get enough protein in their diet. Manufacturers of protein supplements advertise that their products build muscle. However, high amounts of protein in an athlete's diet can lead to higher body fat (because protein-bearing foods usually have a lot of fat), loss of calcium from bones, and dehydration.

HEALTHY DIET

Proper nutrition is vital to a healthy life. Many of the leading causes of death are related to how we eat. According to the United States Department of Agriculture (USDA) dietary guidelines, a healthy diet is one that

- emphasizes fruits, vegetables, whole grains, and fat-free or low-fat milk and milk products;
- includes lean meats, poultry, fish, beans, eggs, and nuts; and
- is low in saturated fat, trans fat, cholesterol, salt (sodium), and added sugar.

A balanced diet provides all of the nutrients necessary to remain healthy. It should contain portions of food from each of the food groups. The food groups identified by the USDA include grains,

Dietary Guidelines

Key recommendations from the USDA dietary guidelines include the following:

- Consume sufficient fruits and vegetables while staying within energy needs. Two cups of fruit and 2.5 cups of vegetables per day are recommended for a reference 2,000-calorie intake, with higher or lower amounts required depending on the calorie level.

- Choose a variety of fruits and vegetables each day. In particular, select from all five vegetable subgroups (dark green, orange, legumes, starchy vegetables, and other vegetables) several times a week.

- Consume three or more 1-ounce (28 g) whole-grain products per day, with the rest of the recommended grains coming from enriched or whole-grain products. At least half of all grain servings should come from whole grains.

- Consume 3 cups per day of fat-free or low-fat milk or equivalent milk products.

- Children and adolescents should consume whole-grain products often; at least half the grains should be whole grains. Also, children aged 2 to 8 years should consume 2 cups per day of fat-free or low-fat milk or equivalent milk products. Children 9 years of age and older should consume 3 cups per day of fat-free or low-fat milk or equivalent milk products.

From: U.S. Department of Health and Human Services & U.S. Department of Agriculture. (2005). Dietary Guidelines for Americans, pg. 24.

Anatomy of MyPyramid

One size doesn't fit all
USDA's new MyPyramid symbolizes a personalized approach to healthy eating and physical activity. The symbol has been designed to be simple. It has been developed to remind consumers to make healthy food choices and to be active every day. The different parts of the symbol are described below.

Activity
Activity is represented by the steps and the person climbing them, as a reminder of the importance of daily physical activity.

Moderation
Moderation is represented by the narrowing of each food group from bottom to top. The wider base stands for foods with little or no solid fats or added sugars. These should be selected more often. The narrower top area stands for foods containing more added sugars and solid fats. The more active you are, the more of these foods can fit into your diet.

Personalization
Personalization is shown by the person on the steps, the slogan, and the URL. Find the kinds and amounts of food to eat each day at MyPyramid.gov.

Proportionality
Proportionality is shown by the different widths of the food group bands. The widths suggest how much food a person should choose from each group. The widths are just a general guide, not exact proportions. Check the Web site for how much is right for you.

Variety
Variety is symbolized by the 6 color bands representing the 5 food groups of the Pyramid and oils. This illustrates that foods from all groups are needed each day for good health.

Gradual Improvement
Gradual improvement is encouraged by the slogan. It suggests that individuals can benefit from taking small steps to improve their diet and lifestyle each day.

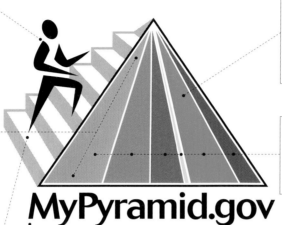

MyPyramid.gov
STEPS TO A HEALTHIER YOU

USDA U.S. Department of Agriculture Center for Nutrition Policy and Promotion April 2005 CNPP-16
USDA is an equal opportunity provider and employer.

GRAINS   VEGETABLES   FRUITS   OILS   MILK   MEAT & BEANS

Figure 28.1   MyPyramid.
U.S. Department of Health and Human Services.

Table 28.3   MyPyramid Daily Servings for 2,000-Calorie Diet

Groups	Daily servings
Fruit group	4 servings or 2 cups
Vegetable group	5 servings or 2.5 cups
Grain group	6 oz (170 g)*
Meat and beans group	5.5 oz (156 g)
Milk group	3 cups
Oils	24 g or 6 tsp
Discretionary calories	No more than 267 calories

*3 oz (85 g) from whole grains

CALORIC BALANCE

For the body to maintain a specific weight, the calories ingested should match the calories burned through daily activity and exercise. If an athlete wishes to gain or lose weight, the **caloric balance** will need to be adjusted. With weight loss, for example, the athlete will need to increase the calories burned, decrease the calories ingested, or, as suggested by the ACSM, both.

Weight Loss

People who need to lose weight should follow the ACSM guidelines for weight loss. These guidelines state that 150 to 250 minutes per week of moderate-intensity physical activity will provide modest

What Would You Do If...

In the locker room a swimmer accidentally drops her purse. All of the contents fall out onto the floor. As you politely help her pick up her things, you notice she has some opened containers of laxatives and diet pills.

weight loss, and more than 250 minutes per week is associated with significant weight loss. It is essential that people looking to lose weight also restrict their caloric intake to a moderate level. Severe limitation of calories will not be more effective than moderate restriction. We recommend consulting with a physician before engaging in a weight-loss program.

Weight Gain

People looking to gain weight should have the goal of increasing their muscle mass; gaining more fat should not be the goal. No more than 1 to 2 pounds (.5-1 kg) per week should be gained. To increase muscle mass, resistance training and conditioning of the muscles should be performed along with slight increase calorie consumption. With more resistance training, an athlete will need slightly more protein in her diet.

Obesity

Obesity is defined as an excessive level of body fat as determined by a person's body mass index (BMI). A person's BMI can be calculated using the following formula: BMI = [weight (lb) ÷ height (in.)^2] × 703. An adult who has a BMI of 30 or higher is considered obese. Obesity is a risk factor for many problems and is associated with higher cholesterol levels, hypertension, kidney disease, joint problems, diabetes, lung diseases, cancer, heart disease, and early death. Obesity is usually caused by a combination of factors, including heredity, overeating, and lack of physical activity.

A tendency toward obesity can begin at birth because of genetic factors. Moreover, a child who is born to parents who are obese is likely to pick up their habits and also become obese. Overeating means that an athlete ingests more calories than the body uses, and the additional calories are stored as fat in the body.

Many people are active in their teenage and college years. Once an athlete takes a job and starts a family, it becomes difficult to maintain the same level of physical activity. The decrease in physical activity coupled with the same eating habits yields additional weight gain. Exercise must be a priority for athletes who have stopped playing sports if they want to avoid gaining weight.

People are born with a certain number of fat cells. As they continue to eat and gain stored fat, the fat cells increase in size until they can hold no more, and then more fat cells are produced. Once a fat cell is produced it does not go away. A weight-loss diet will cause the fat cells to shrink but not go away. People have undergone liposuction to have their fat cells sucked out, but eating habits do not change because of liposuction. People can come home with a body that appears new only to go back to their old eating habits, which will give them their old body back.

Fat is deposited in genetically predetermined areas. In other words, no one can control where the extra calories are deposited or where fat will be burned off with exercise. In females, fat is likely to be deposited in the hips, breasts, abdomen, and thighs. In males, it is likely to be deposited in the abdomen, chest, and thighs.

In some sports obesity is not an issue. For instance, football requires several large players on the line. In wrestling, the various weight classes will accommodate the obese wrestler. Shot-putters, hammer throwers, and sumo wrestlers all tend to be large and sometimes obese.

SPORT NUTRITION

ATs are frequently asked what types of foods an athlete should eat to be the best. The answer is simple—eat a well-balanced meal suggested by the food pyramid. Balanced meals provide all of the nutritional requirements to be healthy and perform well. When designing a program, the AT and dietitian need to know if the athlete wants to gain, lose, or maintain weight.

The AT and dietitian can develop a diet that will ensure all nutritional needs are met based on the nutritional and physical assessment of the athlete. An athlete trying to gain weight will be placed on a diet in which the number of calories

Ramadan is a month of fasting. It is a time for Muslims to remember the suffering of the poor and to appreciate the things that Allah has given them. Fasting occurs during the day and includes no water or food. Food is allowed after dark *(iftar)* and before sunrise *(shurooq)*. If a person is ill, it is acceptable to eat during the fasting hours. A person who is taking medication that requires taking food at the same time may have an upset stomach while fasting.

eaten exceeds the energy expended. An athlete trying to lose weight will be placed on a diet that supplies fewer calories than the amount of energy expended. The athlete's weight loss should not exceed an average of 2 pounds (1 kg) a week. He should never increase room temperatures, sit in a hot tub or sauna, wear rubberized clothing, or work out in high temperatures with lots of clothes in an attempt to lose weight. An exercise and weight-loss plan designed by the AT and the dietitian is the only plan to follow.

Pregame Meals

Pregame meals should be high in carbohydrate and fluids. Carbohydrate is easier to digest than fat and protein, and it can be converted into energy to be used immediately. The pregame meal should be eaten three to four hours before activity. Water is the best liquid to drink, and the athlete should make sure she is well hydrated about one hour before competition.

Athletes who are anxious about an upcoming competition may use carbohydrate-loaded sport drinks. Sport drinks are digested quickly, which helps the anxious athlete avoid feelings of nausea.

When the AT and dietitian are considering a pregame meal, they should remember the diversity of the team. Some athletes may have specific food preferences such as Mexican, Arabic, Greek, or Latin foods. The AT has homework to do—he needs to analyze these diverse foods and determine what types are acceptable before a game. Another consideration is religious holidays. An athlete may observe a holiday by fasting or by not eating meat. The AT and dietitian should be aware of this issue a week in advance to best prepare the athlete for the holiday diet. Vegetarians have special protein needs and should work with the AT and dietitian to make sure their food needs are met. The following box lists the types of vegetarians.

Some good pregame foods include pasta, fruit, plain crackers, rice cakes, cereal, vegetarian foods, potatoes, meatless lasagna, soup, rice, juice, bread, raisins, pancakes, and waffles. Besides eating foods high in carbohydrate, the athlete should eat familiar foods. The pregame meal is no time to experiment.

Postgame Meals

Hopefully the team will do something to celebrate, and food can be there to replenish energy supplies. However, ATs should not use food as a reward (e.g., giving a team pizza, soda, and ice cream if they win) or as a punishment (e.g., driving the team straight home if they lose). Such actions can create an association between eating and pleasurable or miserable experiences that leads to overeating or not eating.

After the event, athletes should eat complex carbohydrate, but some protein, fat, and simple carbohydrate are also fine. Soon after practice and competitions is the best time to replenish the body's energy stores. Water replacement is necessary to compensate for sweating during competition. Several glasses of juice, water, or sport drinks are perfect choices.

Meals During All-Day Events

Many athletic competitions take place over a full day. Athletes may be asked to compete several times during the day, and a full sit-down meal is out of the question. So what should athletes do to keep energy levels up? The answer is to eat small meals many times during the day. The meals should contain little protein and fat and a lot of complex

Types of Vegetarians

- Semivegetarian: vegetable diet with occasional dairy and meats
- Lacto-ovo vegetarian: vegetable diet with dairy and eggs
- Lacto vegetarian: vegetable diet with dairy
- Vegan: vegetable diet

carbohydrate and fluids (not soda). The amount of complex carbohydrate can be half a sandwich six times during the day. When the athlete eats depends on when she must compete; she must provide time to allow the food to digest as much as possible. Good all-day-event foods are bagels (no cream cheese), English muffins, bananas, baked potatoes, soup, fruit, pasta, pancakes, sport drinks, yogurt, cereal, and vegetables.

Carbohydrate Loading

Athletes who participate in endurance events (marathoners, cyclists, triathletes, long-distance swimmers) may benefit from a technique called *carbohydrate loading.* Carbohydrate loading means depleting carbohydrate for seven days and then ingesting large amounts of carbohydrate for three days before the event. The theory behind carbohydrate loading is that carbohydrate stores are used as energy during athletic competition. If the athlete has a lot of stored carbohydrate, he is less likely to run out of energy. Depleting before loading causes the body to store more carbohydrate than usual once carbohydrate consumption resumes. Remember that once carbohydrate stores are used up, the body begins to break down fat. Breaking down fat requires more energy than using readily available carbohydrate, again draining energy from athlete. So the greater the carbohydrate stores, the better the athlete's energy.

If an athlete is involved in an endurance activity, the AT and dietitian should design a program for carbohydrate loading. The athlete's diet will change 10 days before competition. Three days before the event, 70% of what the athlete eats will be carbohydrate. During carbohydrate loading (the three days before the event), the athlete does not exercise. Fat and protein foods are decreased as part of carbohydrate loading.

POPULAR NUTRITIONAL SUPPLEMENTS

Someone is always trying to sell something. Companies hire professional athletes to hype their goods. A good-looking person is used to hype a product while on a beach with a beautiful com-

panion. The advertisement is designed to make potential customers believe that if they use the product they, too, will be someplace warm with a beautiful companion. Some companies claim that certain nutritional items will help an athlete perform better, run faster, or have more energy. When you hear a promise but you don't see independent research evidence to support the claim, keep your money in your pocket.

Herbal Supplements

Over the past several years, herbal dietary supplements derived from natural sources have become popular to reportedly curb the appetite, provide energy, and burn calories. Common herbal supplements include ephedra and hydroxycitric acid. Ephedra was said to suppress the appetite and increase metabolism. Hydroxycitric acid reportedly decreases the appetite as well. Herbal supplements are officially regulated by the FDA, and in 2003 the FDA banned the sale of ephedra because it was possibly associated with death of users and caused serious side effects including high blood pressure, seizures, strokes, and irregular heartbeat. The Mayo Clinic recommends *not* taking an herbal supplement if

- you are taking medications (prescription or over the counter),
- proven medical treatment is already available to address your problem,
- you are having surgery,
- you are pregnant or breastfeeding, or
- you are under age 18 or over age 65.

Creatine

Creatine is a popular nutritional supplement. This substance is found in the body in high levels right after exercise. Creatine is found in fish and in meats. An athlete would have to eat 15 pounds (7 kg) of meat per day to obtain the same amount of creatine recommended as a supplement. Advertisers claim that creatine is an energy source and encourages muscle growth. Athletes who take creatine supplements while strength training appear to have increased power for brief, highly intense exercise.

The long-term effects of creatine are inconclusive; thus, it should be avoided.

Amino Acids

Amino acids are the building blocks of protein. Thus, people have thought that daily amino acid supplements (pills or powder) would make them stronger and faster and increase protein storage. The basis for these ideas was the notion that amino acids cause the release of HGH (see chapter 27). HGH does increase muscle mass, but amino acids do not cause the release of HGH. Amino acids are sold in fitness magazines with pictures of muscular men and women holding the containers. Don't buy it. Amino acid supplements are expensive, and the athlete's daily diet should provide all the necessary amino acids.

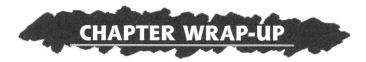

CHAPTER WRAP-UP

Summary

An athlete's daily nutrition plays a critical role in his ability to give an optimal performance. Most athletes meet their daily requirements by eating proper portions of a balanced diet. Some athletes consistently eat foods that are high in fat and cholesterol and low in fiber. This can lead to negative health consequences. As an athlete gets older, her metabolism slows, and she must reduce the number of calories she consumes or she will gain weight. Water intake and fluid replacement are key for athletic participation. The rule for fluid replacement is 1 liter for every 1,000 calories lost. The AT and dietitian should decide on pregame and postgame meals based on the event and the athlete's needs, taking into consideration the athlete's religious and cultural background. Athletes are constantly looking for an edge over their opponents, and fad diets and supplements are hyped as the greatest way to improve performance. Athletes and the AT must research supplements before anyone uses them.

Key Terms

Define the following terms found in this chapter:

amino acids	metabolism
caloric balance	nutrients
cholesterol	trans fat
fiber	

Questions for Review

1. What are the basic nutrients?
2. What are the main food groups?
3. How much water does an athlete need during competition?
4. How can an athlete be sure she is drinking enough fluids?
5. How many servings are needed per day from each food group for a 2,000-calorie diet?
6. A pregame meal should consist of what types of foods?
7. If an athlete desires a postgame meal, what foods should be included?
8. How helpful are food supplements to athletic performance?

Activities for Reinforcement

1. Design a pregame meal for fictitious swim and ice hockey teams.

2. Keep track of what you eat for one week and determine if you have a specific food group from which you eat too much or too little. Make recommendations for improving your eating habits after talking with the AT and school dietitian.

3. Examine the American Heart Association Web page for more information about low-carbohydrate, high-protein diets:

   www.americanheart.org/presenter.jhtml?identifier=11234.

4. Visit the following Web site hosted by the Mayo Clinic and summarize the information provided about herbal supplements:

   www.mayoclinic.com/health/herbal-supplements/SA00044.

5. Visit the Web site of the American Heart Association and learn more about trans fats:

   www.americanheart.org/presenter.jhtml?identifier=3045792.

6. Visit the USDA Web site for information related to food and nutrition: www.usda.gov (click on Food and Nutrition).

7. Check out the tips for vegetarian diets at

   www.mypyramid.gov/tips_resources/vegetarian_diets_print.html.

Above and Beyond

1. Keep a record of your eating habits during a normal day. Examine your record and answer the following: What types of food do you typically eat? What categories in the food pyramid are these foods from? What foods does your diet lack?

2. Read one of the following resources and write a one-page report:

   American College of Sports Medicine (ACSM). 2009. Nutrition and athletic performance. *Medicine and Science in Sports and Exercise* 41(3): 709-733.

   Beltrami, F., T. Hew-Butler, and T. Noakes. 2008. Drinking policies and exercise-associated hyponatraemia: Is anyone still promoting overdrinking? *British Journal of Sports Medicine* 42(10): 496-501.

   Borrione, P., L. Grasso, F. Quaranta, and A. Parisi. 2009. FIMS position statement 2009: vegetarian diet and athletes. *International SportMed Journal* 10(1): 53-60.

   Cialdella-Kam, L., and M. Manore. 2009. Macronutrient needs of active individuals: an update. *Nutrition Today* 44(3): 104-111.

3. Find the food guidelines from another culture and compare them with figure 28.1. What is the biggest difference?

chapter 29

Athletes With Disabilities

Objectives

Upon completing this chapter, the student will be able to do the following:

- Understand the history of sport participation by people with disabilities.
- Understand that athletes with disabilities or disorders have the ability to participate with or without special adaptations.
- Know that there are injury prevention programs based on the needs of each group of disabilities or disorders.

In 1990, the Americans with Disabilities Act defined **disability** as "a physical or mental impairment that substantially limits one or more major life activities." One of those life activities may be participation in athletics. An AT needs to understand each disability and how it is affected by sport participation. Supporting athletes with disabilities is essential to the athlete's positive sport experience.

The first portion of this chapter discusses the growth in sport for people with disabilities. The second part discusses various disabilities and the impact of exercise.

HISTORY OF DISABLED SPORT

After World War II, veterans with spinal cord injuries who used wheelchairs were given an opportunity to participate in the Stoke Mandeville Games in 1948 (Ability v Ability 2006). The games were founded by Sir Ludwig Guttmann, who considered exercise as essential to the recovery of people with spinal cord injuries. Eventually the games branched off into disabled games such as the Paralympics, which includes athletes who have disabilities but who don't necessarily use wheelchairs.

Many organizations run programs for athletes with a specific disability. Organizations include the Dwarf Athletic Association of America (DAAA), Second Wind Lung Transplant Association, Special Olympics, and United States Association of Blind Athletes (USABA). These groups can assist the AT in developing programming, goals, and an understanding of each disability.

A number of students have a disability or disorder that makes sport participation challenging. Very few high schools provide competition exclusively for athletes with physical impairments; athletes with disabilities who participate in high school sport do so against athletes without disabilities. ATs have a great opportunity to work with and support those who face challenges in sport participation.

ORTHOPEDIC DISABILITIES

Orthopedic disabilities are those in which the bones, joints, muscles, tendons, or ligaments are impaired. This section discusses the more common disabilities that affect athletes.

Deformed Limbs

Many athletes who have deformed limbs were born with them. The deformity can be an undeveloped limb or having too many or too few toes or fingers. It can also be constriction from additional webbing between fingers or toes.

The cause of the deformity can be a birth defect caused by a drug or exposure to an illness during pregnancy. It may also result from the constriction of blood flow to the limb during the birth process (Children's Hospital of Wisconsin 2009).

An athlete with a limb deformity can be very successful playing a sport depending on the restriction of the deformity. In some instances no adaptation is necessary and the athlete can readily play. In other cases an athlete may require surgery to obtain the necessary range of motion or may need to learn to adapt to the game.

The important thing for the AT is to learn about restrictions the athlete may have and how the athlete adapts to the game. If the athlete wears a brace or has an artificial limb, the AT needs to learn how to help the athlete stabilize the limb or brace to meet the demands of participation.

One of the most famous athletes with a deformed limb was professional baseball player Jim Abbott. Jim played football and baseball in high school and then went on to play professional baseball. He was born without a right hand. When he played baseball, he would place his glove on his right arm, pitch the ball, and place the glove on his left hand to catch the ball (www.jimabbott.net).

Amputations

An amputee has had a limb or digits removed entirely or partially. Amputations of the lower limb occur as a result of the following: vascular disease (70%), trauma (23%), and congenital deformities (3%) (Durstine and Moore 2003). Depending on the type of amputation, balance and movement may become issues.

The end of the limb is known as the stump. The stump is prone to friction, moisture, and blisters. The athlete and the AT have to watch for degradation of the stump. For the AT, treating a blister on the stump is no different than treating any other blister. The athlete needs to make care of the stump as a part of his regular routine.

Phantom pain is pain felt from the amputated limb. The pain can be mild or severe. In some cases the athlete may require medication to control it (Durstine and Moore 2003).

Athletes with amputations have the ability to compete with those without amputations. For instance, runner Oscar Pistorius was disqualified from participation in the 2008 Olympics because of the belief that his artificial limbs made him too fast for the competition (Topolsky 2008). In some instances being an amputee is a disadvantage; thus there may be a desire to compete against others with the same level of ability. The number of amputations and the amount of limb loss categorize athletes with amputations who compete against each other.

► Understanding Diversity

The Amputee Coalition of America states that Hispanics are three times more likely than non-Hispanic whites to have a foot or leg amputated due to diabetes-related limb problems. Visit www.amputee-coalition.org/fact_sheets/multicultural/all_groups.html for more information.

Lower-limb amputees are classified into three categories (idroscaloclub 2009):

- A1—double-leg amputation above the knee
- A2—single-leg amputation above or through the knee
- A3—bilateral below-the-knee amputation
- A4—single-leg amputation below the knee

Upper-limb amputees are classified into five categories (idroscaloclub 2009):

- A5—bilateral above or through the elbow
- A6—single above or through the elbow
- A7—bilateral below the elbow
- A8—single below the elbow
- A9—bilateral upper and lower limb

Amputees compete in many events without the aid of an artificial limb but with adaptations such as downhill ski poles, wheelchairs built for racing, and bikes for racing. In some instances an artificial limb is designed specifically for the amputee in competition. Carbon-fiber artificial limbs provide the amputee with a prosthetic that is capable of sustaining the rigors of competition. A **prosthetic** is an artificial body part. In some instances the constant intensity causes the carbon-fiber artificial limb to break, so more than one limb may be necessary.

AUDITORY AND VISUAL IMPAIRMENTS

Athletes who have sensory impairments are able to adapt their other senses to accommodate. Athletes are athletes no matter the type of disability. The AT should expect the athlete to be competitive and have the desire to participate regardless of the disability. The AT should also take advantage of opportunities to learn new skills, such as sign language or using a computer that a blind person can read.

Deafness

Deafness can be caused by a number of things, such as trauma, infection, and birth defects. These athletes may have problems with equilibrium if there is injury to the semicircular canals or the vestibular apparatus (Sherry 2007).

What Would You Do If...

You are assisting an AT who is providing medical coverage for a track meet at your school. Among the teams participating, one is from a school for students with hearing loss. One of the athletes from this school is injured during the long jump competition and the AT needs obtain a history of the injury. If you were in the ATs position, what would you do to communicate effectively with the athlete?

Athletes with hearing loss can participate in all sports. Difficulty may come from being unable to react as quickly if the sport requires hearing. In some instances not being able to hear the taunting of unruly fans or other distractions could be beneficial.

Some athletes with hearing loss are able to wear hearing aids. Hearing aids must be cared for to prevent sweat, rain, and water from getting into them. It is best to have extra hearing-aid batteries in the event the device needs a new one.

Blindness

People with vision impairments can be completely blind or partially blind. Sherry (2007) indicates that for an athlete to be eligible to compete in the disabled games (see the following) the athlete's visual acuity has to be 6/60 or less.

Athletes with visual impairments are able to compete in a variety of activities, including running, wrestling, baseball, softball, bowling, and cycling. A number of modifications are made to allow athletes with visual impairments to participate in sport, such as using a ball that beeps, running with another person to assist with the running path, or beginning a wrestling match in contact with the other athlete.

The AT should be aware that athletes with vision impairments are prone to falling and impact injuries. These falls can lead to typical fractures of the limbs (Sherry 2007).

In many instances people talk louder to an athlete with a disability. It sounds obvious, but the AT should realize that talking louder will not improve the athlete's vision.

CARDIOVASCULAR DISORDERS

The cardiovascular system is made up of the heart and blood vessels. To have a normal cardiovascular system, each of the components must be working properly. A disease or an illness may cause the system to not function properly, thus causing the athlete to struggle or even die. In this section, fibrillation of the heart and heart transplants are discussed.

Fibrillation

Fibrillation of the heart means that it is beating rapidly. The fibrillation can be in the upper chambers (atria) or lower chambers (ventricles) of the heart. A good way to visualize a fibrillating heart is as a bag filled with worms moving around. The heart is not able to effectively pump blood to the body, and if fibrillation continues for a long time, it can cause death or a stroke from a blood clot.

Fibrillation in athletes can be caused by alcohol use, an overactive thyroid, a blood clot in the lungs, caffeine intake, or pneumonia. Fibrillation can also be caused by the heart itself via heart valve disease, an enlarged heart, heart disease, high blood pressure, or a faulty electrical node (emedicinehealth 2009).

Athletes suffering from fibrillation may feel as though their heart is coming out of their chest. They may feel weak and anxious, and they may pass out. It is best to call for an ambulance and allow a physician to care for the athlete.

Treatment for the athlete with fibrillation can include dietary changes, medication, resolving other conditions such as high blood pressure, electrical shock to get the heart back to a regular rhythm, a pacemaker, or ablation surgery. An athlete who has fibrillation can return to participation with the permission of a physician.

Heart Transplant

Athletes with heart transplants can participate in athletic activities with the permission of their physician. The AT will need to be aware of the names and types of medications the athlete is using as well as the need for having an AED on hand. Accommodations may be needed for the athlete to participate, such as using a golf cart instead of carrying the golf bag and clubs.

A heart transplant is done because the athlete's heart no longer can function. An athlete who has gone through a heart transplant has likely endured a long process, which may have included having an artificial pump, pacemaker, or defibrillator attached to the heart. When a donor is found, the ineffective heart is removed and replaced with the donor's heart. Approximately 3,500 heart transplants are done worldwide each year (Durstine and Moore 2003).

The transplant patient usually takes antirejection medication so that the new heart is not rejected as a foreign object. The survival rate for adult heart transplants for at least three years was 80% from 1996 to 1999 (Durstine and Moore 2003). Some of the physical changes that occur as a result of the heart transplant include a resting heart rate of 90 to 110, decreased peak heart rate, decreased leg strength from lack of exercise, and increased leg cramps (Durstine and Moore 2003).

NEUROMUSCULAR DISORDERS

A neuromuscular disorder initiates in either the central nervous system (brain, spine) or the peripheral nervous system (nerves that originate at the spine and innervate the muscles and return to the spine). The nervous system sends messages throughout the body to cause the muscles to function. If any part of the nervous system is affected by disease or injury, the muscular system can also be compromised.

What Would You Do If...

A sophomore athlete approaches the AT and explains that she received a heart transplant four years earlier. She wishes to participate in basketball but isn't sure if she is at risk for heart problems if she plays. How do you think the AT should respond?

Paralympic athletes who have neuromuscular disorders are placed in the category of *other* or *les autres* for the purpose of participation. This category includes multiple sclerosis, muscular dystrophy, polio, and spinal bifida (It's the Real Deal 2009).

The following sections explain how the nervous system affects the muscular system in various neuromuscular disorders. They also describe exercise ability and tolerance as each disorder progresses.

The Real World

I had a wrestler who had muscular dystrophy. It wasn't until his second year in our program that I was told that his teammates were carrying him up and down two flights of stairs to get to the wrestling room. His mother, who always advocated for her son, shared that she felt it was unsafe for her son to be carried in such a manner. So I went to work on getting a lift put in so that he could freely move about the athletic area. Shortly after that, we had a ramp and another doorway built so he could lift weights with everyone else. These changes exist today for every student, a legacy of the athlete and his mother.

Anonymous

Multiple Sclerosis

The central nervous system is affected by **multiple sclerosis**. The central nervous system is surrounded by a myelin sheath, a fatty substance that ensures that electrical impulses are conducted through the nervous system to the muscles and organs they are designated to serve. The conduction of the impulses is rapid and coordinated (Durstine and Moore 2003). With multiple sclerosis, the myelin sheath detaches from parts of the central nervous system, making the conduction of impulses erratic.

The athlete with multiple sclerosis can participate in competition with athletes without disabilities, but he may have muscle spasms, balance issues, lack of coordination, fatigue, heat sensitivity, and numbness (Durstine and Moore 2003). Carcione (2006) suggests selecting an exercise that is fun but also meets the needs of the athlete. For example, if the athlete has problems with heat-related illness, swimming may be a good choice.

Over time multiple sclerosis can advance to a point where assistive devices are necessary to support the muscles. Devices may include prosthetics for the ankle joint to support foot drop.

Muscular Dystrophy

Muscular dystrophy is a group of disorders that affect the muscles by replacing muscle cells with connective tissue (Durstine and Moore 2003). With the progression of muscular dystrophy come cognitive deficits and memory loss. If the athlete has cognitive deficits, be sure to convey important ideas (times, place, dates) in writing. The progression

of the disease also causes loss of muscle function, range of motion, and ability to perform activities of daily living.

Muscular dystrophy is genetic. There are many forms of muscular dystrophy, but in general muscular deficits are the commonality. The progression begins with atrophy of muscles, fatigue, muscular spasm, weakness, and eventually cardiac problems (Durstine and Moore 2003).

Contractures caused by muscular dystrophy can be cared for with stretching. Cardiorespiratory exercise and strength training are good ways to maintain health. In addition, helping an athlete maintain a healthy weight is supportive and has therapeutic value (Durstine and Moore 2003).

Durstine and Moore (2003) indicate that it is important to maintain bone strength. In support of bone strength, athletes may add calcium and vitamin D to their diet. On the other hand, the use of corticosteroids can result in thinning of bone mass, thus leading to fractures.

Muscular dystrophy often results in extreme tightness of the muscles, especially at the ankles and hips. Surgery that releases these contractures is most often performed at the ankles and hip adductors as well as at spine when scoliosis is present (Durstine and Moore 2003). Controlling body heat and maintaining fluids are essential.

Exercises that support cardiorespiratory training include walking, cycling, and swimming. If walking is the exercise of choice, a flat surface is essential to preventing falls (University of Illinois at Chicago 2007). Strength training is also beneficial and can be accomplished using weights or therapeutic exercise bands (University of Illinois at Chicago 2007).

Cerebral Palsy

Cerebral palsy (CP) is a disorder that affects the brain before, during, or shortly after birth (Durstine and Moore 2003). CP affects the brain by preventing normal development of the brain, and it is a nonrepairable condition. The CP patient may have poor balance, lack of muscle tone, vision problems, hearing problems, mental retardation, speech impairment, seizures, and lack of control of posture (AAOS, 1991; Durstine and Moore 2003).

The level of CP is based on the extent and site of damage in the brain. CP can be severe enough that the patient needs a wheelchair and an assistant, and it can be mild to the point where the person has some movement problems but for the most part can get around without assistance.

Maintaining a level of fitness is important for people with CP. Some things to watch for are fatigue and increased muscle spasms. Durstine and Moore (2003) indicate that people with CP who participate in regular exercise are able to reduce their antispasm medication. CP athletes may have any number of orthopedic problems, including spinal deformities, hypermobile joints, and frequent subluxations (AAOS 1991).

CP athletes are often inclined to have seizures. Some seizure medications have side effects that can affect exercise, such as depression of the central nervous system, nausea, agitation, and weight loss (Durstine and Moore 2003).

During exercise, the CP athlete may require spotting. An athlete who is in a wheelchair may require restraints, so the AT needs to watch for blisters or pain (Durstine and Moore 2003).

Closed Head Trauma

A closed head injury is caused by an impact to the head that does not fracture the skull. The impact may cause bleeding and swelling within the brain that can lead to brain damage or even death. For those who survive the trauma, there may be permanent damage to the brain. The damage can be minimal or severe.

What Would You Do If...

A wheelchair athlete playing in a basketball competition reports to you with a severe blister on his right hand. He wishes to continue playing, but the tape he used to cover the wound does not stay in place very well.

The impairment caused by the trauma will be related to the portion of the brain that was damaged. Some may have memory deficits, cognitive deficits, mood swings, an inability to move arms and legs on one or both sides, and loss of the ability to speak.

If an athlete with a closed head trauma chooses to participate in sport, the sport may need to be one where falling or head trauma is not possible. In some instances headgear may be worn to protect the head regardless of the sport.

Disabled Sports USA is a group dedicated to helping people with disabilities, including those with head injuries. The sports offered are vast but may require that the athlete use adaptive equipment to participate.

ASSESSING PARTICIPATION CONDITIONS

The AT needs an overview of each athlete's abilities or lack thereof. During the physical examination of a physically challenged athlete, the AT will want to know the following:

- Athlete's strength
- Range of motion at each joint
- Medications used
- Ability to balance
- Appliances worn
- Visual acuity
- Auditory acuity
- Physical reaction to exercise
- Coordination
- Ability to understand direction
- Reaction time

The assessment will assist the AT and coach in establishing realistic goals and expectations for participation. Participation should be a positive experience so that the athlete can pursue the activity throughout a lifetime.

COMMON INJURIES

Competitive athletes with disabilities are similar to other athletes in that they can and do get injured. Some of the injuries that athletes with disabilities suffer are exactly the same, such as a sprained ankle; however, there are also other injuries that are unique to the disability.

The AT may anticipate the following injuries or illnesses based on disability (Sherry 2007):

- Deformed limbs: sprains, strains
- Amputations: blisters, ulcers, fractures
- Fibrillation: stroke, heart attack
- Heart transplant: heart attack
- Multiple sclerosis: fractures
- Muscular dystrophy: fractures

- CP: seizures
- Closed head trauma: additional head injuries
- Visual impairment: fractures, sprains, contusions
- Hearing impairment: fractures, sprains
- Wheelchair athletes: blisters, ulcers, sprains, strains, lacerations, fractures, urinary tract infections, heat regulation, high blood pressure, slow heart rate

The AT should use the standard of care for injuries that occur to an athlete with a disability. This means that a sprain or strain should be treated with PRICES, fractures should be splinted, and all emergency parameters should be used as necessary. Modifications in treatment arise in how an AT communicates with an athlete or how bandages are applied (consider a deformed limb, for example; taping or wrapping may not contour itself the way it does on a nondeformed limb).

The Real World

I had a swimmer who had autism. He was about 280 pounds (127 kg) and loved to swim, but the swim coach was afraid he would drown and she could not save him because of her slight frame and weight of 125 pounds (57 kg). There was an obvious potential for liability and danger but also an obligation to allow the young man to swim. In talking with the parents, we found a compromise. We hired a lifeguard who was designated to be the young man's personal supervisor. The young man enjoyed swimming the entire season and never had any difficulty. The coach felt relieved and the young man had a blast.

Anonymous

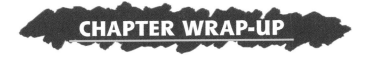

CHAPTER WRAP-UP

Summary

Athletes with disabilities deserve an opportunity to participate in sport. The AT needs to know as much as possible about the athlete and the disability to ensure safe participation. Each disability brings its own concerns such as blisters, ulcers, or possibility of falls. The AT and coach should work together help the athletes obtain their personal goals. Athletes with disabilities can participate in many sports with modification of the game, equipment, or prosthetics.

Key Terms

Define the following terms found in this chapter:

cerebral palsy (CP)
disability
prosthetic

fibrillation
multiple sclerosis
muscular dystrophy

Questions For Review

1. Define *disability*.
2. What was the initial event that led to athletic participation for athletes with disabilities?
3. What types of adaptations are made to allow participation by athletes with disabilities?
4. What are common injuries associated with wheelchair athletes, multiple sclerosis, heart transplants, vision impairments, and closed brain injury?

Activities for Reinforcement

1. Volunteer your time at physical examinations given at a school where students have disabilities.
2. Work at the local paralympic events.
3. Spend one week working with a student with visual or auditory disabilities.
4. Work or attend a wheelchair basketball game or a marathon race that includes wheelchair racers.
5. Invite a prosthetic maker to your class and have her explain how to design an athletic prosthesis.
6. Watch the Paralympic Games and identify a prosthetic device used to accommodate an athlete.

Above and Beyond

1. Invent a game or change the rules of a game to the benefit of an athlete with a disability. For example, wheelchair tennis – the athletes can only hit the ball on one side of the court. Another would be ice hockey games being played the width of the ice rather than the length.
2. Using online research, compare and contrast the sports that are exclusive to athletes with disabilities and the changes in the various rules.
3. Compare the world records of athletes with and without disabilities in Paralympic verses Olympic competition. In what sports do you believed disabled athletes have the advantage?
4. Investigate athletic associations for groups of athletes who are not addressed in this chapter, such as athletes with kidney transplants, arthritis, and AIDS.
5. Visit the Disabled Sports USA Web site and learn more about the programs it offers: www.dsusa.org.

Appendix A

Assumption-of-Risk Form

My child, _____ (print name of athlete),

and I, _____ (print name of parent or guardian), have been warned about the dangers involved with sport participation and are aware that participating in athletics can result in severe injury or even death from a variety of circumstances, which include but are not limited to falls, collisions with other athletes or equipment, and weather conditions, while being involved in the sport of _____

_____. We, the undersigned, understand that athletic participation is inherently dangerous and understand and assume the risks involved.

Student athlete: _____ Date: _____

Parent or guardian: _____ Date: _____

From *Fundamentals of Athletic Training, Third Edition,* by Lorin A. Cartwright and William A. Pitney, 2011, Champaign, IL: Human Kinetics.

Appendix B

Permission-to-Treat Form

I, _____ (name of parent or guardian), give

permission for my child, _____ (name of athlete),

to participate in _____ (sport) during the _____ (year) athletic season. If my child is injured and emergency care is needed, I grant the school's qualified staff permission to provide emergency medical services. Should more advanced treatment be necessary, I give permission to qualified medical personnel to treat him/her with the necessary care with the understanding that every reasonable effort will be made to contact me.

Address: _____

Home phone: ( )_____Work phone: ( )_____

Pager: ( )_____ Cell phone: ( )_____

Other emergency contact name: _____

Address: _____

Home phone: ( )_____Work phone: ( )_____

Pager: ( )_____ Cell phone: ( )_____

Student-Athlete Medical Data

Student ID number: _____

Sex: M ____ F ____

List any and all medical conditions (including allergies):

List any and all medications currently being taken:

Name of insurance company: _____

Address of insurance company: _____

Policyholder name (please print): _____

Policy number: _____ Group number: _____ Type: _____

I attest that the above medical information is accurate and agree to this permission-to-treat form.

Signature of parent or guardian: _____ Date: _____.

From *Fundamentals of Athletic Training, Third Edition*, by Lorin A. Cartwright and William A. Pitney, 2011, Champaign, IL: Human Kinetics. Data obtained from Rankin and Ingersol 1995; Roy and Irvin 1983; and Flegel 1992.

Appendix C

Athletic Injury and Accident Report

Athlete's name: _____ Today's date: _____

Injury date: _____ Body part injured: ❏ L   ❏ R _____ Sport: _____

Was the injury due to athletic participation? ❏ yes   ❏ no   other:_____

Subjective Information

Mechanism of injury: _____

Chief complaint: _____

Type of pain: _____

Other: _____

Objective Information

Inspection (observation): _____

Palpation: _____

Range-of-motion and strength testing: _____

Neurological findings: _____

Special stress tests: _____

Functional testing: _____

Assessment Information

Results of assessment: _____

List of problems: _____

Plan of Action

Initial treatment: _____

The athlete will be: ❏ referred to a physician   ❏ referred to school nurse

❏ treated by a certified athletic trainer

Treatment will be: _____days a week for _____ week(s).

Treatment will consist of: _____

_____

Parents contacted: ❏ yes   ❏ no.

If yes, give date: _____. If no, give reason: _____

Signature of certified athletic trainer: _____

Attach all progress notes to this sheet.

From *Fundamentals of Athletic Training, Third Edition,* by Lorin A. Cartwright and William A. Pitney, 2011, Champaign, IL: Human Kinetics.

Appendix D

Date	Athlete name (Print)	Sport	Ice	Heat	Whirlpool	Ultrasound	Electrical stimulation*	Massage	Exercise	Wound care	Tape wrap	Evaluation	AC[a]

Daily treatment log

*Indicate type (e.g., TENS), [a]Initials

Adapted, by permission, from Pioneer High School, Ann Arbor MI.

From *Fundamentals of Athletic Training, Third Edition,* by Lorin A. Cartwright and William A. Pitney, 2011, Champaign, IL: Human Kinetics.

Appendix E

Treatment Progress Chart

Athlete's name: _____ Injury date: _____

Injury site: _____ Location: ❏ left   ❏ right

Type of injury: ❏ sprain   ❏ strain   ❏ contusion   ❏ other: _____

Sport: _____

Treatment date: _____

Treatment received: _____

Comments or notes: _____

Status: _____ Certified athletic trainer: _____

Treatment date: _____

Treatment received: _____

Comments or notes: _____

Status: _____ Certified athletic trainer: _____

Treatment date: _____

Treatment received: _____

Comments or notes: _____

Status: _____ Certified athletic trainer: _____

Treatment date: _____

Treatment received: _____

Comments or notes: _____

Status: _____ Certified athletic trainer: _____

From *Fundamentals of Athletic Training, Third Edition,* by Lorin A. Cartwright and William A. Pitney, 2011, Champaign, IL: Human Kinetics.

Appendix F

Crisis Plan Practice

Crisis plan for: _____

Address: _____

_____

Written by: _____

Date: _____ Practice date: _____

1. Who is in charge of assessing an injury and beginning first aid until the proper help arrives?

   1. _____
   2. _____
   3. _____
   4. _____

2. Are both an emergency phone number and money for a pay phone available?

   ❑ The numbers have been confirmed before the start of the event.

   ❑ Money for an emergency phone call is inside the training kits.

   ❑ Cellular phone battery is charged and the bill has been paid on time.

   ❑ Home and work phone contacts for all parents have been obtained.

3. Who will call for an ambulance? _____

   Emergency telephone procedures are posted in the following locations:

   _____

   _____

4. Who will control the crowd? _____

5. Who will bring supplies and equipment, and what supplies are needed?

   _____

   _____

6. Who will transport or assist the athlete from the field of play?

   _____

7. Where is the safest and easiest access for emergency services to the area where the injured athlete is?

   Name of area: _____

   Access: _____

From *Fundamentals of Athletic Training, Third Edition*, by Lorin A. Cartwright and William A. Pitney, 2011, Champaign, IL: Human Kinetics.

8. Who will direct the emergency services to the injured athlete?

_____

_____

9. Who will notify the parents that their child has been injured?

_____

_____

10. If more than one athlete is injured, what area will be used to sort the severity of injuries, and how will athletes get to this facility?

    Name of area: _____

    Location: _____

11. What personnel are available in the event of a mass casualty?

_____

_____

12. Who will fill out an accident report form and get statements from other witnesses?

_____

13. Explain how the emergency medical response team work will around known obstacles.

_____

_____

_____

_____

14. What are the evacuation procedures? _____

_____

_____

_____

15. What should be done if someone forgets what to do? _____

_____

_____

16. Who should talk to the press? _____

17. Who will give counseling to those who need it?

_____

_____

_____

_____

Appendix G

Emergency telephone procedures		
Agency	**Information**	**Notes**
Ambulance	1. Give your name and title. Give a phone number where you can be reached. 2. Give the address and exact location of the injured. 3. Explain the nature of the injury and what you need. 4. Tell what is being done for the injured and the qualifications of the person giving care. 5. Give the telephone number from which you are calling. 6. Give the nearest crossroads. 7. Tell how many athletes are injured. 8. Do not hang up first. After the call is completed, be sure to have someone waiting at the door to escort the EMT to the athlete. Document the time of the telephone call.	
Hospital emergency room	1. Give your name and title. 2. Give the reason for your call (be specific about the injury). 3. Estimate the time of arrival of the injured.	
Parents	1. Give your name and title. 2. Document the name of the parent you spoke to and the time. 3. Use the athlete's name and tell the parents what the athlete was doing when she was injured. 4. Tell them what body part was injured and how it is being treated. 5. Give the exact location of the athlete and directions to that location so her parents can find her. 6. Tell the parents what you think is needed. 7. Ask which physician or hospital should be involved. 8. Ask how to transport the injured athlete. 9. Give them the training room phone number in case they need to call.	

Source: Karren, Hafen, Limmer & Mistovich (2004), Prentice (2011), and American Red Cross (2006b).

Glossary

ABCs—Airway, breathing, and circulation. These are the first three things to check after determining that a person is unresponsive.

abduction—Movement away from the midline of the body.

acetabulum—The bones that form the hip socket.

Achilles tendon—Structure that attaches the gastrocnemius muscle to the calcaneus bone of the foot.

acne—A skin condition caused by clogging of the sebaceous glands at the site of hair follicles.

active–assistive range of motion (AAROM)—The range of motion through which the athlete can move her limb with the help of the AT.

active range of motion (AROM)—The range through which the athlete can move his limb unassisted.

adduction—Movement toward the midline of the body.

allergist—A physician who specializes in determining the substances to which a person is allergic and treating such allergies.

allergy—A condition in which a person has a low tolerance for pollen, ragweed, dogs, cats, specific foods, and so on. These often trigger an allergic reaction, typically a sudden runny nose; congestion; red, itchy eyes; and sneezing.

alternating current (AC)—An electrical current that changes direction as it moves back and forth between electrodes.

alveoli—The lung tissue where the gas exchange of oxygen and carbon dioxide occurs.

ambulatory—Able to walk independently or with light support.

amenorrhea—Absence of a menstrual cycle for three or more months.

American Red Cross—A national organization that certifies people in first aid and CPR. The American Red Cross also sponsors services such as disaster relief for communities throughout the world.

amino acid—The basic component of protein.

amnesia—Loss of memory, usually due to a head injury.

amphiarthrodial joint—A joint of cartilage that links bones that don't move much, such as where the ribs join the sternum.

anabolic steroids—A group of synthetic male hormones. Athletes use anabolic steroids to build muscle and recover from workouts more quickly, which allows them to increase their workload.

anatomical position—A standing posture with the arms at the sides and palms facing forward.

anatomy—The science of how the body is organized, concentrating on bones, joints, muscles, and organs and their arrangements.

androstenedione—A steroid that increases one's testosterone level.

anemia—A condition in which fewer red blood cells than normal are in the circulatory system. May be caused by bleeding.

angina pectoris—Pain commonly felt around the heart and chest cavity caused by lack of oxygen to the heart muscle.

annulus fibrosus—The rings of tissue that surround the nucleus pulposus of an intervertebral disk.

anorexia nervosa—A serious eating disorder marked by a pathological fear of weight gain and a loss of appetite. The anorexic has a low body weight and low body fat but may exercise excessively and avoid eating.

anterior—Pertaining to the front of the body.

anterior cruciate ligament (ACL)—A knee ligament that keeps the tibia from moving forward on the femur.

apnea—The temporary cessation of breathing.

appendicular skeleton—The bones of the extremities (shoulders, arms, hands, legs, feet, and pelvis).

arthroscopic surgery—A type of surgery performed on a joint using only small puncture holes to insert instruments, including a camera, to observe and fix injured structures.

articulate—The coming together of two bones to form a joint.

aseptic meningitis—A viral inflammation of the coverings of the brain.

assumption of risk—When an athlete fully understands that she may be injured by participating in sport.

asthma—A condition in which the air passages contract in response to an allergy. The contraction may close the air passage entirely.

ATC—A credential awarded by the BOC after a person has met the AT education requirements and passed the BOC national examination.

athletic trainer—See *certified athletic trainer.*

athletic training—An allied medical profession that is dedicated to maintaining and improving the health and well-being of the physically active population and preventing athletics-related injuries and illnesses.

atrium—One of two upper chambers of the heart that receive blood from the veins and force it into the ventricles.

avascular necrosis—The death of body tissue from lack of blood.

axial load—End-to-end loading of a bone or series of vertebrae. This term is commonly used to denote loading of the cervical spine when a player makes contact with the top of his head.

axial skeleton—The bones of the body that compose the spine, chest, and head.

backboarding—The process of securing an athlete to a spine board in order to stabilize the victim when a spine injury is suspected.

ball-and-socket joint—A joint in which a rounded bone fits into a cuplike socket and swivels. Examples include the hip and shoulder joints. Also called a *multiaxial joint.*

ballistic stretching—A bouncing movement used to lengthen or stretch tissue. Ballistic stretching is not recommended and may cause injury.

battle sign—A discoloration behind the ear resulting from a skull fracture.

beta-adrenergic drugs—Drugs used to control the release of chemicals during an asthma attack by maintaining the airway.

bile—A substance produced by the liver and stored in the gallbladder that assists in the digestion of fat in the small intestine.

biomechanics—The study of the movement of living creatures.

blister—A skin wound characterized by a fluid-filled lesion caused by friction.

blowout—A type of fracture caused when the thin bones beneath the eye absorb the sudden increase in pressure from an impact.

Board of Certification (BOC)—The national organization that examines and certifies athletic trainers so they can practice as ATs.

body temperature—The temperature at which bodily processes take place, normally 98.6° Fahrenheit (37 °C).

boutonniere deformity—A structural irregularity that occurs at the PIP joint of the fingers. A hard impact over the PIP joint can cause a tear in the joint capsule, which will allow the extensor tendons to fall laterally. When the tendons are in the lateral position, they contract and force flexion of the distal interphalangeal joint.

boxer's fracture—A fracture to the metacarpal region, specifically to the fourth or fifth metacarpal as a result of punching.

breathing rate—The number of breaths taken per minute. Normal breathing rate is 12 to 20 breaths per minute.

bronchitis—An inflammation of the bronchial passages, which can be caused by an infection or an allergy.

bulimia nervosa—An eating disorder characterized by bouts of bingeing and self-induced vomiting.

bunion—Excessive deviation or valgus stress at the great toe. Also known as hallux valgus.

burner—A group of symptoms including burning, numbness, tingling, and pain down the arm that results from stretching a group of nerves called the *brachial plexus*. This condition is also called a *stinger.*

bursa—A fluid-filled sac between a tendon and a bone that eases the friction of muscle movement.

bursitis—Inflammation of a bursa sac often characterized by swelling.

calcaneus—The heel bone of the foot.

callus—A mass of connective tissue that forms at the site of a fracture and is converted into bone or a thickening of skin in response to repeated stress.

caloric balance—The relationship between calories ingested and calories expended.

Canadian Standards Association (CSA)—The committee that sets the standards for eye guards and ice hockey helmets.

capillary refill—Blood moving back into the end of a finger or toe after it has been pinched for a moment.

capital femoral epiphysis—The growth plate located between the head and the neck of the femur. It can be fractured, especially in young athletes.

cardiac arrest—When the heart stops beating.

cardiac tamponade—A critical injury whereby fluid fills the sac surrounding the heart.

cardiologist—A physician with specialized knowledge of the cardiovascular system.

cardiopulmonary resuscitation (CPR)—Used when the heart stops. One CPR cycle for an adult is 30 chest compressions and two slow breaths.

cardiorespiratory endurance—The ability to sustain exercise over a long time.

carotid artery—One of two vessels that run from the aorta through the neck and supply the head with oxygenated blood.

carpal tunnel syndrome—A chronic condition caused by compression of the medial nerve where it runs through the carpal tunnel at the anterior aspect of the wrist.

caudal—A point that is lower than another; synonymous with *inferior*.

cauliflower ear—A condition that occurs when the pinna (the projecting portion of the external ear) begins to bleed internally after an impact, causing swelling, redness, and pain. As the ear heals, an excessive growth of reparative tissue distorts the pinna, making it look like a piece of cauliflower.

cephalic—Toward the head; synonymous with *superior*.

cerebral palsy (CP)—A disorder that affects the brain before, during, or shortly after birth and inhibits normal brain development.

cerebrospinal fluid—A liquid from the blood that maintains uniform pressure within the brain, bathes the brain in chemicals for proper functioning, and protects the brain from impacts.

certification—An acknowledgment by an organization or certification board stating that a person possesses specific skills and competencies.

certified athletic trainer (AT)—A person who is concerned with the health and well-being of the physically active and athletic population. The AT's credentials are *ATC*.

cervical spine—The seven vertebrae that compose the uppermost region of the spine.

checkrein—A taping procedure whereby a piece of tape is looped around the thumb and index finger to prevent the thumb from being forcefully abducted.

chicken pox (varicella)—A childhood disease characterized by flulike symptoms and a spotted rash.

chiropractor—Medical personnel who treats mainly musculoskeletal disorders and restores normal function by manipulating bones, specifically at the spinal column.

cholesterol—A fatlike substance produced within the body to perform essential cellular functions.

chondromalacia—The softening or wearing away of the cartilage that lies on the back of the patella.

circuit training—A weight training method whereby a person rotates through a series of 8 to 20 exercises. It is a full-body workout that elevates the heart rate.

circumduction—The movement of a limb in a circular pattern. Occurs when a ball-and-socket joint (shoulder or hip) encompasses several directions with one motion.

closed kinetic chain—When a segment, such as the foot or hand, is in contact with the ground and bearing weight.

code of ethics—A series of behaviors and beliefs that articulate how professionals are to act.

Colles' fracture—A fracture of the radius and ulna whereby the limb bends into extension at the fracture site.

common cold (coryza)—An illness caused by many common viruses and characterized by runny nose, sneezing, and coughing.

concussion—Temporarily impaired brain function caused by a jarring impact to the head or by a rotational force of the head.

conduction—The transfer of heat between two objects in contact with one another.

conjunctiva—The membrane lining of the eye.

conjunctivitis—An infection and inflammatory response affecting the conjunctiva. Often called *pink eye*.

constrict—To narrow an opening or a blood vessel.

contrecoup—An injury that occurs when the head is moving and hits an unyielding surface or object. Upon impact the brain is forced to the side opposite the blow.

convection—The transfer of heat from the movement of a medium. An example of a medium is water.

corneal abrasion—An abrasion or laceration caused by a poke in the eye by a foreign object or by wearing contact lenses too long.

crepitus—A grinding sound that is heard by the athlete, AT, or both. Crepitus can indicate a fracture, cartilage wear, or severe joint inflammation.

crisis plan—The organized action that people should take if an emergency arises. It is also called an *emergency plan*.

cryotherapy—The use of cold on a body part during treatment or rehabilitation.

deep—Away from the body's surface.

DeLorme method—A weight training regimen consisting of three sets of 10 repetitions performed at successively greater intensities.

dentist—A medical specialist who treats primarily teeth and gums.

depression (anatomical)—When a bony segment is moved in an inferior direction.

depression (psychological)—A feeling of hopelessness. Severe depression may need to be observed and treated by a physician, in which case it is referred to as *clinical depression.*

de Quervain's tendinitis—An inflammation that affects the abductor pollicis longus and extensor pollicis brevis as they pass through the wrist.

dermis—A layer that helps hold the skin to underlying bone and muscle tissue.

detached retina—A condition in which the retina of the eye is torn from its normal position. An athlete with a detached retina will have difficulty seeing and requires a physician's care.

diabetes—A disease whereby the pancreas does not secrete insulin effectively or the body is resistant to insulin.

diabetic coma—A condition that occurs when there is not enough insulin to control the sugar in the blood.

diaphragm—The muscle located between the chest and the abdomen that contracts and relaxes to assist with breathing.

diarthrodial joint—A freely movable joint, such as the shoulder. This kind of joint has a joint capsule, a synovial membrane, cartilage, and ligaments.

diastolic pressure—The pressure in the arteries when the heart is resting. Normal diastolic pressure is 80 mmHg.

dietitian (registered)—A specialist concerned with the dietary needs of people.

dilate—To widen an opening or a blood vessel.

dimethyl sulfoxide (DMSO)—A veterinary medicine used to enhance tissue healing. Animal research found that DMSO decreased healing time and wound swelling. Though used by some athletes, there is no indication that it works on humans.

direct current (DC)—Electricity that moves in one direction as it passes through the circuit.

direct pressure—External pressure applied to an open bleeding wound.

disability—A physical or mental impairment that substantially limits one or more major life activities.

dislocation—An injury that disrupts the alignment of bones at a joint, resulting in obvious deformity.

disordered eating—Abnormal eating patterns, often either bulimia or anorexia.

distal—Away from the attachment of a limb.

dorsal—The posterior aspect (back) of a structure.

dorsal aortic rupture—A rupture of the aorta at the dorsal aspect of the heart.

drug—Any substance other than food or water that changes the body's chemistry when it is ingested or applied topically.

duty of care—Having a responsibility to care for an injured person.

dynamic stretching—Moving a limb or part of the body through its range of motion. Swinging the leg forward and backward is an example.

dysmenorrhea—Painful menstrual cycles.

dyspnea—Difficult or labored breathing.

edema—Tissue swelling caused by high levels of protein-based fluid.

effleurage—Massage that involves stroking the tissue with the palm of the hand in a smooth, rhythmical manner.

elastic tape—A flexible tape made of stretchy nylon fibers.

elastic wraps—Stretchy strips of cloth that come in various widths. They are most commonly applied to the body to provide compression around a joint or injured area.

elevation—When a bony segment is moved in a superior direction.

emergency medical technician (EMT)—Someone who is certified to treat and transport people who are ill or injured.

endurance—The ability to withstand fatigue and tolerate prolonged activity.

ephedra—A drug used for weight loss that has been banned by the FDA.

epidermis—The most superficial layer of skin.

epilepsy—A disorder marked by disturbed electrical rhythms of the central nervous system.

epiphysis (growth plate)—The area of the bone where growth occurs.

epistaxis—A bloody nose.

equipment manager—The person responsible for assigning and fitting appropriate playing equipment to athletes.

ergonomics specialist—A person who measures, modifies, and adapts a work environment to prevent injuries.

esophagus—The passage at the back of the throat that carries food from the mouth to the stomach.

evaporation—The process that cools the body.

eversion—A movement that turns the sole of the foot outward, away from the midline of the body.

extension—A straightening movement around a joint to restore it to anatomical position. The anatomical position of the knee, for example, is straight.

extrication—The removal of an injured person from a dangerous situation in order to provide further care without causing more harm.

failure point—The amount of force required to cause a fracture.

fasciitis—Inflammation of the facial tissue.

fat pad syndrome—A condition whereby the fat pad of the knee becomes trapped between the patella and the femur. Often referred to as *Hoffa's syndrome.*

female athlete triad syndrome—A collection of symptoms and decreased bone health caused by disordered eating, amenorrhea, and osteoporosis.

fiber—Indigestible material found in foods high in carbohydrate.

fibrillation—When the heart beats in an extremely rapid fashion and fails to contract properly.

fibroblasts—Connective tissue cells that begin building fibers across an area of injury. They form the scar and take about six weeks to accomplish their task.

fibrous joint—A synarthrodial joint.

flail chest—An injury whereby several consecutive ribs are fractured in two or more places.

flexibility—The ability to move a joint through a full range of motion without restriction.

flexion—A bending movement around a joint in a limb away from its straightened position.

folliculitis—An inflammation of a follicle, especially of a hair follicle.

forward head posture—When the head juts forward so that the athlete's ears are not lined up with the shoulders.

fracture—A break in a bone.

friction massage—Massage using deep, penetrating pressure into the tissue with movement of the finger, thumb, or elbow.

frontal plane—The plane that separates the body into front and back halves.

furuncle—An infection in a skin gland that forms a bright red lump that hurts when touched. It is also known as a boil.

gamma hydroxybutyrate (GHB)—A central nervous system depressant also known as a club drug.

gamekeeper's thumb—An injury to the MCL of the thumb.

ganglion cyst—A pocket of fluid within the sheath of the wrist.

gastrocnemius—A large muscle at the back of the lower leg responsible for pointing the toes.

girth—The distance around a body part.

glenoid labrum—A cartilage disk that surrounds the edge of the scapular fossa and deepens the socket in which the head of the humerus inserts.

goniometer—A device that measures range of motion at joints.

gross negligence—A step beyond negligence whereby a person fails to even minimal care when needed.

gynecologist—A physician who specializes in the diagnosis and treatment of diseases of the female reproductive system.

hallux valgus—Excessive valgus stress at the great toe, also known as a bunion.

hammertoe—A deformity in which the middle joint of the toe is flexed and the metatarsophalangeal and distal phalangeal joints are hyperextended.

hamstrings—The name given collectively to the semimembranosus, semitendinosus, and biceps femoris muscles, which are responsible for flexing the knee and extending the hip.

heart attack—A injury to the heart that occurs when a blocked vessel to the heart, a clot, stress over a period of time, or an injury to the heart muscle itself creates an insufficient blood supply.

heart rate—The number of times the heart beats in a minute; often measured as the pulse in a superficial artery. The normal pulse rate for a teenager is between 60 and 80 beats per minute.

heat cramps—A mild heat-related illness marked by sudden muscular contractions that will not release because the necessary minerals and water are not available.

heat exhaustion—A moderate heat-related illness caused by exercising in a hot, humid environment. Effects are weakness, nausea, dizziness, and profuse sweating, causing dehydration with excessive sodium loss through sweat.

heat index—The combined measurement of air temperature and humidity. It indicates how safe it is to participate in activities and the body's ability to dissipate heat on a particular day.

heatstroke—A severe heat-related illness caused by prolonged exposure to high temperature and humidity and marked by the hypothalamus shutting down, which causes body temperature to rise dangerously. Secondary causes of heatstroke include dehydration, excessive weight loss, obesity, alcoholism, CP, and diabetes.

heat syncope—Fainting due to heat exposure.

heel spur—A small, pointy, bony growth at the bottom of the calcaneus; often caused by plantar fasciitis.

hematoma—A collection of blood at an anatomical site.

hemiplegia—The loss of sensation and muscular function on one side of the body that results from injury to or disease of the motor processes of the brain.

hemophilia—A hereditary blood disorder characterized by delayed clotting of the blood.

hemothorax—Blood in the chest cavity.

hepatitis B virus (HBV)—A virus that tends to persist in the blood and causes an infection in the liver.

hernia—A lump of tissue, usually the intestine, that bulges through a weakness in the abdominal wall.

herpes—A highly contagious skin condition caused by a virus.

hinge joint—An articulation whereby the joint is able to move primarily in flexion and extension. An example of a hinge joint is the knee or elbow.

hip bursitis—Irritation of the greater trochanteric bursa of the hip; often caused by rubbing of the musculature.

hip pointer—A contusion to the iliac crest.

history—The portion of the assessment process consisting of understanding the injured athlete's chief complaint, determining exactly how the injury occurred, assessing functional problems that exist, noting signs and symptoms, and determining preexisting medical conditions.

HIT—An injury assessment process that follows this sequence: **h**istory, **i**nspection, and **t**esting.

Hoffa's syndrome—A condition whereby the fat pad of the knee becomes trapped between the patella and the femur. Often referred to as *fat pad syndrome*.

human growth hormone (HGH)—Protein-based hormone used to stimulate muscle growth.

human immunodeficiency virus (HIV)—A virus known to cause AIDS, which affects the body's ability to fight infection and disease.

hyaline cartilage—A thin layer of cartilage that covers the ends of a bone where it articulates with another bone.

hybrid tape—Tape made from both linen and elastic.

hyperglycemia—A condition in which the blood sugar level is too high.

hypertension—Abnormally high blood pressure, especially arterial pressure.

hyperthermia—Excessive buildup of heat within the body; an exceptionally high fever.

hyperventilation—Excessive rate and depth of breathing (24 breaths or more per minute).

hyphema—An injury to the eye that causes blood to flow into the anterior chamber.

hypoglycemia—A condition in which the blood sugar level is too low.

hyponatremia—Low blood sodium level.

hypotension—Abnormally low blood pressure.

hypothermia—Subnormal body temperature from prolonged exposure to damp cold.

immune system—The internal defense mechanisms of the body.

impetigo—A skin disease characterized by itching and the development of a yellow crusted exterior.

impingement syndrome—A collection of symptoms caused by compression of either the biceps tendon or supraspinatus tendon below the acromion of the shoulder.

infectious mononucleosis—A viral disease, often referred to as *mono*, characterized by headache, extreme fatigue, fever, and body aches. It can result in enlargement of the spleen.

inferior—One point, or structure, being lower than another.

influenza—The medical name for the flu.

informed consent—Permission by parents, after being informed of the possible dangers of participation in athletic activities, for medical staff to treat their child if he is injured.

ingrown toenail—An injury whereby the nail grows into the surrounding soft tissue.

insulin shock—A condition resulting in low blood sugar levels caused by too much insulin.

intermittent compression—A device with a built-in sleeve that fits over a body part. The sleeve periodically fills with air and applies compression to the area to reduce swelling.

intervertebral disks—Structures between the vertebrae that cushion them.

intracranial hematoma—Severe bleeding within the brain caused by a blow to the head.

inversion—A movement that turns the sole of the foot inward toward the midline of the body.

isokinetic contraction—The muscular force applied against a machine that allows the joint to move only at a specific speed.

isometric contraction—A movement that causes the muscle to contract against resistance without changing its length.

isotonic contraction—A movement that causes the muscle fibers to shorten and lengthen against resistance when lifting and lowering a weight.

jersey finger—An injury of the finger in which the flexor tendon tears from the fingertip.

joint capsule—A sac or sleevelike structure that covers a joint. The capsule has a synovial membrane containing synovial fluid to ease joint movement.

Jones fracture—A fracture occurring at the base of the fifth metatarsal bone.

jugular vein—One of two vessels that takes unoxygenated blood from the head to the heart.

Kehr's sign—Pain in the abdomen and the left shoulder that most often indicates injury to the spleen.

kinesiology—The study of human movement.

kyphosis—Excessive roundedness that can occur at the thoracic spine.

labrum—Cartilaginous tissue that deepens the sockets at the hip and shoulder joints.

laryngitis—Inflammation of the larynx.

larynx—An enlarged tube at the top of the trachea made of cartilage and muscle. The voice is created by air passing through the vocal cords in the larynx.

lateral—Away from the midline of the body.

lateral malleolus—The most prominent aspect of the fibula; located on the lateral aspect of the ankle.

Legg-Calvé-Perthes disease—A condition found in some children that is characterized by a disruption of blood flow to the head of the femur, which causes the tissue at the head of the femur to die.

leukocytes—Infection-fighting white blood cells that go to the site of an injury.

leukoplakia—Precancerous cells often found on the cheek, tongue, and gums of those who use smokeless tobacco.

licensure—A state act that specifies who is allowed to practice athletic training and what duties they are allowed to perform.

ligaments—Tissues in the body that connect bone to bone.

linen tape—Tape made from cotton fibers.

Little League elbow—An injury to the medial aspect of the elbow in young throwing athletes, usually from overuse.

local steroid—A drug that is applied to the skin or injected in a joint to reduce swelling and pain; it should not be confused with anabolic steroids.

lordosis—Excessive curvature at the lumbar spine.

lumbar spine—The five vertebrae that compose the low back; located just above the sacrum.

mallet finger—An injury to the fingertip caused by impact that tears the extensor tendon from the bone. Fingertip flexion is the distinguishing feature of this injury.

massage—Kneading and stroking of muscles and other soft tissue by the AT or massage therapist for therapeutic purposes.

massage therapist—A person who administers massage for therapeutic purposes.

medial—Toward the midline of the body.

medial malleolus—The end of the tibia on the medial side.

meniscectomy—A surgical procedure to remove the meniscus from the knee joint.

meniscus—A piece of cartilage within a joint, especially those pieces known as the medial and lateral menisci, which lie between the femur and the tibia.

metabolism—The body's energy system.

metatarsals—The five longest bones of the foot.

microorganism—An organism of microscopic or submicroscopic size such as a virus or bacteria.

moleskin—A thick, soft, sticky tape that cannot be torn by hand.

molluscum contagiosum—A skin condition caused by a virus. It is characterized by the formation of pink lumps.

MRSA—Methicillin-resistant *Staphylococcus aureus* bacterial infection.

multiaxial joint—A joint that has a large range of movement because it can move in a variety of planes.

multiple sclerosis—A condition whereby the myelin sheath detaches from parts of the central nervous system, leading to erratic conduction of electrical impulses.

mumps—A viral illness characterized by swelling around the jawline.

muscular dystrophy—A group of disorders that affect the muscles by replacing muscle cells with connective tissue.

muscular endurance—The ability of a muscle to perform repetitive movements for an extended period. It can be developed by using a high number of repetitions and a small amount of weight.

muscular power—The ability to exert force quickly.

muscular strength—The ability to exert force against a resistance. It can be developed by using a low number of repetitions and heavy weight.

myositis ossificans—The buildup of bone tissue in a muscle following an injury.

myositis—A chronic inflammation of the muscle tissue.

National Athletic Trainers' Association (NATA)—The professional association that recognizes ATs as its primary members and establishes codes of professional conduct.

National Operating Committee on Standards for Athletic Equipment (NOCSAE)—A committee that sets the standards for football, baseball, and softball helmets.

National Safety Council—An organization that certifies people in first aid and CPR procedures.

neck roll—Protective padding that keeps the head within a safe range of motion.

negligence—A legal wrong characterized by the failure to act as a reasonably prudent person would act in a similar situation.

neurocognitive testing—Systematic, objective procedures used to examine the function of the brain. These tests are often computer based and used to create baseline performance measures that are then compared with postconcussion performance to determine if an athlete can return to play.

neurologist—A physician who specializes in the diagnosis and treatment of disease of the nervous system.

neutral spine—Normal cervical, thoracic, and lumbar curvature having neither too much flexion nor too much extension in a position that is comfortable for the athlete.

No HARM—An acronym that denotes using **no** **h**eat, **a**lcohol, **r**unning, or **m**assage to an injury.

nonsteroidal anti-inflammatory drug (NSAID)—A drug used to reduce tissue swelling after an injury.

nonunion—A fracture that does not heal, leaving two pieces of bone where there was one before.

nucleus pulposus—The soft structure at the center of an intervertebral disk.

nutrients—Substances in food that the body uses in metabolism.

nutrition—The processes that use food to fulfill the metabolic needs of the body.

one-repetition maximum (1RM)—The amount of weight an athlete can lift for only one repetition.

open kinetic chain—When a segment, such as the foot or hand, is moving freely in space (not in contact with the ground) and not bearing weight.

opposition—Occurs when you move your thumb across your hand to meet your smallest finger, or fifth digit.

organization and administration—An aspect of athletic training that emphasizes management.

orthopedist—A physician who deals primarily with conditions and injuries of the musculoskeletal system.

Osgood-Schlatter disorder—A condition characterized by an irritation or loosening of the patellar tendon at its attachment at the top anterior aspect of the tibia, usually seen in younger athletes who perform a great deal of running and jumping.

osteoporosis—Deterioration of the bone.

overload principle—A strength and conditioning principle based on the idea that in order for muscles to get stronger, they must be challenged to lift more than they are used to lifting.

palpation—Examination of an injured area by touch to determine the type of injury, such as fracture, swelling, muscle ruptures, and tendinitis. Palpation also gives an indication of the athlete's pain level.

paraffin bath—Heated wax that is used to warm a body area, such as a hand or foot.

paralysis—The inability to move.

paraplegia—The loss of sensation and muscular function in the lower extremities caused by an injury of the spinal cord.

partial airway obstruction—When a portion of the airway is closed off by an object in the throat.

passive range of motion (PROM)—The extent to which an injured body part can be moved by the AT without pain to or exertion from the athlete.

patellar tendinitis—Inflammation of the patellar tendon; often called *jumper's knee.*

pediatrician—A specialist in the medical treatment of children.

percussion massage—Massage using light chopping motions to the tissue.

petrissage—A massage stroke that squeezes the skin, muscles, and fasciae between the hands; it is often described as kneading the tissue.

phagocytes—Specialized white blood cells that clear dead cells from the site of an injury.

phalanges—The small bones that make up the fingers and toes.

pharmacology—The science of drugs and their effects on the body.

phlegm—A thick mucus secreted in the respiratory passages in response to allergy or infection. The body expels it by coughing.

physical therapist—An allied medical professional who specializes in rehabilitation of orthopedic and nonorthopedic conditions.

physician assistant—An allied medical professional works directly under the supervision of a physician and conducts examinations, orders diagnostic tests, writes prescriptions, and diagnoses and treats injuries and illnesses.

physics—A science that deals with energy and matter.

physiology—A branch of biology that deals with cells and organ systems and how they function.

plantar fasciitis—Inflammation of the plantar fascia of the foot.

plantar surface—The bottom of the foot.

plantar warts—A skin disorder caused by HPV that commonly affects weight-bearing portions of the foot.

platelets—Blood cells that carry blood-clotting materials.

pneumothorax—Air in the chest cavity, commonly referred to as a *collapsed lung*.

podiatrist—A specialist in foot disorders.

posterior—The back of the body.

posterior cruciate ligament (PCL)—A knee ligament that prevents the tibia from moving posteriorly on the femur.

post-traumatic response—An emotional disorder resulting from a traumatic experience.

PREMIER model—A framework for thinking about being a professional: **P**romote a professional image. **R**emember your vision. **E**ngage in learning. **M**aximize your strengths. **I**nnovate and create. **E**nlist the help of others. **R**eflect on your actions.

pressure point—A place on the body where arteries, such as the brachial artery and the femoral artery, are easily accessed and pressure can be applied with the hand to slow the blood flow to a body part.

PRICES—An acronym for **p**rotection, **r**est, **i**ce, **c**ompression, **e**levation and **s**upport of an injured body part that represents the initial steps of care for musculoskeletal injuries such as ligament sprains or muscle strains.

primary assessment—The aspect of assessment devoted to determining if an athlete has a clear airway, is breathing, and has a pulse.

primary care physician—The athlete's primary doctor. She must be notified after an athlete is injured.

progression—The advancement of an exercise or activity from simple to complex, slow to fast, and less aggressive to more aggressive.

progressive resistive exercise (PRE)—The gradual progression of an exercise from easy to more difficult from one set to the next and over time.

pronation—A movement that turns the palm of the hand down as if it were emptying a bowl of soup.

proprioception—The ability of the body to give information to the brain regarding the body's position, movements being performed, and forces acting on it.

prosthetic—An artificial body part.

protraction—Movement of the scapulas away from one another; the opposite of retraction.

proximal—Toward the attachment of the limb to the trunk.

proximate cause—A close connection between the act of a certified AT and resulting injury to an athlete.

psychology—The science of human mental processes such as behavior and personality.

pulse points—Areas where arteries lie close to the skin.

pulse pressure—The difference between the diastolic and systolic pressures.

pulse rate—The number of times the heart beats per minute, normally 60 to 80 per minute, taken at the wrist or neck.

pyramid method—A strength training regimen that involves multiple sets whereby the first set is low intensity, the second set is moderate intensity, the third set is intense, then the fourth set is back to moderate intensity, and the fifth set is low intensity.

quadriplegia—The inability to move the arms and legs.

reconditioning—Getting the athlete back into shape for athletic participation.

recreational drug—A drug that has no medical purpose.

registration—The step of contacting state authorities before acting in the capacity of an AT. It is required by law in some states.

rehabilitation—The process or means of getting a person back to his normal level of function following an injury or illness.

reposition—means simply returning your thumb and fifth digit to their starting position.

resistance training—An organized program to work the muscles, usually by lifting weights.

retraction—When the scapulas are moved, or pulled, together.

rotation—The spinning or turning movement of a bony segment around an axis.

rotator cuff—A group of muscles around the shoulder joint. The muscles of the rotator cuff are the supraspinatus, infraspinatus, teres minor, and subscapularis.

rubella—A form of measles often referred to as *German measles*. It is characterized by a rash and itching.

rubeola—A form of measles characterized by high fever, chills, rash (even inside the mouth), and coughing.

ruptured eardrum—A tear of the tympanic membrane.

sacrum—The bottommost segment of the spine, which consists of bones that are fused.

sagittal plane—A plane that divides the body into left and right halves.

school nurse—A licensed nurse who provides services to a school or school district.

scoliosis—Excessive side-to-side curvature of the spine.

second-impact syndrome—A set of symptoms resulting from more than one concussion or blow to the head in a relatively short time.

seizure—Uncontrollable shaking resulting from a brain chemical imbalance or head injury.

shin splints—A term for pain of the lower leg, often along the tibia. It is often called *medial tibial stress syndrome*.

shoulder separation—A sprain of the acromioclavicular joint.

sickle cell anemia—An inherited disease in which the red blood cells become shaped like sickles with points on each end, which causes the cells to hook onto the sides of the blood vessels, creating a logjam of cells in a particular area. The result is that oxygen is not carried efficiently to all parts of the body.

sign—Objective evidence that a rescuer can measure or sense, such as sweating, breath odor, temperature, blood pressure, breathing rate, heart rate, and so on.

SITS—An acronym for the muscles of the rotator cuff—**s**upraspinatus, **i**nfraspinatus, **t**eres minor, and **s**ubscapularis.

SOAP note—A document outlining the findings of an injury assessment using **s**ubjective, **o**bjective, **a**ssessment, and **p**lan-of-action components.

soleus—a posterior lower leg muscle that plantar flexes the foot.

specificity—The principle stating that the type of activity a person performs in training is the type of activity she will get better at performing.

spondylolisthesis—A spondylolysis degeneration of a vertebra that fails to heal, therefore separating and causing the spine to become unstable. The resulting instability allows a vertebra to shunt, or slip, forward on the vertebra below it.

spondylolysis—A stress fracture or bone degeneration of the vertebrae.

sport psychologist—A professional who works with athletes who may need help with goal setting, anxiety, frustration, self-esteem, family issues, and more.

sport psychology—The science of how variables such as life stress, mood, and motivation affect sport performance and sport-related injury.

sports medicine—A broad term that refers to the care of the physically active who have suffered an athletics-related injury or illness.

sports medicine team—All of the people who might work with and care for an athlete at one point or another during his participation in athletics.

sport-specific function—Specific exercises and activities that are similar to the activities that the athlete will face upon return to participation.

sprain—Injury to a ligament.

standards of professional practice—The way an AT is expected to act while doing her job.

static stretching—Holding a stretched muscle in one position for a short length of time.

stinger—A group of symptoms including burning, numbness, tingling, and pain down the arm that results from stretching a group of nerves called the *brachial plexus*. This condition is also called a *burner*.

strain—An injury that occurs to a muscle or tendon.

strength and conditioning coach—A person who works with athletes to ensure that each is in shape to meet the demands of athletic competition.

student assistant—A student who volunteers to observe (and assist when deemed appropriate) a certified AT in order to learn more about the profession.

subconjunctival hemorrhage—An athlete may cough hard repeatedly, which causes the small vessels in the eye to rupture, turning the conjunctiva red. An athlete may also get poked in the conjunctiva or hit by a ball, which causes the same result.

sucking chest wound—A puncture injury to the wall of the chest that causes air to be drawn noisily into the chest cavity.

superficial—Close to the body's surface.

superior—One point, or structure, being higher than another.

supination—A movement that turns the palm of the hand up as if it were holding a bowl of soup.

swimmer's ear—An infection that results from water in the ear.

symptom—What the athlete feels but cannot see, smell, or hear, such as pain, nausea, or anxiousness.

synarthrodial joint—A type of joint in which bones are held together by tough connective tissue, making the joint essentially immovable.

syncope—Fainting caused by a lack of blood flow to the brain, such as from standing up quickly.

syndesmosis—The soft tissue that binds the distal ends of the tibia and fibula together.

synovial membrane—A tissue that completely surrounds diarthrodial joints and secretes a slippery fluid.

synovitis—Inflammation of the synovial lining of diarthrodial joints.

systolic pressure—The pressure in the arteries when the heart is beating. Normal systolic pressure is 120 mmHg.

talus—Ankle bone located directly above the calcaneus.

team physician—The medical authority of the sports medicine team whose role is to work with the AT to oversee the entire sports medicine team.

temporomandibular joint (TMJ) dysfunction—A condition in which the muscles surrounding the joint spasm.

tendinitis—Chronic inflammation of a tendon.

tendons—Tissues in the body that connect a muscle to a bone.

tennis elbow—Inflammation of the lateral epicondyle of the elbow, usually from overuse of the wrist extensor muscles.

therapeutic drug—A drug that has a medical purpose.

thoracic—Pertaining to the chest region of the body.

tinea corporis—A red, scaly, ring-shaped abnormality that appears on the skin. It is a fungal skin condition commonly called *ringworm*.

tinea pedis—A fungal infection of the foot commonly called *athlete's foot*.

tinnitus—Ringing in the ears.

total airway obstruction—Complete blockage of the airway by an object that prevents the athlete from speaking, coughing, or breathing.

trachea—A cartilage tube that allows passage of air from the larynx in the throat to the bronchial tube of the lungs.

traction—A pulling force used deliberately to separate joints of the body that have been compressed or gotten stiff.

transcutaneous electrical nerve stimulation (TENS)—The application of an electrical current to the surface of the skin that is designed to stimulate the region.

trans fat—Fatty acids that are created when hydrogen is added to vegetable oil so they are more solid.

transverse plane—The plane that divides the body into top and bottom halves.

triage—The determination of the order in which to send injured patients to the hospital; the most seriously hurt go first.

triangular fibrocartilage complex (TFCC)—An anatomical structure located at the medial aspect of the wrist that supports the carpal bones.

ultrasound—A thermal modality because it can produce a deep-heating effect, break down tissues, or image soft tissues on a screen (used to determine the sex of an unborn baby, for example).

universal choking sign—Grabbing the throat with both hands to indicate choking. People who are choking instinctively do this no matter what their nationality.

universal precautions—A set of procedures designed to prevent the spread of bloodborne diseases.

urologist—A physician who deals with problems of the urinary tract such as painful urination.

vaccinations—Injections of tiny amounts of viruses (sometimes live and sometimes dead) into the body to create an immunity to specific viruses.

valgus—An outward deviation of a body segment.

ventral—The anterior aspect of a structure.

ventricle—A chamber of the heart that receives blood from a corresponding atrium and from which blood is forced into the arteries.

vibration massage—A massage stroke that causes the tissue to tremble or shake vigorously.

vital signs—Signs of life observed and measured during the secondary assessment to determine the seriousness of an injury, including body temperature, skin color, breathing rate, heart rate, response to pain, pupillary reaction, ability to move, and capillary refill.

whirlpool—A tub in which jets of air circulate hot or cold water.

X rays—Electromagnetic waves used to make a picture to aid in diagnosing injuries to bones and joints.

Bibliography

Ability v Ability. 2006. The Stoke Mandeville Games—1948. www.abilityvability.co.uk/files/factsheets/FS3%20-%20The%20Stoke%20Mandeville%20Games%201948.pdf

Academy for eating disorders. 2010. About eating disorders. www.aedweb.org/About_Eating_Disorders/1857.htm

Adams, B.B. 2002. Dermatologic disorders of the athlete. *Sports Medicine* 32(5): 309-321.

Adams, N. 2004. Knee injuries. *Emergency Nurse* 11(10): 19-27.

Abián-Vicén, J., L. Alegre, J. Fernández-Rodríguez, and X. Aguado. 2009. Prophylactic ankle taping: elastic versus inelastic taping. *Foot and Ankle International* 30(3): 218-225.

Aleccia, J. 2010. Smokeless products 2nd most common source of accidents: Tobacco 'mints' tied to kids' poisoning. www.msnbc.msn.com/id/36564107/ns/health-kids_and_parenting/.

Altizer, L. 2003a. Hand and wrist fractures, part I. *Orthopaedic Nursing* 22(2): 131-138.

Altizer, L. 2003b. Hand and wrist fractures, part II. *Orthopaedic Nursing* 22(3): 232-239.

Amato, H.K., and M.J. Warner. 1996. Athletic trainers: leaders in sports. *Athletic Therapy Today* 1(1): 30-32.

American Academy of Orthopaedic Surgeons. 1999. *Emergency care and transportation of the sick and injured.* 7th ed. Boston: Jones and Bartlett.

American Academy of Orthopaedic Surgeons. 1991. *Athletic training and sports medicine.* 2nd ed. Park Ridge, IL: Author.

American Academy of Pediatrics. 2004. Protective eyewear for young athletes. www.sportseyeinjuries.com/docs/Protective_eyewear.pdf.

American College of Sports Medicine. 2007. Exercise and fluid replacement position stand. www.acsm.org/AM/Template.cfm?Section=Home_Page&template=/CM/ContentDisplay.cfm&ContentID=6862.

American College of Sports Medicine (ACSM). 2009. Nutrition and athletic performance. *Medicine and Science in Sports and Exercise* 41(3): 709-733.

American Heart Association. 2010. AHA guidelines for CPR & ECC. *Circulation* 122(318).

American Medical Association. 2001. Principles of medical ethics. www.ama-assn.org/ama/pub/physician-resources/medical-ethics/code-medical-ethics/principles-medical-ethics.shtml.

American Red Cross. 2006a. *CPR/AED for the professional rescuer.* Yardley, PA: Staywell.

American Red Cross. 2006b. *First aid/CPR/AED for schools and the community.* Yardley, PA: Staywell.

Americans with Disabilities Act of 1990 (ADA). 2005. A guide to disability rights laws. www.ada.gov/cguide.htm.

Andersen, J.C., R.W. Courson, D.M. Kleiner, and T.A. McLoda. 2002. National Athletic Trainers' Association position statement: emergency planning in athletics. *Journal of Athletic Training* 37: 99-104.

Anderson, B., and E. Swann. 2009. Insurance and reimbursement: addressing the bottom line. In *Administrative topics in athletic training: concepts to practice*, ed. G.L. Harrelson, G. Gardner, and A.P. Winterstein. Thorofare, NJ: Slack.

Anderson, M.K., S.J. Hall, and M. Martin. 2000. *Sports injury management.* 2nd ed. Philadelphia: Lippincott Williams & Wilkins.

Andrews, J.R., and J.A. Whiteside. 1993. Common elbow problems in the athlete. *Journal of Orthopaedic and Sports Physical Therapy* 17(6): 289-295.

Anthony, C.P., and G.A. Thibodeau. 1983. *Textbook of anatomy and physiology.* St. Louis: Mosby.

Armstrong, L.E., Casa, D.J, Maresh, C. M, and Ganio, M. S. 2007. Caffeine, fluid-electrolyte balance, temperature, and exercise-heat tolerance. *Exercise Sport Science Review* 35(3): 135-140.

Bahr, R., and S. Maehlum, eds. 2004. *Clinical guide to sports injuries.* Champaign, IL: Human Kinetics.

Bailes, J.E., and V. Hudson. 2001. Classification of sport-related head trauma: a spectrum of mild to severe injury. *Journal of Athletic Training* 36(3): 236-243.

Barh, R., and S. Maehlum, eds. 2004. *Clinical guide to sports injuries: an illustrated guide to the management of injuries in physical activity.* Champaign, IL: Human Kinetics.

Barleson, J.B. 2010. Back pain. www.mayoclinic.com/health/acupuncture-for-back-pain/AN02055.

Bauer, A., E. Bluman, M. Wilson, and C. Chiodo. 2009. Injuries of the distal lower extremity syndesmosis. *Current Orthopaedic Practice* 20(2): 111-116.

Beattie, P. 2008. Current understanding of lumbar intervertebral disc degeneration: a review with emphasis upon etiology, pathophysiology, and lumbar magnetic resonance imaging findings. *Journal of Orthopaedic and Sports Physical Therapy* 38(6): 329-340.

Bechtel, M., A. Bechtel, and M. Zirwas. 2009. Skin infections in wrestlers and other athletes. *Emergency Medicine* 41(1): 25-29.

Beduschi, G. 2003. Current popular ergogenic aids used in sports: a critical review. *Nutrition and Dietetics* 60(2): 104-118.

Behnke, R. 2001. *Kinetic anatomy.* Champaign, IL: Human Kinetics.

Behrens, D. 2006. Treatment of epistaxis in the emergency department. *Emergency Medicine Journal* 23(3): 241.

Beltrami, F., T. Hew-Butler, and T. Noakes. 2008. Drinking policies and exercise-associated hyponatraemia: Is anyone still promoting overdrinking? *British Journal of Sports Medicine* 42(10): 496-501.

Binkley, H.M., J. Beckett, D.J. Casa, D.K. Kleiner, and P.E. Plummer. 2002. National Athletic Trainers' Association position statement: exertional heat illnesses. *Journal of Athletic Training* 37(3): 329-343.

Binningsley, D. 2003. Tear of the acetabular labrum in an elite athlete. *British Journal of Sports Medicine* 37(1): 84-88.

Bittencourt, N., L. Mendonca, A. Silva, and S. Fonseca. 2008. Correlation between patellar anatomical alignment and patellar tendinosis. *British Journal of Sports Medicine* 42(6): 509-10.

Blauvelt, C.T., and F. Nelson. 1994. *A manual of orthopaedic terminology*. 5th ed. St. Louis: Mosby.

Boden, B., and C. Jarvis. 2009. Spinal injuries in sports. *Physical Medicine and Rehabilitation Clinics of North America* 20(1): 55-68.

Bonci, C.M., L.J. Bonci, L.R. Granger, C.L. Johnson, R.M. Malina, L.W. Milne, R.R. Ryan, and E.M. Vanderbunt. 2008. National Athletic Trainers' Association position statement: preventing, detecting, and managing disordered eating in athletes. *Journal of Athletic Training* 43(1): 80-108.

Bonza, J., S. Fields, E. Yard, and R. Comstock. 2009. Shoulder injuries among United States high school athletes during the 2005-2006 and 2006-2007 school years. *Journal of Athletic Training* 44(1): 76-83.

Borelli, A. 2009. Engineering a strong pitching elbow: an off-season training plan. *Journal of Strength and Conditioning* 31(2): 64-73

Borrione, P., L. Grasso, F. Quaranta, and A. Parisi. 2009. FIMS position statement 2009: vegetarian diet and athletes. *International SportMed Journal* 10(1): 53-60.

Boyd, J. 1997. *Research update: the PCL-deficient knee*. Paper presented at the Great Lakes Athletic Trainers Association Annual Meeting and Symposium, Minneapolis, March 13, 1997.

Bradley, T., C. Baldwick, D. Fischer, and G. Murrell, G. (2009). Effect of taping on the shoulders of Australian football players. *British Journal of Sports Medicine* 43(10): 735-738.

Brockenbrough, G. 2009. Prescribe less play to prevent elbow injuries in pediatric/adolescent athletes. *Orthopedics Today* 29(6): 28.

Broglio, S., and T. Puetz. 2008. The effect of sport concussion on neurocognitive function, self-report symptoms and postural control: a meta-analysis. *Sports Medicine* 38(1): 53-67.

Bunton, E.E., W.A. Pitney, A.W. Kane, and T.A. Cappaert. 1993. The role of limb torque, muscle action, and proprioception during closed kinetic chain rehabilitation of the lower extremity. *Journal of Athletic Training* 28(1): 10-20.

Bureau of Labor Statistics. 2010. Occupational outlook handbook, 2010-11 edition: athletic trainers. www.bls.gov/oco/ocos294.htm#outlook.

Burnett, R., G. Rocca, H. Prather, M. Curry, W. Maloney, and J. Clohisy. 2006.

Clinical presentation of patients with tears of the acetabular labrum. *Journal of Bone and Joint Surgery, American Volume* 88A(7): 1448-1457.

Cantu, R.C. 2001. Posttraumatic retrograde and anterograde amnesia: Pathophysiology and implications in grading and safe return to play. *Journal of Athletic Training* 36(3): 244-248.

Carcione, J. 2006. Multiple sclerosis exercise. www.webmd.com/multiple-sclerosis/guide/multiple-sclerosis-exercise.

Carlisle, J.C., C.A. Goldfarb, N. Mall, J.W. Powell, and M.J. Matava. 2008. Upper extremity injuries in the National Football League, part II: elbow, forearm, and wrist injuries. *American Journal of Sports Medicine* 36(10): 1945-1952.

Cassidy, R., W. Shaffer, and D. Johnson. 2005. Sports medicine update: spondylolysis and spondylolisthesis in the athlete. *Orthopedics* 28(11): 1331-1333.

Casterline, M., S. Osowski, and G. Ulrich. 1996. Femoral stress fractures. *Journal of Athletic Training* 31(1): 53-56.

Caswell, S.V., and R.G. Deivert. 2002. Lacrosse helmet designs and the effects of impact forces. *Journal of Athletic Training* 37(2): 164-171.

Chew, K., H. Lew, E. Date, and M. Fredericson. 2007. Current evidence and clinical applications of therapeutic knee braces. *American Journal of Physical Medicine and Rehabilitation* 86(8): 678-686.

Children's Hospital of Wisconsin. 2009. Congenital limb defects. www.chw.org/display/PPF/DocID/22566/router.asp.

Chisholm, M.M. 1993. Anxiety. In *Mental health: psychiatric nursing*, ed. R.P. Rawlins, S.R. Williams, and C.K. Beck (3rd ed.). St. Louis: Mosby.

Cialdella-Kam, L., and M. Manore. 2009. Macronutrient needs of active individuals: an update. *Nutrition Today* 44(3): 104-111.

Coleman, E. 1984. Nutrition principles for the child athlete. *Sports Medicine Digest* 6(12): 6.

Collins, C., and R. Comstock. 2008. Epidemiological features of high school baseball injuries in the United States, 2005-2007. *Pediatrics* 121(6): 1181-1187.

Colston, M.A. 2004. Professionalism and ethics. Informed consent: review and implementation. *Athletic Therapy Today* 9(1): 29-31.

Connor, C. 2003. Injury management update: use of an ultrasonic bone-growth stimulator to promote healing of a Jones fracture. *Athletic Therapy Today* 8(1): 37-39.

Cooper, J., J.A. Ellison, and M.M. Walsh. 2003. Spit (smokeless)-tobacco use by baseball players entering the professional ranks. *Journal of Athletic Training* 38(2): 126-132.

Courson, R., and V.N. Mosesso. 2008. Emergency planning for sudden cardiac arrest in athletic programs. *Coaching Women's Basketball* (July): 12-14.

Covassin, T., C.B. Swanik, and M. Sachs. 2003. Sex differences and the incidence of concussions among collegiate athletes. *Journal of Athletic Training* 38(3): 238-244.

Crenshaw, D.A. 1990. *Bereavement*. New York: Continuum.

Croisier, J. 2004. Factors associated with recurrent hamstring injuries. *Sports Medicine* 34(10): 681-695.

Croisier, J., S. Ganteaume, J. Binet, M. Genty, and J. Ferret. 2008. Strength imbalances and prevention of hamstring injury in professional soccer players: a prospective study. *American Journal of Sports Medicine* 36(8): 1469-1475.

Dartmouth University. 1997. *A guide to suicide prevention.* www.dartmouth.edu/~chd/resources/suicide/index.html.

Delahunt, E., J. O'Driscoll, and K. Moran. 2009. Effects of taping and exercise on ankle joint movement in subjects with chronic ankle instability: a preliminary investigation. *Archives of Physical Medicine and Rehabilitation* 90(8): 1418-1422.

Delavier, F. 2001. *Strength training anatomy.* Champaign, IL: Human Kinetics.

Del Rossi, G., M. Horodyski, and M.E. Powers. 2003. A comparison of spine-board transfer techniques and the effect of training on performance. *Journal of Athletic Training* 38(3): 204-208.

Denegar, C.R. 2000. *Therapeutic modalities for athletic injuries.* Champaign, IL: Human Kinetics.

Denegar, C.R., E. Saliba, and S. Saliba. 2006. *Therapeutic modalities for musculoskeletal injuries.* 2nd ed. Champaign, IL: Human Kinetics.

Diaz, J.A., D.A. Fischer, A.C. Rettig, T.J. Davis, and K.D. Shelbourne. 2003. Severe quadriceps muscle contusions in athletes: A report of three cases. *American Journal of Sports Medicine* 31(2): 289-293.

Dick, T. 2004. Professional etiquette: how you show your respect for people. *Emergency Medical Services* 33(4): 91-96.

Donnelly, J., Blair, S., Jakicic, J., Manore, M., Rankin, J., & Smith, B. 2009. American College of Sports Medicine position stand: appropriate physical activity intervention strategies for weight loss and prevention of weight regain for adults. *Medicine and Science in Sports and Exercise* 41(2): 459-471.

Dougherty, T.M. 2003. Physician perspective. Sports dermatology: what certified athletic trainers and therapists need to know. *Athletic Therapy Today* 8(3): 46-48.

Downes, N.J. (1997). *Ethnic Americans for the health professional* (2nd ed.). Dubuque, IA: Kendall/Hunt

Drezner, J.A., R.W. Courson, W.O. Roberts, V.N. Mosesso, M.S. Link, and B.J. Maron. 2007. Inter-Association Task Force recommendations on emergency preparedness and management of sudden cardiac arrest in high school and college athletic programs: a consensus statement. *Journal of Athletic Training* 42(1): 143-158.

Drowatzky, J.N., and C.W. Armstrong. 1984. *Physical education: career perspectives and professional foundations.* Englewood Cliffs, NJ: Prentice Hall.

Drummond, J., K. Hostetter, P. Laguna, A. Gillentine, and G. Del Rossi. 2007. Self-reported comfort of collegiate athletes with injury and condition care by same-sex and opposite-sex athletic trainers. *Journal of Athletic Training* 42(1): 106-112.

Durstine, L., and G. Moore. 2003. *Exercise management for persons with chronic diseases and disabilities.* Champaign, IL: Human Kinetics.

Easterbrook, M. 1981. Eye protection for squash and racquetball. *Physician and Sportsmedicine* 9(2): 79-82.

Eichelberger, M.R. 1981. Torso injuries in athletics. *Physician and Sportsmedicine* 9(3): 87-92.

Eichner, E. 1989. Sickle cell trait and exercise-related death. *Sports Medicine Digest* 11(2): 4.

Ellenbecker, T.S., and A.J. Mattalino. 1997. *The elbow in sport.* Champaign, IL: Human Kinetics.

emedicinehealth. 2009. Atrial fibrillation. www.emedicinehealth.com/atrial_fibrillation/page2_em.htm.

Erickson D'Avanzo, C., & Geissler, E. (2003). *Pocket guide to cultural health assessment* (3rd ed.). St. Louis, MO: Mosby.

Erne, H., I. Zouzias, and M. Rosenwasser. 2009. Medial collateral ligament reconstruction in the baseball pitcher's elbow. *Hand Clinics* 25(3): 339-346

Field, L.D., and D.W. Altchek. 1995. Elbow injuries. *Clinical Sports Medicine* 14(1): 59-78.

Field, R.W., and S.O. Roberts. 1999. *Weight training.* Boston: McGraw-Hill.

Flegel, M.J. 1992. *Sport first aid.* Champaign, IL: Human Kinetics.

Food and Drug Administration (FDA). 2009. Fortify your knowledge about vitamins. www.fda.gov/ForConsumers/ConsumerUpdates/ucm118079.htm.

Fox, E.L., R.W. Bowers, and M.L. Foss. 1993. *The physiological basis for exercise and sport.* 5th ed. Madison, WI: Brown and Benchmark.

Gale, S., L. Decoster, and E. Swartz. 2008. The combined tool approach for face mask removal during on-field conditions. *Journal of Athletic Training* 43(1): 14-20.

Gaudard, A., E. Varlet-Marie, F. Bressolle, and M. Audran. 2003. Drugs for increasing oxygen transport and their potential use in doping: a review. *Sports Medicine* 33(3): 187-192.

Gebhard, J.S., D.H. Donaldson, and C.W. Brown. 1994. Soft-tissue injuries of the cervical spine. *Orthopedic Review* (May Suppl.): 9-17.

Gerberich, S.S., J.D. Priest, J. Boen, C.P. Straub, and R.E. Maxwell. 1983. Concussion incidence and severity in secondary school varsity football players. *American Journal of Public Health* 73: 1370-1375.

Giza, C.C., and D.A. Hovda. 2001. The neurometabolic cascade of concussion. *Journal of Athletic Training* 36(3): 228-235.

Glass, A.L. 1994. *Weight training.* Dubuque, IA: Kendall/Hunt.

Glover, D.W., B.J. Maron, and G.O. Matheson. 1999. The preparticipation physical examination: steps toward consensus and uniformity. *Physician and Sportsmedicine* 27(8).

Goitz, R.J., and M.M. Tomaino. 2002. Traumatic hand injuries evaluation and management: Understanding of the complex anatomy is the key to diagnosis. *Journal of Musculoskeletal Medicine* 19(5): 204-206, 208-210.

Goldstein, T.S. 1995. *Functional rehabilitation in orthopaedics.* Gaithersburg, MD: Aspen.

Graham, L.S. 1985. Ten ways to dodge the malpractice bullet. *Journal of the National Athletic Trainers' Association* 20(2): 117-119.

Gray, R.S. 1997. The role of the clinical athletic trainer. In *Clinical athletic training*, ed. J.J. Konin. Thorofare, NJ: Slack.

Greenstein, J.S., and D.M. Kleiner. 2000. Guidelines for the pre-hospital management of the spine-injured athlete. *Journal of Sports Chiropractic and Rehabilitation* 14(4): 105-110, 134-135.

Griggs, P. 2008. Hyphema. www.nlm.nih.gov/medlineplus/ency/article/001021.htm.

Gross, M.T., and H. Liu. 2003. The role of ankle bracing for prevention of ankle sprain injuries. *Journal of Orthopaedic and Sports Physical Therapy* 33(10): 572-577.

Guskiewicz, K.M., S.L. Bruce, R.C. Cantu, M.S. Ferrara, J.P. Kelly, M. McCrea, M. Putukian, M., and T.C. Valovich McLeod. 2004. National Athletic Trainers' Association position statement: management of sport-related concussion. *Journal of Athletic Training* 39(3): 280-297.

Guskiewicz, K., D. Perrin, and B. Gansneder. 1996. Effects of mild head injury on postural stability in athletes. *Journal of Athletic Training* 31(4): 300-306.

Hadzic, V., T. Sattler, E. Topole, Z. Jarnovic, H. Burger, and E. Dervisevic. 2009. Risk factors for ankle sprain in volleyball players: a preliminary analysis. *Isokinetics and Exercise Science* 17(3): 155-160.

Hass, C., M. Feigenbaum, and B. Franklin. 2001. Prescription of resistance training for healthy populations. *Sports Medicine* 31: 953-964.

Heck, J.F., M.P. Weis, J.M. Garland, and C.R. Weis. 1994. Minimizing liability risks of head and neck injuries in football. *Journal of Athletic Training* 29(2): 128-139.

Heck, J.F., Clarke, K.S.,Peterson, T.R., Torg,J.S., and M.P.. Weis. 2004. NATA Position Statement: head Down Contact in Football. *Journal of Athletic Training* 39(1): 101-111

Hegarty, V. 1988. *Decisions in nutrition.* St. Louis: Times Mirror/Mosby.

Heinzman, S.E. 1991. Quality physicals that generate funds for the training room. *Journal of the National Athletic Trainers' Association* 26(1): 66-69.

Henderson, J., and W. Carroll. 1993. The athletic trainer's role in preventing sport injury and rehabilitating injured athletes: a psychological perspective. In *Psychological bases of sport injuries*, ed. D. Pargman. Morgantown, WV: Fitness Information Technology.

Hertling, D., and R.M. Kessler. 1996. *Management of common musculoskeletal disorders.* 3rd ed. Philadelphia: Lippincott Williams & Wilkins.

Honsik, K. 2004. Emergency treatment of dentoalveolar trauma: Essential tips for treating active patients. *Physician and Sportsmedicine* 32(9): 23.

Houglum, P.A. 2010. *Therapeutic exercise for musculoskeletal injuries.* 3rd ed. Champaign, IL: Human Kinetics.

Houglum, P.A. 1992. Soft tissue healing and its impact on rehabilitation. *Journal of Sport Rehabilitation* 1: 19-23.

Housner, J.A., and J.E. Kuhn. 2003. Clavicle fractures: individualizing treatment for fracture type. *Physician and Sportsmedicine* 31(12): 30-36.

Hunt, V.K. 1997. Fitness centers: untapped job market for ATCs? *NATA News* (October 4-5): 20.

Idroscalo Club. 2009. Physical disability categories. www.idroscaloclub.org/campionati/form/Physical_Disability_Categories.pdf.

Itagaki, M., and N. Knight. 2004. Kidney trauma in martial arts: A case report of kidney contusion in jujitsu. *American Journal of Sports Medicine* 32(2): 522-524.

It's the Real Deal Petro-Canada Paraylmpic Schools Program. 2009. www.paralympiceducation.ca.

Jim Abbott Official Web Site. 2010. Biography. www.jimabbott.info/biography.html.

Jimenez, C.C., M.H. Corcoran, J.T. Crawley, W.G. Hornsby, K. Peer, R.D. Philbin, and M.C. Riddell. 2007. National Athletic Trainers' Association position statement: management of the athlete with type 1 diabetes mellitus. *Journal of Athletic Training* 42(4): 536-545

Johnson, J.D., and W.W. Briner, Jr. 2005. Primary care of the sports hernia. *Physician and Sportsmedicine* 33(2): 35.

Johnson, B.C., and L.A. Klabunde. 1995. The elusive slipped capital femoral epiphysis. *Journal of Athletic Training* 30(2): 124-127.

Kaeding, C.C, A.D. Pedroza, and B.C. Powers. 2007. Surgical treatment of chronic patellar tendinosis: a systematic review. *Clinical Orthopedic Related Research* 455: 102-106.

Karren, K.J., B.Q. Hafen, D. Limmer, and J.J. Mistovich. 2004. *First aid for colleges and universities.* 8th ed. San Francisco: Pearson Benjamin Cummings.

Katch, F.I., and W.D. McArdle. 1993. *Nutrition, weight control, and exercise.* Philadelphia: Lea & Febiger.

Kaut, K.P., R. DePompei, J. Kerr, and J. Congeni. 2003. Reports of head injury and symptom knowledge among college athletes: Implications for assessment and educational intervention. *Clinical Journal of Sport Medicine* 13(4): 213-221.

Kelly, J.P. 2001. Loss of consciousness: Pathophysiology and implications in grading and safe return to play. *Journal of Athletic Training* 36(3): 249-252.

Kendall, P.F., E.K. McCreary, and P.G. Provance. 1993. *Muscles, testing and function.* 4th ed. Baltimore: Williams & Wilkins.

Kenna, K. 1983. The diabetic athlete. *Athletic Training* 18(2): 131-134.

Kennedy, R. 1995. *Taping guide.* St. Louis: Mosby.

Kennett, F. (1976). *Folk medicine fact and fiction.* New York: Marshall Cavendish.

Khoo, D., W. Carmichaels, and R.J. Spinner. 1996. Ulnar nerve entrapment. *Orthopedic Clinics of North America* 27(2): 317-338.

Kibler, W.B. 2003. Rehabilitation of rotator cuff tendinopathy. *Clinics in Sports Medicine* 22(4): 837-847.

Kibler, W., and A. Sciascia. 2008. Rehabilitation of the athlete's shoulder. *Clinics in Sports Medicine* 27(4): 821-831.

Kisner, C., and L.A. Colby. 1996. *Therapeutic exercise.* 3rd ed. Philadelphia: Davis.

Kloth, L.C., and J.M. McCulloch, eds. 2002. *Wound healing: alternatives in management.* 3rd ed. Philadelphia: Davis.

Knapik, J., S. Marshall, R. Lee, S. Darakjy, S. Jones, T. Mitchener, et al. 2007. Mouthguards in sport activities: history, physical properties and injury prevention effectiveness. *Sports Medicine* 37(2): 117-144.

Knight, K.L. 1996. Interview by the author. Orlando, FL, June.

Knight, K.L. 1995. *Cryotherapy in sport injury management.* Champaign, IL: Human Kinetics.

Knight, K.L., and D.O. Draper. 2008. *Therapeutic modalities: the art and science.* Philadelphia: Lippincott Williams & Wilkins.

Kocher, M., R. Solomon, B. Lee, L. Micheli, J. Solomon, and A. Stubbs. 2006. Arthroscopic debridement of hip labral tears in dancers. *Journal of Dance Medicine and Science* 10(3-4): 99-105.

Koester, M.C. 1995. Refocusing the adolescent preparticipation physical evaluation toward preventive health care. *Journal of Athletic Training* 30(4): 352-360.

Konin, J.J. 1997a. Communication skills in clinical athletic training. In *Clinical athletic training,* ed. J.J. Konin. Thorofare, NJ: Slack.

Konin, J.J. 1997b. The roles of allied health care providers. In *Clinical athletic training,* ed. J.J. Konin. Thorofare, NJ: Slack.

Kozanek, M., E. Fu, S.K. Van de Velde, T. Gill, and G. Li. 2009. Posterolateral structures of the knee in posterior cruciate ligament deficiency. *American Journal of Sports Medicine* 37(3): 534-541.

Kraemer, W.J. 2003. Strength training basics: designing workouts to meet patients' goals. *Physician and Sportsmedicine* 31(8): 39-45.

Kratina, K. 2005. Tips for coaches: preventing eating disorders in athletes. Westbury, NYNational Eating Disorders Association.

Kubler-Ross, E. 1969. *On death and dying.* New York: Macmillan.

Labella, C.R., B.W. Smith, and A. Sigurdsson. 2002. Effect of mouthguards on dental injuries and concussions in college basketball. *Medicine and Science in Sports and Exercise* 34(1): 41-44.

Lahti, H., J. Sane, and P. Ylipaavalniemi. 2002. Dental injuries in ice hockey games and training. *Medicine and Science in Sports and Exercise* 34(3): 400-402.

Larson, J.P. 1993. Massage as a modality in trauma and sports medicine. *Trauma* 35(4): 81-94.

Larson, C.M., L.C. Almekinders, S.G. Karas, and W.E. Garrett. 2002. Evaluating and managing muscle contusions and myositis ossificans. *Physician and Sportsmedicine* 30(2): 41-44, 49-50.

Lavallee, L., and F. Flint. 1996. The relationship of stress, competitive anxiety, mood state, and social support to athletic injury. *Journal of Athletic Training* 31(4): 296-299.

Leong, S.C., R.J. Roe, and A. Karkanevatos. 2005. No-frills management of epistaxis. *Emergency Medicine Journal* 22: 470-472.

Lephart, S.M., D.M. Pincivero, J.L. Giraldo, and F.H. Fu. 1997. The role of proprioception in the management and rehabilitation of athletic injuries. *American Journal of Sports Medicine* 25(1): 130-137.

Leverenz, L.J., and L.B. Helms. 1990. Suing athletic trainers: part II. *Journal of the National Athletic Trainers' Association* 25(3): 219-226.

Luke, A., and P. d'Hemecourt. 2007. Prevention of infectious diseases in athletes. *Clinical in Sports Medicine* 26(3): 321-344.

Luscombe, M.D., and J.L. Williams. 2003. Comparison of a long spinal board and vacuum mattress for spinal immobilization. *Emergency Medicine Journal* 20(5): 476-478.

Lyman, S., G.S. Fleisig, J.R. Andrews, and E.D. Osinski. 2002. Effect of pitch type, pitch count, and pitching mechanics on risk of elbow and shoulder pain in youth baseball pitchers. *American Journal of Sports Medicine* 30(4).

Magee, D.J. 1997. *Orthopedic physical assessment.* 3rd ed. Philadelphia: Saunders.

Maitland, M.E. 2003. Best of the literature: Neuromuscular training helps prevent ACL injuries. *Physician and Sportsmedicine* 31(12): 8-9.

Marchessault, J., M. Conti, and M. Baratz. 2009. Carpal fractures in athletes excluding the scaphoid. *Hand Clinics* 25(3): 371-388.

Martin, T.J. 2001. Technical report: knee brace use in the young athlete. *Pediatrics* 108: 503-507.

Massie, J., D. Donnelly, and K. Ricker. 2009. Liver laceration sustained by a college football player. *Athletic Therapy Today* 14(2): 23-26.

McCrea, M. 2001. Standardized mental status testing on the sideline after sport-related concussion. *Journal of Athletic Training* 36(3): 274-279.

McCulloch, J.M., L.C. Kloth, and J.A. Feedar. 1995. *Wound healing: alternatives in management.* 2nd ed. Philadelphia: Davis.

McGavock, J.M., N.D. Eves, S. Mandic, and N.M. Glenn. 2004. The role of exercise in the treatment of cardiovascular disease associated with type 2 diabetes mellitus. *Sports Medicine* 34(1): 27-48.

McGuine, T. 1996. Recognizing abdominal injuries in high school athletes. *Sports Plus.* Winter/Spring: 2-3.

McLeod, T., R. Bay, J. Parsons, E. Sauers, and A. Snyder. 2009. Recent injury and health-related quality of life in adolescent athletes. *Journal of Athletic Training* 44(6): 603-610.

Meana, M., L.M. Alegre, J.L. Elvira, and X. Aguado. 2008. Kinematics of ankle taping after a training session. *International Journal of Sports Medicine* 29(1): 70-76.3.

Meyers, W., E. Yoo, O. Devon, N. Jain, M. Horner, C. Lauencin, et al. 2007. Understanding "sports hernia" (athletic pubalgia): the anatomic and pathophysiologic basis for abdominal and groin pain in athletes. *Operative Techniques in Sports Medicine* 15(4): 165-177.

Michigan High School Athletic Association. (MHSAA). 2010. Fall sport coaches preseason alerts sports medicine, heat illness, concussions. *www.mhsaa.com/LinkClick.aspx?fileticket=5WLj8XfvBiE%3D&tabid=38.*

Mickleborough, T.D., and R.W. Gotshall. 2003. Dietary components with demonstrated effectiveness in decreasing the severity of exercise-induced asthma. *Sports Medicine* 33(9): 671-681.

Midgley, A.W., L.R. McNaughton, and M. Sleap. 2003. Infection and the elite athlete: a review. *Research in Sports Medicine* 11(4): 235-259.

Miller, A.E. 1996. Creatine supplements in athletics. *Sports Medicine Update* 11(3): 12-16.

Miller, M., D. Berry, G. Gariepy, and J. Tittler. 2006. Attitudes of high school ice hockey players toward mouthguard usage. *Internet Journal of Allied Health Sciences and Practice* 4(4).

Moeller, J.L., and S.F. Rifat. 2003. Identifying and treating uncomplicated corneal abrasions. *Physician and Sportsmedicine* 31(8): 15.

Moeller, J.L., and S.F. Rifat. 2001. Spondylolysis in active adolescents: Expediting return to play. *Physician and Sportsmedicine* 29(12): 27-32.

Mottram, D.R. 1988. *Drugs in sport.* Champaign, IL: Human Kinetics.

Moylan, F. 2003. Swimmer's ear mystery. *Physician and Sportsmedicine* 31(9): 48.

Mueller, F.O., R.C. Cantu, and S.P. Van Camp. 1996. *Catastrophic injuries in high school and college sports.* Vol. 8. Sport Science Monograph Series. Champaign, IL: Human Kinetics.

Mullen, J.E., and M.J. O'Malley. 2004. Sprains: residual instability of subtalar, Lisfranc joints, and turf toe. *Clinics in Sports Medicine* 23(1): 97-121.

Myer, G.D., K.R. Ford, and T.E. Hewett. 2004. Rationale and clinical techniques for anterior cruciate ligament injury prevention among female athletes. *Journal of Athletic Training* 39(4): 352-364.

National Athletic Trainers' Association (NATA). 2009. The facts about athletic trainers. www.nata.org/sites/default/files/AT_Facts.pdf.

National Athletic Trainers' Association (NATA). 1998. *1998 membership directory: NATA code of ethics.* Dallas: Author.

National Registry of Emergency Medical Technicians. 2008. General information: overview. www.nremt.org/nremt/about/gen_info_overview.asp.

National Safety Council. 2001. *First aid and CPR.* 4th ed. Boston: Jones and Bartlett.

National Safety Council. 1997. *First responder.* Boston: Jones and Bartlett.

Nicholls, R.L., B.C. Elliott, and K. Miller. 2004. Impact injuries in baseball: prevalence, aetiology and the role of equipment performance. *Sports Medicine* 34(1): 17-25.

Niedfeldt, M.W. 2001. Managing hypertension in athletes and physically active patients. *American Family Physician* 66(3): 445-452, 457-458.

Oakley, J.C. 2003. An update on the treatment of chronic low back pain. *Critical Reviews in Physical and Rehabilitation Medicine* 15(2): 113-140.

Ollivierre, C.O., R.P. Nirschl, and F.A. Peltrone. 1995. Resection and repair for medial tennis elbow. *American Journal of Sports Medicine* 23(2): 214-221.

Olsen, S.J., G.S. Fleisig, S. Dun, J. Loftice, and J.R. Andrews. 2006. Risk factors for shoulder and elbow injuries in adolescent baseball pitchers. *American Journal of Sports Medicine* 34: 905-912.

Osborne, B. 2001. Principles of liability for athletic trainers: managing sport-related concussion. *Journal of Athletic Training* 36(3): 316-321.

Palmer, D. 2007. Assessment and management of patients with Achilles tendon rupture. *Advanced Emergency Nursing Journal* 29(3): 249-259.

Papanek, P.E. 2003. The female athlete triad: an emerging role for physical therapy. *Journal of Orthopaedic and Sports Physical Therapy* 33(10): 594-614.

Pargman, D. 1993. Sport injuries: an overview of psychological perspectives. In *Psychological bases of sport injuries,* ed. D. Pargman. Morgantown, WV: Fitness Information Technology.

Park, M.C., T.A. Blaine, and W.N. Levine. 2002. Shoulder dislocation in young athletes: Current concepts in management. *Physician and Sportsmedicine* 30(12): 41-48, 55-56.

Paris, S.V. 1990. The spine and swimming. In *The spine in sports,* ed. S.H. Hochschuler. Philadelphia: Hanley and Belfus.

Pauls, J.A., and K.L. Reed. 1996. *Quick reference to physical therapy.* Gaithersburg, MD: Aspen.

Pease, J., M. Miller, and R. Gumoc. 2009. An easily overlooked injury: Lisfranc fracture. *Military Medicine* 174(6): 645-646.

Peterson, M., and K. Peterson. 1988. *Eat to compete: a guide to sports nutrition.* Chicago: Year Book Medical.

Pfeiffer, R.P., and B.C. Mangus. 2002. *Concepts of athletic training.* 3rd ed. Boston: Jones and Bartlett.

Pohl, M., J. Hamill, and I. Davis, I. 2009. Biomechanical and anatomic factors associated with a history of plantar fasciitis in female runners. *Clinical Journal of Sport Medicine* 19(5): 372-376.

Porterfield, J.A., and C. DeRosa. 1991. *Mechanical low back pain.* Philadelphia: Saunders.

Prentice, W.E. 2011. *Rehabilitation techniques for sports medicine and athletic training.* 5th ed. Boston: McGraw-Hill.

Prentice, W.E. 2009. *Arnheim's principles of athletic training: a competency-based approach.* 13th ed. Boston: McGraw-Hill.

Prentice, W.E. 2009. *Therapeutic modalities for sports medicine and athletic training.* 6th ed. Boston: McGraw-Hill.

Purnell, L.D., & Paulanka, B.J. (2003). *Transcultural health care: A culturally competent approach* (2nd ed.). Philadelphia: Davis.

Purnell, L.D., & Paulanka, B.J. (2005). *Guide to culturally competent health care.* Philadelphia: Davis.

Putukian, M., and R. Echemendia. 1996. Managing successive minor head injuries. *Physician and Sportsmedicine* 24(11): 25-38.

Quillen, W.S., and F.B. Underwood. 1995. *Laboratory manual to accompany therapeutic modalities in sports medicine.* 3rd ed. St. Louis: Mosby.

Ramirez, M., J. Yang, L. Bourque, J. Javien, S. Kashani, M. Limbos, and C. Peek-Asa. 2009. Sports injuries to high school athletes with disabilities. *Pediatrics* 123: 690-696.

Rankin, J.M., and C. Ingersoll. 1995. *Athletic training management.* St. Louis: Mosby.

Rawlins, R.P. 1993. Hope-hopelessness. In *Mental health: psychiatric nursing,* ed. R.P. Rawlins, S.R. Williams, and C.K. Beck (3rd ed.). St. Louis: Mosby.

Ray, R. 1994. *Management strategies in athletic training.* Champaign, IL: Human Kinetics.

Ray, R., and D.M. Wiese-Bjornstal, eds. 1999. *Counseling in sports medicine.* Champaign, IL: Human Kinetics.

Refshauge, K., J. Raymond, S. Kilbreath, L. Pengel, and I. Heijnen. 2009. The effect of ankle taping on detection of inversion-eversion movements in participants with recurrent ankle sprain. *American Journal of Sports Medicine* 37(2): 371-375.

Rettig, A.C. 2003. Athletic injuries of the wrist and hand, part I: Traumatic injuries of the wrist. *American Journal of Sports Medicine* 31(6): 1038-1048.

Rodriguez, J.O., A.M. Lavina, and A. Agarwal. 2003. Prevention and treatment of common eye injuries in sports. *American Family Physician* 67(7): 1433-1435, 1481-1488, 1494-1496.

Rosenthal, M.D., and D.J. McMillan. 2004. Injury management update. Hamstring-strain rehabilitation: a functional stepwise approach for return to sports, part II. *Athletic Therapy Today* 9(1): 44-45.

Rosenthal, M.D., and D.J. McMillan. 2003. Injury management update. Hamstring-strain rehabilitation: a functional stepwise approach for return to sports, part I. *Athletic Therapy Today* 8(6): 34-35.

Roy, S., and R. Irvin. 1983. *Sports medicine: prevention, evaluation, management, and rehabilitation.* Englewood Cliffs, NJ: Prentice Hall.

Ruchelsman, D.E., and S.K. Lee. 2009. Neurovascular injuries of the hand in athletes. *Current Orthopaedic Practice* 20(4): 409-415.

Sandrey, M.A. 2003. Acute and chronic tendon injuries: Factors affecting the healing response and treatment. *Journal of Sport Rehabilitation* 12(1): 70-91.

Saunders, H.D., and R. Saunders. 1993. *Evaluation, treatment and prevention of musculoskeletal disorders.* 3rd ed., vol. 1. Bloomington, MN: Educational Opportunities.

Schrefer, S. (Ed.). (1994). *Quick reference to cultural assessment.* St. Louis, MO. Mosby.

Seaward, B.L. 1997. *Managing stress.* 2nd ed. Boston: Jones and Bartlett.

Seeley, R.R., T.D. Stephens, and P. Tate. 1992. *Anatomy and physiology.* 2nd ed. St. Louis: Mosby.

Shea, K.G., P.J. Apel, and R.P. Pfeiffer. 2003. Anterior cruciate ligament injury in paediatric and adolescent patients: a review of basic science and clinical research. *Sports Medicine* 33(6): 455-471.

Sherry, E., ed. 2007. World ortho textbook, sports medicine section, chapter 84: the disabled athlete. www.worldortho.com/dev/index.php?option=com_content&view=article&id=2233.

Shiel, W.C. 2008. Osteoarthritis. www.medicinenet.com/osteoarthritis/article.htm.

Sluijs, E.A. 1991. Checklist to assess patient education in physical therapy practice: development and reliability. *Physical Therapy* 71(4): 561-569.

Solari, A. 1997. Interview by the author. Ann Arbor, MI, February 10.

Solari, A. 1998. Interview by the author. Ann Arbor, MI, January 14.

Spector, R.E. 2004. *Cultural diversity in health and illness.* 6th ed. Upper Saddle River, NJ: Prentice Hall.

Standaert, C.J. 2002. Practice management: spondylolysis in the adolescent athlete. *Clinical Journal of Sport Medicine* 12(2): 119-122.

Starkey, C. 1999. *Therapeutic modalities.* Philadelphia: Davis.

Starkey, C. 2004. *Therapeutic modalities.* 3rd ed. Philadelphia: FA Davis.

Starkey, C., and J. Ryan. 1996. *Evaluation of orthopedic and athletic injuries.* Philadelphia: Davis.

Steele, M.K. 1996. *Sideline help.* Champaign, IL: Human Kinetics.

Stiller-Ostrowski, J., D. Gould, and T. Covassin. 2009. An evaluation of an educational intervention in psychology of injury for athletic training students. *Journal of Athletic Training* 44(5): 482-489.

Stith, W.J. 1990. Exercise and the intervertebral disk. In *The spine in sports*, ed. S.H. Hochschuler. Philadelphia: Hanley and Belfus.

Stone, J.A., N.B. Partin, J.S. Lueken, K.E. Timm, and E.J. Ryan. 1994. Upper extremity proprioceptive training. *Journal of Athletic Training* 29(1): 15-18.

Stopka, C. 2003. Disability and special needs. Athletic therapy for athletes with disabilities, part 2: special conditions. *Athletic Therapy Today* 8(3): 23-25.

Storms, W.W. 2003. Review of exercise-induced asthma. *Medicine and Science in Sports and Exercise* 35(9): 1464-1470.

Straub, S.J. 1993. Working with adolescents in a high school setting. *Journal of Athletic Training* 28(1): 75-80.

Street, S.A., and D. Runkle. 2000. *Athletic protective equipment: care, selection, and fitting*. Boston: McGraw-Hill.

Susco, T.M. 2003. Injury management update. Establishing concussion-assessment guidelines: on-field, sideline, and off-field. *Athletic Therapy Today* 8(4): 48-50.

Swart, J., R. Tucker, R.P. Lamberts, Y. Albertus-Kajee, and M.I. Lambert. 2008. Potential causes of chronic knee pain in a former winner of the Tour de France. *International SportMed Journal* 9(4): 162-171.

Swartz, E., S. Norkus, T. Cappaert, and L. Decoster. 2005. Football equipment design affects face mask removal efficiency. *American Journal of Sports Medicine* 33(8): 1210-1219.

Templin, J.M. 1992. *Anatomy and physiology laboratory manual*. 2nd ed. St. Louis: Mosby.

Thomas, C.L., ed. 1985. *Taber's cyclopedic medical dictionary*. 13th ed. Philadelphia: Davis.

Thorogood, L. 2003. Proprioception exercises following ankle sprain. *Emergency Nurse* 11(8): 33-36.

Tierney, R.T., C.G. Mattacola, M.R. Sitler, and C. Maldjian. 2002. Head position and football equipment influence cervical spine-cord space during immobilization. *Journal of Athletic Training* 37(2): 185-189.

Tolbert, R.S. 2004. Emergency planning for high school athletics. *Coach and Athletic Director* 74(3): 58-59.

Tomberlin, J.P., and H.D. Saunders. 1994. *Evaluation, treatment and prevention of musculoskeletal disorders*. 3rd ed., vol. 2. Chaska, MN: Saunders Group.

Tommasone, B., and T. Valovich McLeod. (2006). Contact sport concussion incidence. *Journal of Athletic Training* 41(4): 470-472.

Topolsky, J. 2008. Prosthetic runner disqualified from Olympics. www.engadget.com/2008/01/17/prosthetic-limbed-runner-disqualified-from-olympics/.

Torg, J., ed. 1991. *Athletic injuries to the head, neck, and face*. 2nd ed. St. Louis: Mosby.

Tortora, G.J. 1999. *Principles of human anatomy*. 8th ed. Menlow Park, CA: Addison Wesley Longman.

Ubell, M.L., J.P. Boylan, J.A. Ashton-Miller, and E.M. Wojtys. 2003. The effect of ankle braces on the prevention of dynamic forced ankle inversion. *American Journal of Sports Medicine* 31(6): 935-940.

University of Illinois at Chicago, Department of Disability and Human Development. 2007. Disability/condition: muscular dystrophy. http://www.ncpad.org/disability/fact_sheet.php?sheet=73&view=all

Unverzagt, C., T. Schuemann, and J. Mathisen. 2008. Differential diagnosis of a sports hernia in a high-school athlete. *Journal of Orthopaedic and Sports Physical Therapy* 38(2): 63-70.

U.S. Department of Health and Human Services. 1992 *Important information about hepatitis b, hepatitis b vaccine, and hepatitis b immune globulin*. Washington, DC: GPO.

U.S. Department of Labor Occupational Safety and Health Administration. 2009. Bloodborne pathogens and needlestick prevention. www.osha.gov/SLTC/bloodbornepathogens/index.html.

Vaccaro, P. 1987. Thoracic and vascular injuries in athletes. *Athletic Training* 22(4): 290-294.

Valance, M. 2007. Quick clinic, swimmer's ear: Submerge yourself in the facts. *CMA Today* 40(3): 16-17.

Tamara C. Valovich McLeod, R. Curtis Bay, John T. Parsons, Eric L. Sauers, Alison R. Snyder. 2009. Recent Injury and Health-Related Quality of Life in Adolescent Athletes. *Journal of Athletic Training*: Vol. 44, No. 6, 603-610.

Vela, L., T.W. Tourville, and J. Hertel. 2003. Physical examination of acutely injured ankles: an evidence-based approach. *Athletic Therapy Today* 8(5): 13-19, 36-37.

Velasquez, B.J. 2002. When is a skin rash more than just a rash? Sexually transmitted diseases: a dermatological perspective. *Athletic Therapy Today* 7(3): 16-23, 38-39, 64.

Vinci, D.M. 2002. Nutrition notes: athletes and type 1 diabetes mellitus. *Athletic Therapy Today* 7(6): 48-49.

Vinger, P.F. 2000. A practical guide for sports eye protection. *Physician and Sportsmedicine* 28(b).

Vorvick, L. 2008. Conjunctivitis. www.nlm.nih.gov/medlineplus/ency/article/001010.htm.

Walker, N., J. Thatcher, and D. Lavallee. 2007. Psychological responses to injury in competitive sport: a critical review. *Journal of the Royal Society for the Promotion of Health* 127(4): 174-180.

Walsh, K.M., B. Bennett, M.A. Cooper, R.L. Holle, R. Kithil, and R.E. Lopez. 2000. National Athletic Trainers' Association position statement: lightning safety for athletics and recreation. *Journal of Athletic Training* 35(4): 471-477.

Waman, D., and M. Khelifa. 1996. Psychological issues in sport injury rehabilitation: current knowledge and practice. *Journal of Athletic Training* 31(3): 257-261.

Wann, D.L. 1997. *Sport psychology*. Upper Saddle River, NJ: Prentice Hall.

Watkins, R.C. 2002. Lumbar disc injury in the athlete. *Clinics in Sports Medicine* 21(1): 147-165.

Watkins, J. 1999. *Structure and function of the musculoskeletal system.* Champaign, IL: Human Kinetics.

Weaver, T.D., M.V. Ton, and T.V. Pham. 2004. Ingrowing toenails: management practices and research outcomes. *International Journal of Lower Extremity Wounds* 3(1): 22-34.

Weber, T.S. 2003. Environmental and infectious conditions in sports. *Clinics in Sports Medicine* 22(1): 181-196.

Weidner, T., and T. Sevier. 1996. Sport, exercise, and the common cold. *Journal of Athletic Training* 31(2): 154-159.

Whittle, R., and B. Crow. 2009. Prevention of ACL injuries in female athletes through early intervention. *Sport Journal* 12(3).

Wilkerson, G.B. 2002. Biomechanical and neuromuscular effects of ankle taping and bracing. *Journal of Athletic Training* 37(4): 436-444.

Williams, M.H. 1992. Alcohol and sport performance. *Gatorade Sports Science Exchange* 4(40).

Williams, M. 1989. *Beyond training: how athletes enhance performance legally and illegally.* Champaign, IL: Human Kinetics.

Wilmore, J.H. 2003. Aerobic exercise and endurance: improving fitness for health benefits. *Physician and Sportsmedicine* 31(5): 45-51.

Winokur, R., and W. Dexter. 2004. Fungal infections and parasitic infestations in sports: expedient identification and treatment. *Physician and Sportsmedicine* 32(10): 23.

Woodmansey, K. 1999. Athletic mouth guards prevent orofacial injuries: a review. *General Dentistry* 47(1): 64-71.

Wright, K.E., and W.R. Whitehill. 1991. *The comprehensive manual of taping and wrapping techniques.* Gardner, KS: Cramer Products.

Yehieli, M., & Grey, M. (2005). *Health matters.* Yarmouth, ME: Intercultural Press.

Index

PLEASE NOTE: Page numbers followed by an italicized *f* or *t* indicate a figure or table on that page, respectively. Page numbers followed by italicized *ff* or *tt* indicate multiple figures or tables on that page, respectively.

of the knee 147-149, 148ff
of the lower leg and ankle 159, 159f
oblique 95
pectoralis 114
quadriceps 148f
relaxation 214
rotator cuff 114f
skeletal 35-36
sphincter 35
spinal 106
sternocleidomastoid 101
strains 180t
and tendon injuries 144-145, 151-153
tissue 35
two-joint 126
of the wrist and hand 132
muscle spasm 177t, 180t-181t, 185t
muscle-spasm stitch 95
muscle weakness 115, 185t
muscular development programs 192-193, 193f
muscular dystrophy 351-352
muscular endurance 190, 192-193
muscular power 193
muscular strength 192
myelin sheath 351
myocardial contusion 88
myositis 44
myositis ossificans 144, 145f
MyPyramid 341ff

N

nasal bones 55f, 65f, 68
nasal fracture 76
NATA. See National Athletic Trainers'
  Association
NATA Educational Competencies 8-9, 9t
National Athletic Trainers' Association
  (NATA)
  about 3, 12
  on asthma in athletes 308
  on concussion management 60
  on disordered eating 314
  on emergency planning 219
  ethical guidelines 12
  on exertional heat illnesses 255
  on fluid replacement 257
  on lightning safety 261
  on management of concussions 58
  on management of diabetes 312
  membership data 9-10
  position statements 12
  on preexercise hydration 336
  salary survey 10-12
National Athletic Training Month 12
National Center for Early Defibrillation 233
National Operating Committee on Standards
  for Athletic Equipment (NOCSAE) 17,
  291
National Registry for Emergency Medical
  Technicians 7
National Safety Council 4
Native American food pyramid 340
natural lighting 19
Nautilus method of weight training 192
navicular bones 158f
nearsighted 67
neck of a tooth 68f
neck range-of-motion activities 199
neck rolls 292
neck rolls, removing 266-267
neck stretches 199, 200f
negligence 16

neoprene sleeves 299
nerve root
  compression 181t
  impingement 184
nerve tissue 44
neurocognitive testing 61
neurological problems 245-246
neurological shock 246t-247t
neurologists 6
neuroma 44
neuromuscular disorders 350-352
neutral spine 99
NexTT Solutions Injury Management software
  23
nicotine 329
NOCSAE. See National Operating
  Committee on Standards for Athletic
  Equipment
nonsteroidal anti-inflammatory drugs
  (NSAIDS) 327-328
nonunion fractures 50
normal posture 102, 102f
nose 68
  guards 292
  injuries 75-76
nosebleed 75-76
nucleus pulposus 100
nutritional aspects of injuries and illness 8
nutritional supplements 344

O

obesity 342
objective data 172
oblique fractures 47f
oblique muscles 95
obstructed airway 231-232, 232f
occipital bone 55f
Occupational Safety and Health Administration (OHSA) 236
office or record-keeping areas 18, 19
one-repetition maximum (1RM) 191
open basket weave 283, 283f
open kinetic chain 192
open wounds 177t
opposition 38
optic nerves 66, 66f
orbital foramen 66
orbital roof fracture 72-73
organization and administration 4
organized athletics 9-10
orthopedic clinical examination and diagnosis
  8
orthopedic disabilities 348-349
orthopedists 5
Osgood-Schlatter disorder 152
OSHA. See Occupational Safety and Health
  Administration
osteogenesis 50
osteoporosis 33, 50, 315, 337
otitis externa 74
ovaries 94
overeating 342
overload principle 190
Oxford technique 193f
oxygenated, definition of 82
oxygenated blood 82-83
oxygen tanks 309

P

padding, removing 268
pain 175, 177t, 181t, 185t, 242, 348
palate 68
palmaris longus muscle 132

palpation 244
pancreas 94, 94f
pancreas injury 96
paraffin bath 178, 179f
Paralympic athletes 351
Paralympics 3477
paralysis 242
paraplegia 242
parietal bone 55f
partial airway obstruction 232
participation conditions, assessing 352-353
passive range of motion (PROM) 175
patella 34f, 147, 148f
patella brace 299
patellar dislocation 151
patellar ligament 149f
patellar tendinitis 151
patellofemoral joint 147
patellofemoral syndrome 151
pathological fractures 48f
pathology of injury and illnesses 8
PCL. See posterior cruciate ligament
pectoralis major 36f
pectoralis muscles 114
pediatric cardiopulmonary resuscitation 231
pediatricians 6
pelvis 34f, 95, 141
  anatomy of 141-142, 142ff
  injuries 142-144, 144f
pendulum exercises 200-201, 202f
peptide hormones 332
performance enhancing drugs 330-331
periodontitis 68
peripheral vascular disease 177t
peristalsis 94
permission to treat 16-17
peroneus ligaments 160f
peroneus longus muscle 159f
petrissage 183, 183f
phagocytes 44kmyositis
phalanges 132f, 157, 158f
phantom pain 348
pharmacology 8
phases of treatment. See also therapeutic
    modalities
  endurance 176
  initial injury phase 174-175
  mobility restoration phase 175-176
  proprioception 176
  resistance training 176
  sport-specific function 176
phlegm 83, 307
phone numbers, emergency 220
phosphorus 338t
physical environment 214
physical examinations, preparticipation 17
physical fitness 20
physical function 172
physical therapists 6
physician. See team physician
physician assistants 6
physician-owned clinics 10-11
pink eye 70
pinna 67f
pinna laceration 75
Pistorius, Oscar 348
Pitney, Bill 8, 151, 243
Pitney, Lisa V. 151
plan of action 172
plantar fasciitis 163
plantar flexion 148, 159, 195f
plantarsurface 158

About the Authors

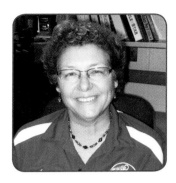

Lorin A. Cartwright, MS, ATC, is assistant principal and athletic director at Pioneer High School in Ann Arbor, Michigan. As a teacher and the school's head athletic trainer for more than 15 years, she has extensive experience with all aspects of instruction of student athletic trainers. She was an adjunct professor in athletic training at the University of Michigan for three years. Cartwright earned a bachelor's degree in physical education from Grand Valley State University and a master's degree in education from the University of Michigan.

Cartwright is the author of three books, including the popular *Preparing for the Athletic Trainers' Certification Exam,* and was the first woman and first high school athletic trainer to serve as the president of the Great Lakes Athletic Trainers' Association. She served as the investigative chair on the Ethics Committee for the National Athletic Trainers' Association (NATA) from 1998 to 2004 and was also an active member of NATA's National Membership Committee and the National Review Committee for Misconduct from 1988 through 1992. Highly regarded in her field, Cartwright was the recipient of the Great Lakes Athletic Trainers' Association Outstanding Educator Award in 2010, the Athletic Trainer Award from the Great Lakes Athletic Trainers' Association in 2002, the Most Distinguished Athletic Trainer Award from the Michigan Athletic Trainers' Society in 1999, and the Distinguished Service Award from the National Athletic Trainers' Association in 1998.

Her travels have taken her to Alaska, Italy, Nova Scotia, Sweden, Finland, and the Caribbean. Cartwright has been the athletic trainer for the amateur and semipro summer basketball league and the Michigan men's basketball all-star team, and she worked at the Olympic Trials for wrestling.

Cartwright resides in Ann Arbor, Michigan, where she enjoys woodworking, creating stained glass, and gardening in her free time.

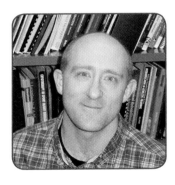

William A. Pitney, EdD, ATC, FNATA, is an associate professor in the department of kinesiology and physical education at Northern Illinois University. Dr. Pitney is a recognized leader in qualitative research in the athletic training profession and is a fellow of the National Athletic Trainers' Association. He has authored more than 25 peer-reviewed articles and two textbooks and is a section editor for the *Journal of Athletic Training,* in which he published one of the first articles on qualitative research. He is also the editor in chief for the *Athletic Training Education Journal* and the author of *Qualitative Research in Physical Activity and the Health Professions*, and he has served on the Great Lakes Athletic Trainers' Association Research Assistance Committee.

Dr. Pitney earned a bachelor's degree in physical education with a specialization in athletic training from Indiana State University in 1988, a master's degree in physical education from Eastern Michigan University in 1992, and an EdD in adult continuing education from Northern Illinois University in 2000. In his leisure time, he enjoys mountaineering, bicycling, and running.

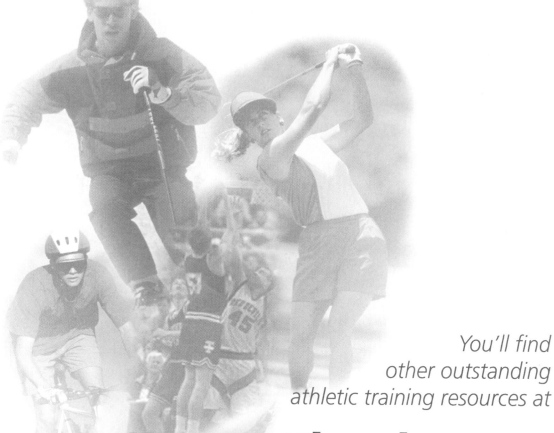